S0-BSN-251

A COMMONSENSE GUIDE TO SEX, BIRTH & BABIES

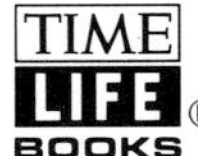

Other Publications:

PLANET EARTH
COLLECTOR'S LIBRARY OF THE CIVIL WAR
CLASSICS OF THE OLD WEST
THE EPIC OF FLIGHT
THE GOOD COOK
THE SEAFARERS
THE ENYCLOPEDIA OF COLLECTIBLES
THE GREAT CITIES
WORLD WAR II
HOME REPAIR AND IMPROVEMENT
THE WORLD'S WILD PLACES
THE TIME-LIFE LIBRARY OF BOATING
HUMAN BEHAVIOR
THE ART OF SEWING
THE OLD WEST
THE EMERGENCE OF MAN
THE AMERICAN WILDERNESS
THE TIME-LIFE ENCYCLOPEDIA OF GARDENING
LIFE LIBRARY OF PHOTOGRAPHY
THIS FABULOUS CENTURY
FOODS OF THE WORLD
TIME-LIFE LIBRARY OF AMERICA
TIME-LIFE LIBRARY OF ART
GREAT AGES OF MAN
LIFE SCIENCE LIBRARY
THE LIFE HISTORY OF THE UNITED STATES
TIME READING PROGRAM
LIFE NATURE LIBRARY
LIFE WORLD LIBRARY

FAMILY LIBRARY:
HOW THINGS WORK IN YOUR HOME
THE TIME-LIFE BOOK OF THE FAMILY CAR
THE TIME-LIFE FAMILY LEGAL GUIDE
THE TIME-LIFE BOOK OF FAMILY FINANCE

This volume is one of a series designed to familiarize readers with the latest advances in medical science as a guide in maintaining their own health and fitness.

A COMMONSENSE GUIDE TO

SEX, BIRTH & BABIES

BY THE EDITORS OF TIME-LIFE BOOKS

LIBRARY OF HEALTH / TIME-LIFE BOOKS / ALEXANDRIA, VIRGINIA

THE CONSULTANTS:
Dr. Harvey P. Katz is associate professor of pediatrics at the Johns Hopkins School of Medicine in Baltimore, and heads the Departments of Pediatrics and Health Education of the Columbia Medical Plan in Columbia, Maryland. Dr. Katz is a specialist in pediatric endocrinology and has organized numerous workshops and conferences in the area of child health services.

Dr. James E. Jordan is assistant professor of obstetrics and gynecology at the Johns Hopkins Hospital in Baltimore, and is Chief of Obstetrics-Gynecology and Medical Director of the Columbia Medical Plan in Columbia, Maryland. He was formerly Chief of Obstetrics-Gynecology at Columbia's Howard County General Hospital.

Dr. Joseph V. Collea is associate professor of obstetrics and gynecology at the Georgetown University School of Medicine in Washington, D.C. A specialist in maternal and fetal medicine, Dr. Collea has written extensively on the subject of breech presentation in childbirth.

Dr. Donald P. Jenkins is associate professor of anatomy at the Georgetown University School of Medicine and directs the Gross Anatomy Teaching Program in the university's dental, medical and graduate schools. His principal research has been in cellular and molecular biology; his most recent work deals with the application of anatomical concepts to diagnostic procedures.

For information about any Time-Life book, please write:
Reader Information, Time-Life Books,
541 North Fairbanks Court, Chicago, Illinois 60611.

First printing. Printed in U.S.A.
Published simultaneously in Canada.
School and library distribution by Silver Burdett Company, Morristown, New Jersey.

Library of Congress Cataloguing in Publication Data
The Editors of Time-Life Books
A Commonsense Guide to SEX, BIRTH & BABIES
(Library of Health)
Bibliography: p.
Includes index.
1. Pregnancy. 2. Childbirth. 3. Child development. 4. Pediatrics—Popular works.
I. Time-Life Books. II. Title. III. Series.
RG525.C685 612.6 82-168822
ISBN 0-8094-3826-7
ISBN 0-8094-3827-5 (lib. bdg.)

CONTENTS

CHAPTER 1

An internal epic of creation

A female cycle ruled by hormones
The male contribution: sperm cells by the million
Controlling disorder in the systems
Elusive causes of infertility
Surgery to aid conception
Solving problems by sex therapy

"A baby," wrote the poet Carl Sandburg, "is God's opinion that life should go on."

The arrival of a new family member does indeed signify continuity—if not on a cosmic level, certainly on a personal one for the parents. No human experience carries the dramatic impact and symbolic meaning of childbearing. Each infant, whether brought forth in a modern hospital or in a mud-thatched hut, affirms that this family will now live on in another generation.

In a sense, the creation of a new life is a grand gesture of optimism, the ultimate act of commitment. It brings with it a staggering array of physical, emotional, social and financial repercussions. For many men and women, becoming parents is a watershed event, the central fact around which the rest of their lives is arranged.

However unprepared they may be at the outset, the new mother and father soon find awakened in themselves some of the most basic and powerful of human instincts—the drive to nourish, to protect, to love a child. Over the years, child rearing will challenge their wits and energies and test their adaptive abilities as nothing else can. There will be times when some might second Mark Twain's wry assessment: "A baby is an inestimable blessing and bother." Yet rare indeed is the mother or father who fails to acknowledge, after the children are grown and gone from the household, the deeply gratifying sense of fulfillment in parenthood.

Such fulfillment is denied to some. As many as 15 per cent of all couples who want to conceive are unable to. Others may have more children than they can care for, or must cope with youthful illness. Today these problems can often be prevented or overcome, and the rewards of parenthood are attainable to a degree once undreamed of.

Medical progress has proceeded on many fronts. A variety of birth-control techniques has made it simple for couples to plan their families. Better understanding of sex has shown men and women how to find mutual fulfillment in physical love, while new knowledge of reproductive processes has enabled many who thought themselves infertile to conceive the children they want. Pregnant women, once looked upon as suffering a kind of temporary illness, are now encouraged to pursue their normal activities as long as possible. Programs to prepare couples for childbirth have done much to dispel the ignorance and myth that formerly made it a fearful prospect; by learning in advance what happens during labor and delivery, many mothers and fathers are able to participate more actively—and happily—in the process.

With new techniques and equipment, potential problems for mother and infant are detected increasingly early in pregnancy, and great strides in the care of newborn babies and mothers have saved the lives of thousands. As recently as 1915, nearly 100 out of every thousand infants died before they were a year old; in that same year, 608 of every hundred thousand mothers died in childbirth. By 1980, the United States infant mortality rate was down to 15.2 per thousand, and maternal mortality was 9.9 per hundred thousand; in Sweden these key death rates were even lower: 6.9 and 6.

In an anonymous painting done about 1830, Adam and Eve take their ease in a lush Garden of Eden. The Bible links sexuality and procreation in the statement, "Male and female created He them," and in the command, "Be fruitful and multiply."

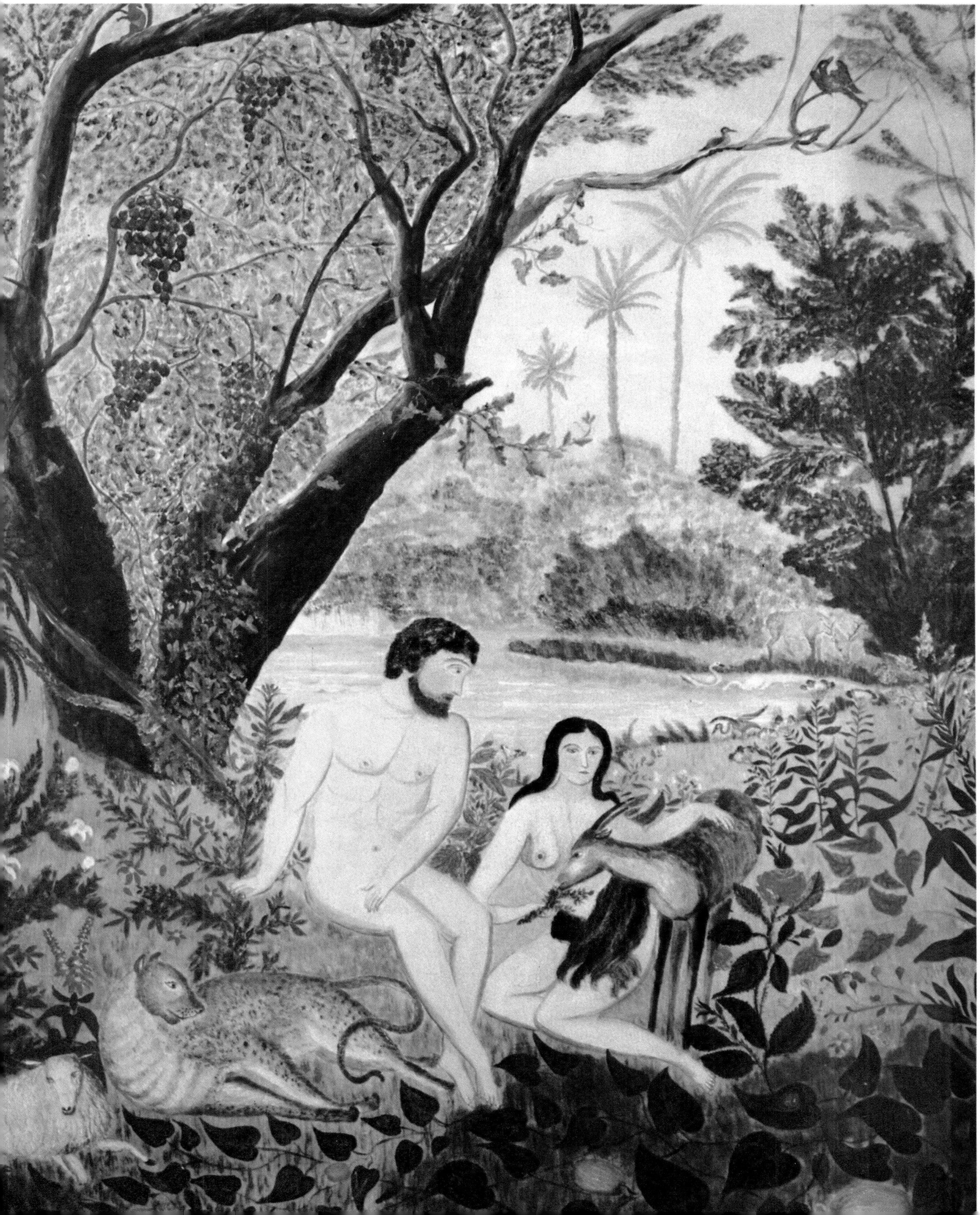

The diseases that threatened the health and lives of children a century ago—typhoid fever, smallpox, diphtheria and rickets, to name a few—are all but eliminated. As a result, the concerns of parents have shifted dramatically: Instead of worrying about keeping their sick children alive, they now can focus on the intellectual, emotional and social development of healthy youngsters, and lead them comfortably through the inevitable minor ills and traumas of growing up.

Attitudes toward sexuality and reproduction have not remained untouched by the findings of scientific research. Where there are psychological barriers to healthy sexual functioning, sex therapists may show a couple how to find natural enjoyment in the mating process.

Human societies have invested sexuality with a provocative load of secondary purposes beyond its biological goal of reproduction. It can bring fear or pleasure, guilt or self-confidence, discord or harmony. How many notes of music, strokes of painting, lines of poetry and pages of prose have been produced in the effort to describe the vexations and delights of this physical union of man and woman?

In Ernest Hemingway's novel *For Whom the Bell Tolls,* the American Robert Jordan and his young Spanish comrade Maria were so awed by the power of their love-making that they "felt the earth move."

Wrote Hemingway, "Then they were walking along the stream together and he said, 'Maria, I love thee and thou art so lovely and so wonderful and so beautiful and it does such things to me to be with thee that I feel as though I wanted to die when I am loving thee.'

" 'Oh,' she said. 'I die each time. Do you not die?'

" 'No. Almost. But did thee feel the earth move?'

" 'Yes. As I died. Put thy arm around me, please.' "

Later Jordan gently dismisses Maria's queries about his previous women: " 'It was a pleasure but it was not thus.'

" 'And then the earth moved. The earth never moved before?'

" 'Nay. Truly never.'

" 'Ay,' she said. 'And this we have for one day.' "

A prosaic explanation of their passion begins with a look at the male and female anatomy: The two bodies are made to fit together like a lock and key, with features designed expressly for the purpose of making and nurturing babies. The male's most prominent characteristic is a slender penis, an organ shaped so it may directly insert sperm into the narrow female vagina leading to the womb. The woman's distinguishing feature, large breasts, are there to nourish a newborn child.

The anatomical differences so noticeable in adults are actually present long before birth, from an early embryonic stage. Boy and girl begin in the same way, as a mother's egg cell unites with a father's sperm cell; their structures are identical for the first 40 days of development. Then the sexual organs of the male or the female begin to take shape, following the individual's genetic blueprint.

In both male and female embryos there are two duct systems, the Müllerian ducts and the Wolffian ducts, which initially function as embryonic kidneys. Eventually these duct systems develop into the elaborate apparatus of reproduction. In the male, the Müllerian duct atrophies while the Wolffian duct develops into parts of the male sex organs. In the female, the reverse occurs: The Wolffian duct degenerates while the Müllerian duct becomes the Fallopian tubes, the uterus and the upper third of the vagina.

These organs, essentially in finished form at birth, now enter a long period of dormancy within the growing boy and girl. They remain virtually unchanged until puberty, when they are reawakened by hormones that prepare them for their biological purpose—producing more children. Around the age of 12, the boy's voice deepens, his muscle becomes more solid, and he develops a beard. At this time, his genital organs begin to produce sperm, and erections occur.

The girl's reproductive system becomes active at about the same age, with the onset of the menstrual cycle—the monthly process of releasing an egg, preparing the body for its nurture in the event fertilization occurs, and then eliminating unneeded tissue from the system if the egg is not fertilized.

A female cycle ruled by hormones

The menstrual cycle is one of nature's most intricate compositions. Through a minutely orchestrated production of hormones, it readies a woman's reproductive organs for possible

Plotting the menstrual rhythms

Menstruation, the periodic shedding of the lining of the uterus, or womb, is but one part of an intricately choreographed cycle in which interdependent shifts in the levels of chemical messengers called hormones produce dramatic physical changes. The true climax of these changes is not menstruation but ovulation *(page 24)*, the release of an egg from an ovary, generally midway through the menstrual cycle. For several hours then, the egg can be fertilized by a sperm and the nine-month nurturing of pregnancy can begin.

If any part of the synchronized pattern fails—if, for example, a hormone is not released, or an organ does not respond to it—the woman may be infertile. Yet despite the cycle's inherent vulnerability, it is successfully completed at least 400 times during an average woman's lifetime.

The four graphs below trace an average 28-day cycle, beginning with the first day of menstruation; ovulation usually occurs on day 14. The first two graphs trace the changing levels of hormones released by the pituitary gland at the base of the brain and by the ovaries. The last two trace significant physical effects stimulated by the fluctuating hormones: changes in body temperature and in the thickness of the lining of the womb.

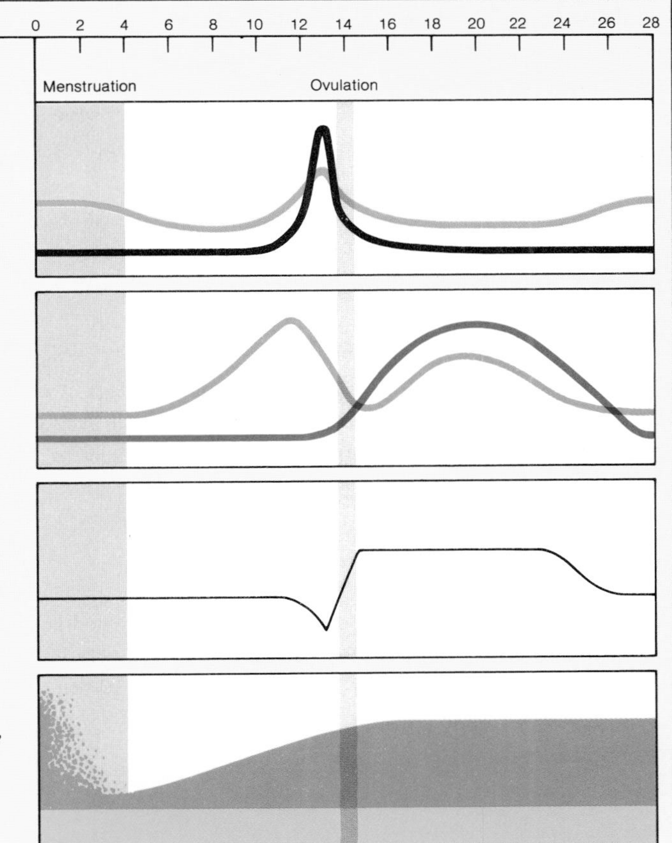

THE PITUITARY'S HORMONES
Early in the cycle, follicle-stimulating hormone (green) fosters the growth of the egg and its surrounding capsule, called a follicle. Just before ovulation, luteinizing hormone (black) triggers the egg's release from the ovary and transforms follicle cells into a hormone-secreting mass, the corpus luteum.

THE OVARY'S HORMONES
Estrogen (blue) and progesterone (red) act throughout a woman's body, adapting reproductive organs for fertilization and the nurture of a fertilized egg. Successive secretions from the follicle and the corpus luteum produce the double peak of the estrogen curve; progesterone is produced by the corpus luteum alone.

TEMPERATURE CLUES TO THE COURSE OF THE CYCLE
Resting body temperature, taken upon waking each morning, is about 97.4° F. at the beginning of the cycle. It dips slightly before ovulation; then, stimulated by progesterone, it rises to about 98.4° and stays there until the progesterone level drops. This pattern can be used to detect the imminent onset of ovulation.

UPS AND DOWNS IN THE LINING OF THE WOMB
At menstruation, the upper layers of the lining of the womb are shed and discharged from the body. Rising levels of estrogen make new cells grow, thickening the lining; increased progesterone levels stimulate the growth of nutritive glands and blood vessels. Falling hormone levels trigger the next menstruation.

motherhood each month; it is as if her body were hoping for a baby with every menstrual cycle. Its rhythm varies widely among individuals and with circumstances. Although the average cycle is 28 days, healthy women may have cycles that range from 15 to 45 days, and in some individuals or in some circumstances the pattern may be variable.

The menstrual process begins when one of the body's main control centers, the pituitary gland beneath the brain, signals the female reproductive system with two hormones, follicle-stimulating hormone (FSH) and luteinizing hormone (LH). The destination of these chemical messengers is the ovaries, two pecan-sized sacs that nestle on either side of the uterus and contain a lifetime supply of eggs. Each egg is enclosed in its own wrapper, a hollow sphere called an ovarian follicle. Every month, under the influence of FSH, some 20 follicles begin to develop and grow. After about a week, however, hormonal shifts make all but one of the follicles stop growing and regress, leaving the front runner to develop fully. In rare cases, more than one follicle will ripen—and fraternal twins, triplets, quadruplets or even quintuplets may be born.

The select follicle grows until about the 14th day of the menstrual cycle, when it bursts at the surface of the ovary, pouring out a cloud of follicular liquid. Within minutes the egg floats free, surrounded by a sticky entourage of follicular fluids that nourish it and also enable tiny hairlike projections, called cilia, to grasp it and move it on a three-day journey to the womb. To begin this odyssey, the egg must pass briefly through the open space of the abdominal cavity and into the end of the nearby Fallopian tube; then it continues slowly through this passageway to the uterus.

Only now can normal fertilization take place. If a baby is to be conceived during this menstrual cycle, a sperm must reach the egg and penetrate it during the few days it spends passing through the Fallopian tube. Immediately before ovulation, one hormone, estrogen, stimulates the secretion of sperm-welcoming mucus; immediately after ovulation, another hormone, progesterone, stimulates the development of the lining of the uterus, softening it and lacing it with blood vessels in preparation for the arrival of a fertilized egg.

For most women in most cycles, fertilization does not take place, and instead menstruation occurs—the womb's monthly gesture of resignation. About 14 days after ovulation the uterus begins to shed its newly built-up padding, discharging fluids and cellular debris through the vagina.

The menstrual cycle brings several distinct psychological and physical experiences—some pleasant, others annoying or painful. *Mittelschmerz*—German for "middle pain"—may accompany ovulation, at the mid-point of the cycle. This temporary aching or cramping is believed to be caused by irritation from the follicular fluid ejected with the egg. At ovulation some women also experience heightened senses of sight, hearing and smell, and a decreased sensitivity to pain, as well as greater feelings of sexuality, creativity and well-being. During the week or so before menstruation, tension and mood shifts may result from hormonal changes.

In many women the onset of menstrual flow is accompanied by cramps. Most often the cramping begins in puberty and is chronic; this condition, known as primary dysmenorrhea, is not dangerous. Until recently, many doctors dismissed the problem as largely psychosomatic, but now it is viewed as purely physical. The pain is thought to result from uterine spasms or from menstrual clots that block the lower opening of the womb, the cervix. The pain can be eased by aspirin or acetaminophen, but simpler measures also provide relief—exercise or heat applied to the abdomen.

Menstrual cramps that arise suddenly in adulthood or abruptly worsen years after the menstrual cycle has been established are called secondary dysmenorrhea. They may signal a serious disorder such as endometriosis, which frequently causes infertility. In this condition, tissues from the lining of the uterus migrate into the abdominal cavity, become implanted there and react to hormones in much the same fashion as the regular uterine lining. Building up each month, these remote colonies are unable to slough off as the lining of the uterus does; but they bleed, with considerable pain, then heal—only to build up again during the next menstrual cycle. The malady is commonly treated with hormones, although surgery may be needed to remove large sections of tissue. Many women find that these menstrual cramps—as well as those of primary dysmenorrhea—are less severe after they have had a baby or if they take birth-control pills, which mimic pregnancy in their hormonal effects.

The normal menstrual cycle repeats its inexorable sequence perhaps 400 times over a lifetime. Approximately every month from puberty to menopause, a few eggs—from an initial supply of some two million present at birth—are stimulated to grow, the uterus is prepared, and then unneeded materials are discharged. The sequence can be interrupted by illness—or by fertilization of the egg by a man's sperm cell.

The male contribution: sperm cells by the million

Sperm, or spermatozoa, are constantly manufactured in the male in a pair of organs called testicles, which are suspended between the thighs in a fleshy sac called the scrotum. Compared to the seclusion and security of the female reproductive organs, the vulnerable exposure of the testicles seems incongruous but apparently serves for cooling. At 98.6° F., the normal body temperature, sperm will not be produced; located in a sac just outside the trunk of the body, the testicles are kept at a more favorable temperature, a fairly constant 94° F. When the surrounding temperature falls, or when danger threatens, the testicles are automatically withdrawn closer to the body for warmth or protection.

Packed into this pair of organs is some of the most delicate ductwork to be found in nature. Inside each testicle are seminiferous, or "sperm-carrying," tubules the diameter of sewing thread—each is about 24 inches long, but they are so compactly coiled that some 800 fit into a space barely an inch across. Cells on the inner walls of the tubules divide to form spermatids, rudimentary sex cells that mature into sperm after about 60 days. This process, beginning during puberty and continuing throughout a lifetime, reaches peak production during early adulthood—averaging about 72 million sperm cells a day—and then begins to taper off.

Each sperm cell is two to three thousandths of an inch long—too small to be seen with the naked eye—and consists of a rounded head that narrows sharply into a long tail. Like the much larger and heavier egg, it contains exactly half the genetic material needed to produce the body cells of a new individual; but within the male half is the genetic marker, or chromosome, that determines sex. Roughly half of all sperm bear the chromosome, designated type X, that will produce a baby girl; the remainder have a so-called Y chromosome, which will produce a boy. Whether an X-bearing sperm or a Y-bearing one fertilizes an egg seems to be a matter of chance, and equality of the sexes is a happy reality at this earliest stage of human existence; X-bearing sperm and Y-bearing sperm unite with eggs in roughly equal numbers to produce a worldwide balance of boy and girl babies.

The overall balance does not, of course, balance an individual family; five daughters may be born to one couple, while the parents across the street seem able to produce nothing but sons. In recent years, as more parents have elected to limit the size of their families, researchers have sought to improve the odds of conceiving a child of a chosen gender.

Several techniques have been tried. One is based on a report that boy-producing sperm are smaller and faster-moving than the girl-producing kind. By fixing the exact time of ovulation and then calculating the timing of intercourse, couples attempt to ensure that the egg will be positioned to meet a faster or a slower sperm, depending on the desired gender of the offspring. Altering the acid-alkaline balance in the woman's vagina by douching is also claimed to influence sperm movement—acid (from vinegar) favoring a girl, alkaline (from baking soda) a boy. In the laboratory, attempts have been made to separate the two types of sperm from a sample of the father's semen; then the desired type could be used to artificially inseminate the mother.

All of these methods are controversial and unproved. Said Dr. Ervin Nichols of the American College of Obstetricians and Gynecologists, "There is no strong evidence to substantiate anybody's theory about sex selection. This doesn't mean it can't happen, but we haven't seen it yet."

Between the time a mature sperm becomes capable of determining the gender of a baby and the day it finally has an opportunity to do so, many weeks may pass. After sperm mature, they move out of the testicles into the epididymis, a collector in the scrotum composed of as much as 20 feet of tubing coiled into a length of 1½ inches. From there they pass on into the vas deferens, where they may remain stored

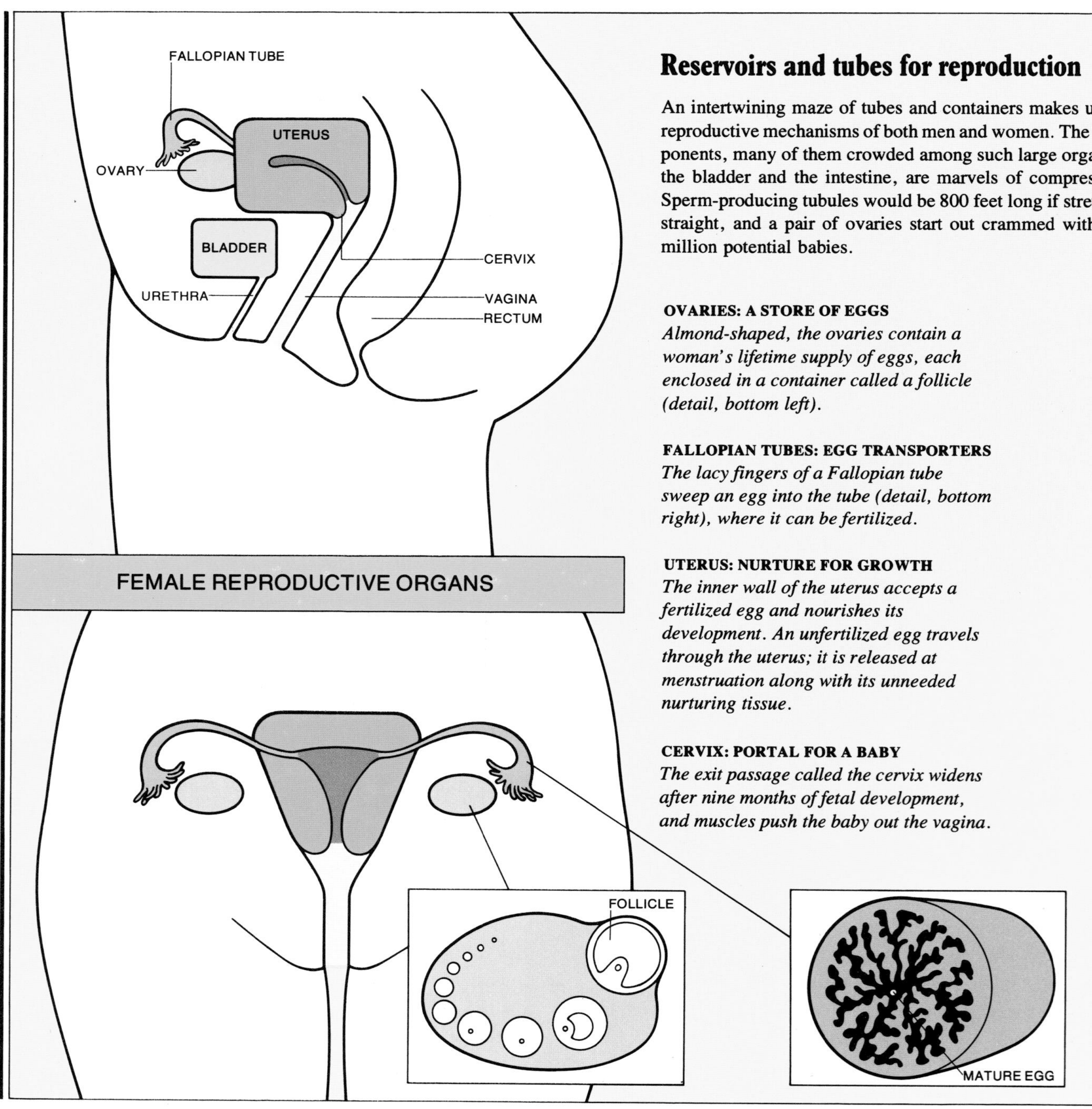

Reservoirs and tubes for reproduction

An intertwining maze of tubes and containers makes up the reproductive mechanisms of both men and women. The components, many of them crowded among such large organs as the bladder and the intestine, are marvels of compression: Sperm-producing tubules would be 800 feet long if stretched straight, and a pair of ovaries start out crammed with two million potential babies.

OVARIES: A STORE OF EGGS
Almond-shaped, the ovaries contain a woman's lifetime supply of eggs, each enclosed in a container called a follicle (detail, bottom left).

FALLOPIAN TUBES: EGG TRANSPORTERS
The lacy fingers of a Fallopian tube sweep an egg into the tube (detail, bottom right), where it can be fertilized.

UTERUS: NURTURE FOR GROWTH
The inner wall of the uterus accepts a fertilized egg and nourishes its development. An unfertilized egg travels through the uterus; it is released at menstruation along with its unneeded nurturing tissue.

CERVIX: PORTAL FOR A BABY
The exit passage called the cervix widens after nine months of fetal development, and muscles push the baby out the vagina.

Inside an ovary, about 20 egg-bearing follicles (circles) begin to mature each month. Only one ripens enough to expel a fertile egg from the ovary (upper right); the others shrivel up as their fluid contents are absorbed into the circulatory system.

This cross-section view of a Fallopian tube at a point close to the ovary reveals the convoluted folds of tissue inside it that hold the ripened egg (white dot in center). Hairlike projections from the folds help sweep the egg along to the uterus.

These drawings depict the components spread out in highly stylized form. Thus one egg-producing ovary and an egg-collecting Fallopian tube are shown in front of the uterus, or womb, in the side view *(far left, top),* while in the front view *(far left, bottom)* the pair are at either side of the uterus. In reality, the ovaries sit close to the upper sides of the uterus, toward its back, and the Fallopian tubes loop around them.

TESTICLE: FACTORY FOR SPERM
Suspended in the scrotum, the testicles produce sperm to fertilize an egg. The sperm collects in the epididymis, a 20-foot tube coiled and twisted in a small space.

VAS DEFERENS: PIPELINE FOR SPERM
This pair of long tubes stores sperm and also carries it across the bladder to the ejaculatory ducts.

GLANDS TO MAKE SEMEN
Seminal vesicles add a nourishing sugar to the sperm as it enters the ejaculatory ducts. The prostate adds an alkaline fluid, and Cowper's glands supply a lubricant that completes the semen mixture.

URETHRA: PIPELINE FOR SEMEN
This tube, which takes either semen or urine through the penis, is switched between reproductive and eliminative functions by muscles at the bladder.

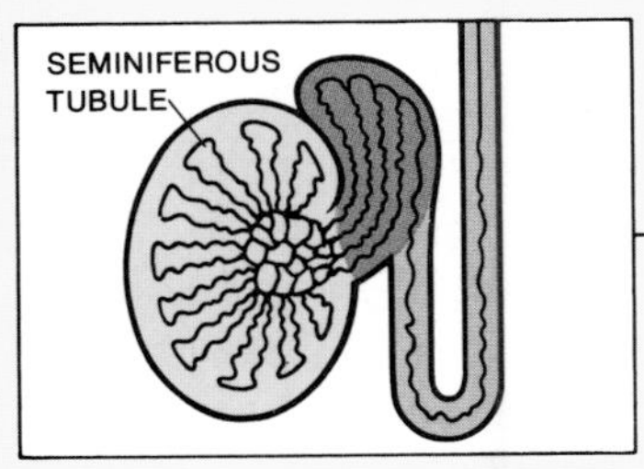

Each of the testicles, seen here in cross section with its epididymis and vas deferens, is packed with seminiferous tubules, invisibly thin sperm-producing tubes. Beginning in puberty, the tubules continuously supply sperm cells.

for several months. The vas is a much straighter tube, about 16 inches long, that winds upward from the scrotum into the pelvic cavity and passes on to the urethra, the tube that channels sperm through the penis and out of the body. When a man is sterilized, it is generally the vas deferens that is cut and tied off to block sperm—a vasectomy. While in the epididymis, the sperm develop the capacity to move by wiggling their long, thin tails in a swimming action that they will use after they leave the male body and enter the woman's vagina during intercourse.

In that climactic event, the most intensely intimate of all human relationships, the erotic sensations of intercourse clearly eclipse the purely physical mechanics. No two acts of love-making are ever exactly the same, for each partner brings to the union a unique combination of physical, mental and emotional ingredients. But the physiological processes nearly always operate according to the same pattern.

In the man, a combination of emotional excitement and tactile stimulation causes the penis to become erect. In a matter of seconds, or perhaps minutes, it is transformed from its normally flaccid state—averaging three or four inches in length—to a stiff member 6 to 6½ inches long. This tumescence occurs as nerve signals dilate arteries that supply the penis with blood, simultaneously constricting the veins that carry blood away. At the same time, nerve signals contract the epididymis, the vas deferens and the ampulla, a small chamber at the end of the vas. The squeezing action propels sperm from the vas into the urethra; this is the same channel through which urine ordinarily passes, but the sexual reflex automatically blocks off urine for the moment.

When the urethra begins to fill, other nerve signals trigger muscles around the erect penis to pulse rhythmically. The sequence climaxes in ejaculation, a pleasurable muscular spasm that sends the semen into the vagina. The discharge of physical and mental tension that occurs with the orgasmic burst is widely regarded as one of life's most satisfying sensations; women, too, may experience the pleasurable release of orgasm, although it plays no direct role in reproduction.

Each ejaculation produces about a thimbleful of semen, but less than half is sperm—100 million cells on the average. The rest of the semen is fluids the sperm has picked up along the way from supplementary organs. Some of these substances serve as a transport medium; others balance acidity.

If intercourse occurs at the time of ovulation, hormones in the female body have created conditions that are hospitable for sperm and conducive to conception. The vagina and lining of the uterus at that time are bathed in a thin mucus that possesses a remarkable capacity: It forms itself into channels that lead straight through the cervix and into the innermost recesses of the womb. Once sperm cells are deposited within this beckoning medium, they swim along the convenient channels into the uterus and from there through the inner end of the Fallopian tubes toward their destined target, the egg; most sperm make this journey in 60 to 90 minutes.

But the dropout rate is high: Of the millions of sperm released during sexual intercourse, only about 50 ever reach the egg. Many perish in the vagina, succumbing to acid secretions there. The survivors face an ingenious series of obstacles that are apparently designed to modulate sperm movement, regulating their flow so that they progress in a slow and steady stream toward the egg. This assures a gradual but continuous assault on the egg, a pattern that is much more likely to lead to conception than a system allowing all the sperm to flood through the Fallopian tubes at once.

The first of these regulating obstacles is the cervix. The sperm that enter it do so one at a time, following single file. Once into the cervix, most sperm are detained in tiny storage cavities along its inside wall, reservoirs from which they are slowly released farther into the uterus. Sperm reach another bottleneck at the openings to the Fallopian tubes, where once again they are allowed to pass through gradually. Only about 400 make it past this point—half of them into the wrong tube—and they then must swim upstream against strong currents of mucus; kept in motion by the ceaseless beating of cilia in the tube, the mucus flows in the direction of the uterus, bearing the egg toward its own destination.

Throughout the reproductive process the odds are heavily loaded in favor of conception. Hormonal signals create physical and psychological incentives for mating; sperm are available in plentiful supply; the ovaries and Fallopian tubes come in duplicate, to provide a backup system should one be damaged. Still, things can go awry. Disease, either contagious or inherent, may disrupt the process at almost any juncture. Congenital disorders and malformations may keep sperm from following the necessary path through the female tract; psychological inhibitions may interfere with conception by throwing the finely tuned hormonal machinery out of balance. Fortunately, there is much medical assistance available to treat all these ills and to help couples keep their genital systems in order and achieve a healthy conception and birth.

Controlling disorder in the systems

The fact that reproductive systems are the source of life and of many of its rewards also makes them a source of trouble, physical and psychological. In men and women, structures that are designed to nurture and safeguard delicate cellular life unfortunately can nurture disease bacteria and viruses as well. Some of the infections are contagious—these are the venereal, or sexually transmitted, diseases (STD). They afflict an estimated one in 20 Americans each year, the chief offenders being syphilis, gonorrhea and herpes.

Syphilis, caused by bacteria, first appears as an oozing sore in the area of sexual contact. If untreated, it can cause permanent damage to the heart and nervous system in both men and women. A pregnant woman who has syphilis puts her unborn child in great danger. The chances are high that the baby will be stillborn or severely deformed.

More common, but also a bacterial infection, gonorrhea causes urinary discomfort and a thick yellow-green discharge in men, and sometimes a vaginal discharge in women, although as many as 90 per cent of female cases produce no symptoms. Gonorrhea can cause permanent sterility and crippling arthritis, and if a pregnant woman is infected at the time of delivery, she can pass the disease on to her child. The baby's eyes may be permanently damaged, despite protective measures now routinely applied to the newborn.

Both syphilis and gonorrhea can be cured by antibiotics. Far more difficult to treat is the most common sexually transmitted disease, genital herpes, which is caused by a virus related to the less dangerous one of the common cold sore.

A stained smear of vaginal material from a patient with candidiasis, a common vaginal infection, reveals the disease's cause and the body's defenses against it. The red filaments are cells of Candida albicans, a yeastlike fungus; the red circles are spores from which new filaments will grow; and the small blue circles are white blood cells mobilized to destroy the invaders.

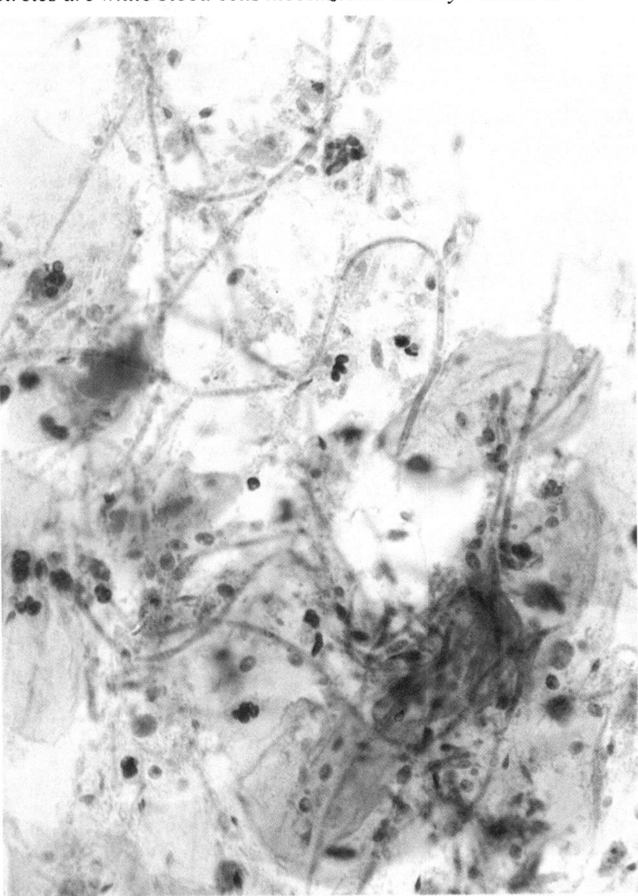

The virus takes up permanent residence in the nerve cells of the body after the initial infection, and it has been linked to an array of complications, from diseases of newborns to cervical cancer. An infant who contracts herpes in the birth canal of an infected mother may die. If a pregnant woman has an active case of genital herpes as she approaches labor, the baby should be delivered by cesarean section.

Because of the serious damage that sexually transmitted diseases can bring to victims and their children, a careful examination for them ought to be a part of a medical checkup before childbirth—preferably before conception.

In addition to these contagious diseases, there also are

several noncontagious infections of the sex organs. Most have in their names the medical syllable *itis*—which means inflammation or irritation—and all require medical attention. A variety of bacteria, fungi and protozoa, for example, cause the annoying infections of the vagina known collectively as vaginitis. These and other genital disorders are described in the Encyclopedia of Symptoms *(pages 160-171)*.

Because the ills of the reproductive systems do not always signal their presence with warning symptoms, regular medical examinations are necessary to detect problems in the early, treatable stages. For men, an annual examination beginning at the age of 40 is recommended; a woman's complex, vulnerable system requires regular monitoring from the age of 20—or sooner if she is already sexually active.

Elusive causes of infertility

Subtle disorders of the reproductive tract may be missed in a routine check-up, prompting concern only when a couple has tried and failed to conceive. Infertility troubles one in every six American couples; the causes, when they can be identified, are about evenly divided between men and women.

Male infertility is the simplest to diagnose; most often it results from a lack of effective sperm. Although the number of sperm released can vary by as much as a factor of five without noticeably affecting the ability to father a child, the number and viability are important, for the greater the number of healthy sperm that enter the woman's body, the greater the likelihood that at least one can wriggle its way to an egg and fertilize it. To test for adequate sperm, a sample obtained by masturbation is placed under a microscope to see how many cells there are and how actively they move. Even when sperm counts are low, pregnancy can occur if the cells are normal in size and shape and are able to move energetically.

Some causes of male infertility are simple and easily countered. The culprit may be a drug; some drugs lower sperm count. Extreme heat may be a factor—from a fever, from a job requiring work near a furnace, or simply from tight underwear that squeezes the testicles too close to body heat.

Generally, however, chronically low levels of sperm are caused by hormonal disturbance, by blockage in the sexual tubing or by some malfunction in the sperm-producing tubules. Most hormone deficiencies can be remedied with drugs, and faulty sperm manufacture or duct blockage is generally repairable by surgery.

Infertility in the female is more difficult to pinpoint because the reproductive mechanisms are so complex. Sometimes the search for solutions continues for years.

"Month after month, the day after my menstrual period ended, there I was back in the gynecologist's office, saying, 'Okay doctor, what do we try next?' " a New York magazine writer said, recalling the four exasperating years she and her husband spent trying to conceive a child following five years of carefully planned childlessness.

Because her husband had fathered children by a previous marriage, she was almost certainly the source of the problem. A history of irregular menstrual cycles—frequently a clue to hormonal malfunctioning—suggested that this common abnormality might be the cause of infertility, as it is for many women. Too little estrogen and progesterone, for example, may interfere with preparation of the uterine lining for the implantation of the fertilized egg. A sample of tissue scraped from the lining of the uterus can show whether it has developed sufficiently for implantation, but even simpler techniques often suffice to evaluate hormone production.

To determine whether estrogen and progesterone are being released on schedule, the woman may be asked to keep a daily chart of her body's basal—its very lowest—temperature. She must take this reading every morning before she gets up, since the slightest activity can raise the temperature. Basal temperature is an index of hormone production and ovulation because it jumps at least .8 degree, and perhaps as much as 1.5 degrees, when the egg is released, and it remains that high until menstruation begins—or, should conception take place, throughout the subsequent pregnancy.

The temperature change is caused by opposite effects of the two hormones. Estrogen, manufactured while the egg follicle is developing during the first half of the menstrual cycle, depresses temperature. Progesterone, manufactured as soon as an egg is released, raises body temperature.

Temperature charts can be a helpful but tedious exercise in

a couple's quest for fertility. "You can't get away from it," the New York woman reflected. "It's on your mind every morning the minute you open your eyes: You've got to take that temperature before you can even sit up. When I traveled on business, the first thing I packed was that thermometer."

The woman's chart did indeed reveal irregular hormone levels. Her basal temperature did not jump at mid-cycle to indicate ovulation and preparation for pregnancy; apparently no viable egg was being released or the accompanying hormonal activity was inadequate. Her doctor found that at the time ovulation should have occurred, her cervical mucus, also controlled by hormones, was too thick to permit proper transport of her husband's sperm. Its *spinnbarkeit*—"ability to be spun" in German—was low, unlike that of healthy mid-cycle mucus, which can be stretched to as much as 20 times its unstressed dimensions. Also below normal was its "ferning": Healthy mucus dries in a fernlike pattern.

Medicines to alter the quality and quantity of cervical mucus and hormones to stimulate the ovaries were among several therapies the New York woman's doctor prescribed over three years. And like many stories of long-childless parents, this couple's eventually had a happy—and inadvertent—ending. Conception occurred at a seemingly impossible point in the woman's menstrual cycle, on a July day long past the presumed time of ovulation, when she and her husband were vacationing and not dutifully trying to conceive.

When her menstrual period did not begin on schedule, she noted a new temperature pattern: The chart had gone up during the vacation and then stayed at the higher level, the usual signal of pregnancy. "When I showed my doctor the chart he smiled and said, 'Well, hello, Mama! These charts almost never lie!' " A healthy baby girl was born in April of the following year.

In a positive test for one aspect of female fertility, a dried sample of the mucus that protects the cervix, or neck of the womb, exhibits a fine, fernlike pattern at the time of ovulation. The pattern indicates that the mucus is relatively thin and clear, permitting sperm to move easily through the cervix and into the womb; during the rest of the month, the mucus is dense and impenetrable.

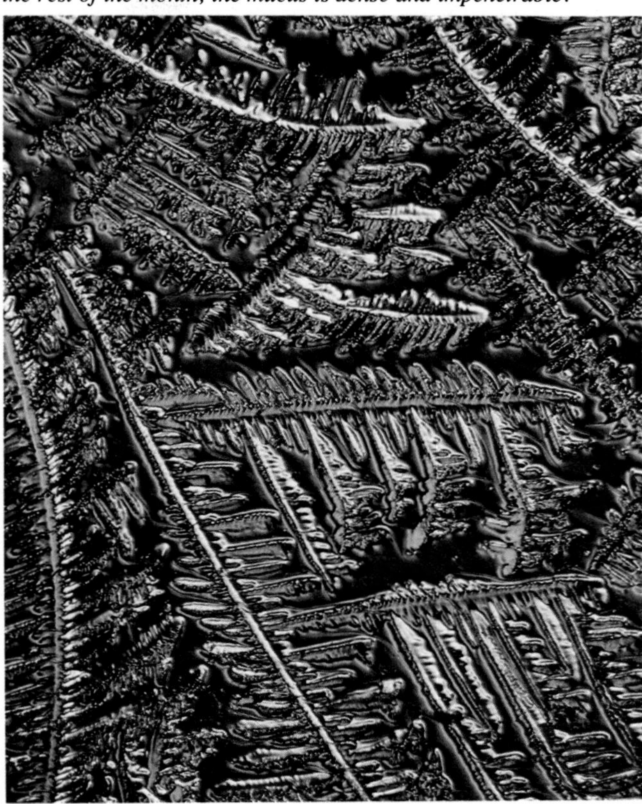

Surgery to aid conception

In many cases of infertility, the fault is not chemical but structural. Malformations of the ovaries, Fallopian tubes or uterus, either from disease or from some trauma—for example, scar tissue stemming from an appendectomy—can be to blame. Surgical repair may permit conception, though such intervention brings some risk of further complications.

Today, physicians can look directly into cloistered internal organs with instruments employing optical fibers, pencil-thin bundles of glass fibers that transmit light into the body and bring images out to an eyepiece. One such instrument is an optical-fiber laparoscope, which is inserted through a tiny incision in the abdomen. While performing such an examination, a doctor may carry out a test that gauges the ability of the tubes to transport the egg to the uterus. He inserts grains of sterilized starch through the incision and deposits them into the upper ends of the Fallopian tubes. The cilia should bring the grains to the uterus; from here the grains will move out into the vagina, where they are easily detected. The laparoscope and similar devices enable the doctor to check

Methods of family planning

Many doctors recommend that couples space the births of their children at least two or three years apart. The advice has a medical basis: The mother's body needs time to recover from the physical stress of childbirth and to regain nutrients lost in pregnancy and breast-feeding. Her health, of course, helps determine the health of the children she bears.

Many methods for contraception, or birth control, are available to couples who wish to plan their families in this way. Eight common methods are described on these pages. All are safe, but they vary widely in effectiveness. In the statistics given here, based on compilations by Dr. Robert A. Hatcher of Emory University and Dr. Gary K. Stewart of the University of California, each effectiveness figure represents the success rate of 100 couples who used the method for a year. Theoretically, maximum effectiveness is somewhat higher, but even to attain the rates given below, the methods must be used correctly and consistently. Be sure you fully understand the method you select, and be prepared to use a backup method if one is called for.

Several widely practiced methods of birth control are not included here. Some, such as sterilization, are essentially irreversible and therefore can play only a final role in family planning. Others have been found ineffective or unsafe; douching after intercourse, for example, may actually promote pregnancy by forcing sperm upward into the uterus.

RHYTHMIC ABSTINENCE

This method of birth control has three variations, all based on abstinence from intercourse during the most fertile days of the menstrual cycle: the three days before ovulation and the two after it. A woman may use one or a combination of the variations. Calendar rhythm is best used by a woman with extremely regular periods. The day of ovulation is predicted by counting back 14 days from the expected onset of the next menstruation. Temperature rhythm relies on identifying the slight rise in basal body temperature that generally accompanies ovulation (page 9). To predict ovulation, a woman must take her temperature daily upon arising and chart the readings. Mucus rhythm requires the daily examination of cervical mucus for changes in quantity and texture that indicate ovulation; thin, clear mucus produced in abundance is characteristic of the days of fertility.

EFFECTIVENESS: 76 per cent. The low success rate has several causes. Because ovulation can occur at any time during the menstrual cycle, the possibility of pregnancy always exists. Temperature changes and mucus changes are often difficult to detect and may be produced by factors other than ovulation, such as semen in the vagina or a fever.

ADVANTAGES: The method has no side effects. It is the only method acceptable to the Roman Catholic Church.

DISADVANTAGES: The method increases the likelihood of fertilizing an overripe ovum, which in turn carries an increased risk of fetal abnormalities.

COITUS INTERRUPTUS

In this ancient method, the man prevents sperm from entering the vagina by completely withdrawing the penis before ejaculation. A spermicide should be available for immediate use if a couple believes semen has escaped into the vagina, and a backup method of birth control should be used if intercourse is repeated soon.

EFFECTIVENESS: 77 per cent. The low success rate is mainly due to failures in the control of ejaculation.

ADVANTAGES: This method has no side effects and is always available.

DISADVANTAGES: Besides the need to control ejaculation, the method carries intrinsic hazards. Semen can leak into the vagina in small amounts without the man's knowledge, especially if he has already had an orgasm. If ejaculation occurs near the woman's external genitals, sperm may migrate into the vagina.

CONDOM

A condom is a rubber or animal-skin sheath that covers the penis; the exterior of the sheath is often lubricated before intercourse. During ejaculation, semen collects in the condom. To prevent this collected semen from spilling into the vagina, the penis and condom must be withdrawn before erection is lost. A spermicide should be available for immediate use if a couple believes that semen has escaped into the vagina.

EFFECTIVENESS: 90 per cent. The most likely cause of failure is improper use, such as withdrawing the penis after erection is lost; using a rubber-weakening lubricant, such as petroleum jelly or cold cream; reusing a condom, or using one that is either heat-damaged or more than five years old.

ADVANTAGES: Condoms are easy to use and readily available without a prescription. They provide partial protection against venereal diseases and infections. They are often recommended when a woman is breast-feeding, because they do not introduce chemicals that can adversely affect breast milk.

DISADVANTAGES: Rubber condoms can provoke an allergic reaction; this can be avoided by using condoms made of animal skin.

DIAPHRAGM

A diaphragm is a dome-shaped device made of soft latex or rubber. Held in place by the tension of a flexible metal rim, it covers the inner end of the vaginal canal, including the cervix, and keeps sperm out of the uterus. It must always be accompanied by a spermicide. After intercourse, the diaphragm must remain in place at least six hours before removal. If intercourse is repeated during that time, a backup method such as a spermicide or a condom should be used.

EFFECTIVENESS: 81 per cent. Failure is most likely to occur if the diaphragm is incorrectly fitted or inserted, if it is used without a spermicide, or if a backup method is not used when intercourse is repeated.

ADVANTAGES: A diaphragm, with instruction, is fairly easy to use. It offers some protection from venereal diseases and infections.

DISADVANTAGES: Diaphragms cannot be inserted correctly by women with certain vaginal conformations. The devices may cause urinary and vaginal infections, constipation and allergic reactions. Some women have difficulty in inserting or removing a diaphragm.

CERVICAL CAP

The cervical cap is similar to the diaphragm, but covers the cervix alone, and is held in place by suction rather than tension. It is used with a spermicide and must be left in place at least six hours after intercourse.

EFFECTIVENESS: 87 per cent. Although studies are incomplete, failure seems to come primarily from incorrect fitting or insertion, from slippage due to an excess of spermicide, and from spermicides that become ineffective during the relatively long time a cap is worn.

ADVANTAGES: The cervical cap can safely remain in place up to three days. Women unable to wear diaphragms can often be successfully fitted for a cap. Because it does not press on the bladder, it is less likely to contribute to urinary-tract infections.

DISADVANTAGES: For some women the cap is harder to insert and remove than a diaphragm. It may also carry a greater risk of cervical irritation than the diaphragm. Although cervical caps have been used in Europe for more than a century, they do not yet have the approval of the Food and Drug Administration and are available only through clinics and doctors who have special FDA permission to dispense them.

SPERMICIDES

Spermicides are chemicals that prevent conception by blocking the cervix and by releasing an agent that immobilizes and kills sperm. They come in many forms: creams, jellies, aerosol foams, suppositories and tablets. Each must be inserted deep in the vagina near the cervix shortly before intercourse.

EFFECTIVENESS: 82 per cent. Spermicides fail primarily because of inconsistent or improper use. Manufacturer's directions must be followed with special care.

ADVANTAGES: Available without a prescription, spermicides are especially useful as a temporary, backup or emergency method of birth control. They provide partial protection from venereal diseases and infections and have few proven side effects.

DISADVANTAGES: Spermicides must be reinserted before each act of intercourse. On rare occasions, they have caused allergic reactions. Suppositories and tablets sometimes fail to dissolve completely, causing irritation and decreasing their effectiveness.

HORMONAL CONTRACEPTIVES

Hormonal contraceptives are drugs available in two varieties, both by prescription only. A combined oral contraceptive (the Pill), containing the hormones estrogen and progestin, prevents pregnancy mainly by suppressing ovulation. A progestin-only oral contraceptive (the Minipill) creates a uterine environment that is hostile to both sperm and ovum. The Minipill must be taken daily; the Pill is taken on 21 days of the menstrual cycle, but many manufacturers package it with seven dummy tablets to encourage a one-a-day regimen. Backup methods of birth control are recommended for the first month of Pill use, the first two months of Minipill use, and whenever a sequence of doses is broken.

EFFECTIVENESS: Pill: 98 per cent; Minipill: 97.5 per cent. Most failures occur because pills are skipped or because the prescribed levels of hormones are too low.

ADVANTAGES: These are easy to use. They tend to ease premenstrual tension, reduce menstrual flow and relieve cramps.

DISADVANTAGES: Some women experience one or more of the following side effects: nausea, vomiting, dizziness, headache, enlarged or tender breasts, fluid retention, weight gain or bleeding. These contraceptives have been linked to cancer of the cervix and skin, and tend to raise blood pressure and thus increase the risk of stroke and coronary-artery disease. The Minipill increases the risk of a dangerous ectopic pregnancy, in which the fertilized ovum is implanted outside the uterus.

INTRAUTERINE DEVICE

The intrauterine device (IUD) is a small, flexible device that is inserted into the uterus, where it can stay for up to three years. It prevents pregnancy, according to one theory, by keeping the uterine wall constantly irritated and thus preventing the implantation of a fertilized egg in the wall of the uterus. IUDs come in a variety of sizes and shapes and must be inserted and removed by a doctor.

EFFECTIVENESS: 95 per cent. Failure usually results from the improper insertion or undetected expulsion of the device.

ADVANTAGES: Once the IUD is inserted, the user need only periodically check strings that extend from the device and through the cervical opening.

DISADVANTAGES: Many women expel the devices spontaneously or suffer from repeated infections, pain, severe menstrual cramps or increased blood loss during menstruation. The IUD also increases the risk of pelvic inflammatory disease and ectopic pregnancies.

for malformations of the uterus—which often cause repeated miscarriages—and to look for tumors and the misplaced uterine tissue of endometriosis.

In cases of seemingly intractable infertility—whatever the cause—radical remedies are sometimes possible, although their use is the subject of moral and medical controversy. Since the 1770s, women have been artificially inseminated with sperm from their husbands; since the 1890s, with sperm from donors more fertile than their husbands. Today a living egg can be removed from a woman's ovary with a laparoscope, fertilized in a laboratory with her husband's sperm, then implanted directly into her uterus for growth. This technique enabled Mrs. Lesley Brown of Bristol, England, to give birth, on July 25, 1978, to a healthy daughter, the world's first test-tube baby.

A more elusive impediment to fertility than either disease or physical abnormality—and one affecting women and men alike—is the psychological and physical impact of tension. Stress influences not just a man's short-term ability to perform the sex act; in women stress can sometimes affect hormone levels and cause organs to function improperly.

Ironically, stress at times can be an unintended by-product of a childless couple's desperate attempts to conceive a child. One woman who tried with her husband for years to become pregnant, carefully timing intercourse according to her individual hormonal calendar, summed up the dilemma this way: "You just can't make love on schedule month in and month out, and then watch your efforts fail every time, without it taking a toll on the loving relationship," she said. "After a while, one does begin to question one's femininity. 'Everybody else can do it, why can't I?' is the way you begin to feel. Then, because you feel inadequate, you start thinking maybe your husband thinks you're inadequate, and a kind of spiral of doubting yourself and your husband begins. These feelings can really turn a marriage inside out."

Solving problems by sex therapy

The stressful effects of futilely trying to become parents are generally transient; most couples who want children this badly have relationships strong enough to withstand their inability to conceive. Other aspects of sex may be a greater threat to a marriage. Many people manage to have children with no difficulty at all, yet cannot seem to achieve the same successful results with the loving intimacy, playfulness and erotic pleasure that are essential to a well-adjusted sex life. For more than a century, sexual incompatibility has been treated with lengthy, expensive psychoanalysis, but only after World War II was direct, simple sexual therapy developed. By the 1980s, it was being provided by an estimated 2,500 practitioners.

Sex therapy is brisk and short-term, a direct confrontation with the particular problems affecting a couple. It has come under fire for those very qualities, often criticized as mechanical, superficial and capable only of short-term benefits. Some therapists who treat individuals rather than couples have been accused of practices bordering on prostitution. For obvious reasons, the success—or failure—of sex therapy programs is very difficult to evaluate.

Couples who seek this kind of counseling often suffer from one of two types of sexual dissatisfaction: problems of desire or problems of response. Both types trouble both men and women and, with one important exception, seem to be largely psychological in origin. The exception is a man's failure to achieve or maintain an erection during intercourse—impotence. Any man may suffer this minor malfunction from time to time, but for some it happens so frequently—and brings with it so much emotional fallout—that sex life is disrupted. A lack of the hormone testosterone may reduce the sex drive. And in recent years doctors have noted a variety of physical substances and disturbances that affect male erection—among them diabetes, fatigue, reduced blood flow to the penis and drugs such as tranquilizers and blood-pressure medicines. Some experts believe that at least half of all impotence has physical causes, and treating the known causes generally eliminates the impotence.

When physical abnormality is ruled out, the treatment of sexual problems is simple and straightforward, although the patients may not find the prescriptions easy to follow. Techniques vary with the practitioners, but all aim to teach the couple ways to attain loving pleasure through sexual intercourse and other expressions of physical closeness. At the St. Louis clinic of pioneer sex therapists Dr. William H. Masters and Virginia E. Johnson, couples are usually required to stay for two weeks. One wife, who credits the program with saving her marriage, reflected on the great changes wrought in her relationship with her husband within those two weeks: "We were finally able to give each other what we needed and wanted, after so many years of antagonism. We were discovering a whole new basis for our life together. Together is an important word here," she added. "We stopped thinking of *me* and thought in terms of *us*."

This basic shift in attitude was brought about through counseling—plus, surprisingly, an embargo on sexual activity for the first 48 hours of the program. Even discussing the problem was forbidden. In one counseling session, the woman recalled, Dr. Masters explained that "giving pleasure and satisfaction to another person can be one of the most satisfying acts in the whole human experience. There is a pleasant emotion in simply holding and loving and being close to someone. The sexual act, to be fully satisfying emotionally, should be an act of commitment to another person, even if only for a short time."

To introduce the couple to this relaxed notion of sex, Dr. Masters instructed them to set aside two periods of about 20 minutes during the next 24 hours, and to use them as practice sessions in purely giving pleasure to each other. "If I wanted my hair combed, or my back rubbed, or my face caressed, this is what my husband was to do," the woman explained. "He was to concentrate on the pleasure-giving aspects of the moment, enjoying the feeling of texture under his fingers."

During these periods, there was to be no sex or sexual stimulation; the idea was to avoid emphasis on that part of the relationship and concentrate on the sheer pleasure of bodily communication. Gradually, the woman said, "We were able to look at each other as pleasure-giving individuals, whereas before, our relationship was so full of pain we avoided almost all contact." In an atmosphere of pleasure-giving, Masters and Johnson have found, sex naturally flourishes.

When it does, and when conception is not blocked by contraceptives or physical defects, things happen fast. Minutes after sperm have entered the vagina during intercourse, they begin to penetrate the cervical mucus and swim on into the womb, moving along at a speed of about an eighth of an inch per minute. Within half an hour of ejaculation, sperm can be in the Fallopian tubes, where fertilization is to occur. When the sperm encounters the egg, chemicals in the head of the male sex cell dissolve the egg's protective coating—and at the moment the sperm penetrates, the two cells fuse and form a casing impenetrable to other sperm. The journey continues, and if all goes well the fertilized egg reaches the uterus within a few days.

Inside this minute structure, still no larger than a pinpoint, the identity of the new individual has already been established. The parents' joined chromosomes, a genetic blueprint for the growth of their child, have helped determine the color of the eyes and skin, the shape of the nose and the ultimate height of the body. Here too is the chromosome that determines whether the baby will be a boy or a girl, with the capacity to become a father or mother in turn some day. The epic of sex and procreation has begun once again. ❋

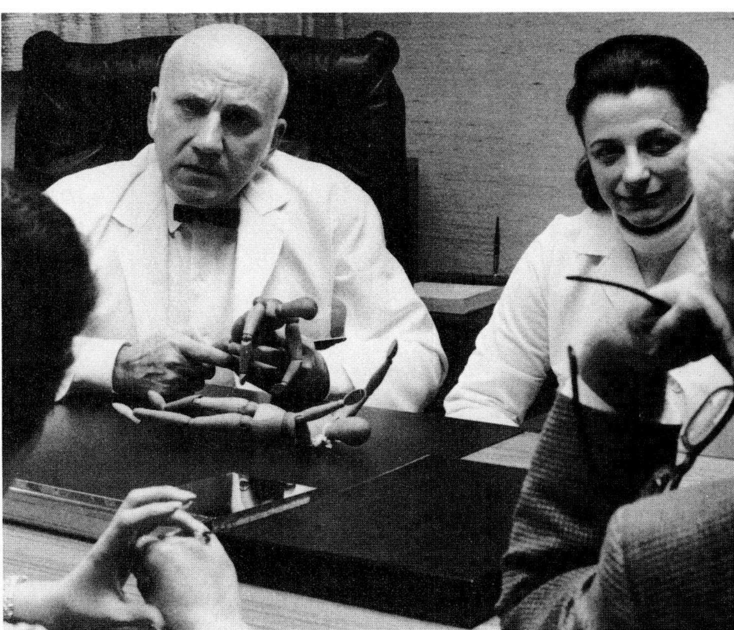

At their clinic in St. Louis, Missouri, sex researchers William H. Masters and Virginia E. Johnson use wooden models in counseling a couple in therapy. In addition to compiling studies of sexual behavior, Masters and Johnson pioneered techniques for dealing with infertility, impotence and sexual incompatibility—problems that may afflict as many as half of American marriages.

The startling beauty of life's primal scenes

The drama of life's opening act unfolds in places of intricate and unexpected beauty, but only in recent years have photographic techniques brought the details of this fundamental human event within the range of the human eye. The pictures shown here and on the following pages—some taken inside living bodies, others in dissected tissue, still others in laboratory glassware—are among the first images ever recorded of an egg's long, slow journey to the womb. The journey begins in the ovary, where eggs are stored and released. It ends in the uterus, where a single egg is nurtured and grows. But its climax takes place between the two, in the lining of a Fallopian tube *(right),* where sperm and egg meet and conception occurs.

The courtship of sperm and egg is a cat-and-mouse affair, conducted against barriers of time and distance. Sperm cells, ejected by the millions during intercourse, live only 48 hours; the object they struggle to reach, a ripened egg in the Fallopian tube, dies within 18 hours if it is not fertilized. And though the distance from the vagina to the farthest reaches of the Fallopian tube is only a few inches, the minute, single-celled sperm takes up to an hour and a half to traverse it. Consisting of little more than a lashing tail for propulsion and a head bearing genetic information, a sperm cell makes its way upstream in the female genital tract, fighting against currents of mucus and other fluids to fulfill its mission—the fateful meeting that marks the beginning of new life.

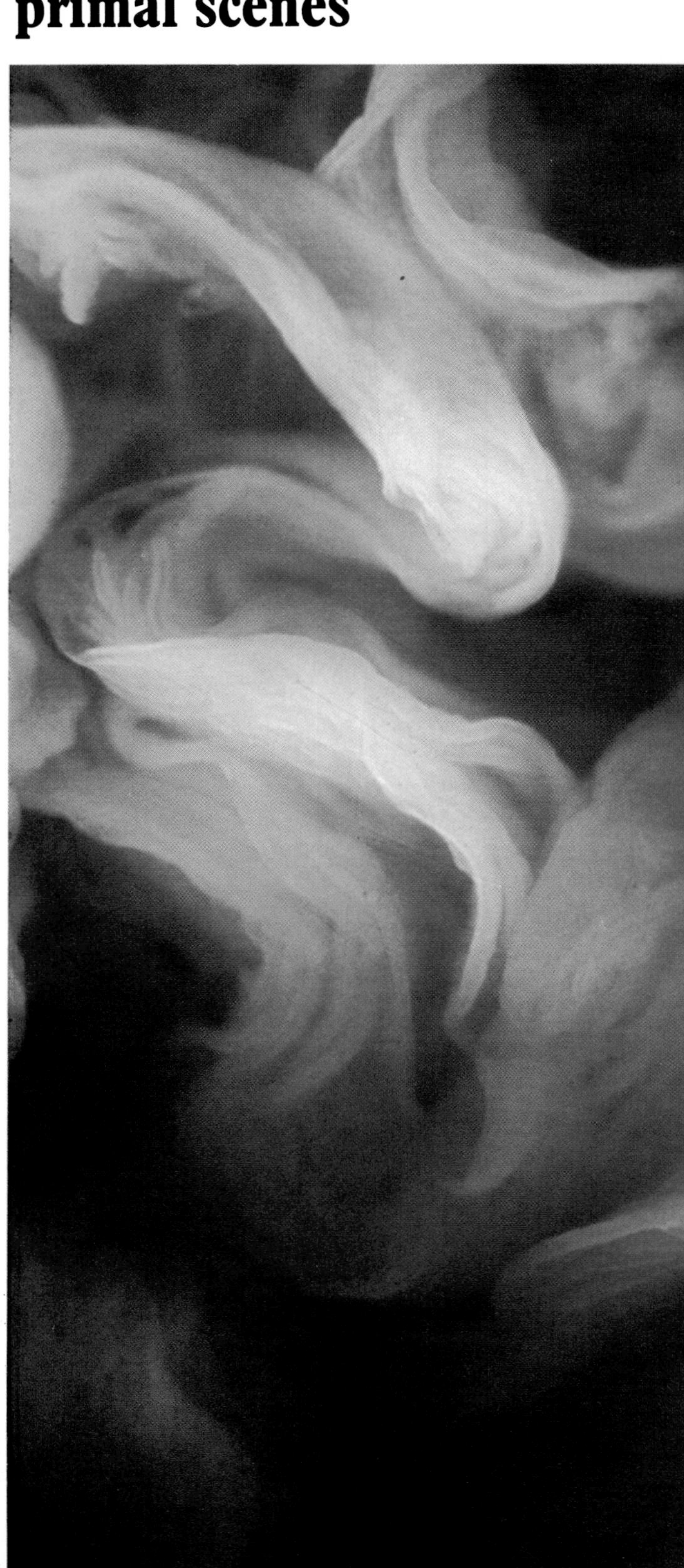

A section of tissue removed from a Fallopian-tube lining, magnified 25 times, suggests a cloudscape in constant motion. Within these folds and filaments, sperm and egg come together for a three-day journey to the womb, inched along by rhythmic contractions and undulations of the Fallopian wall.

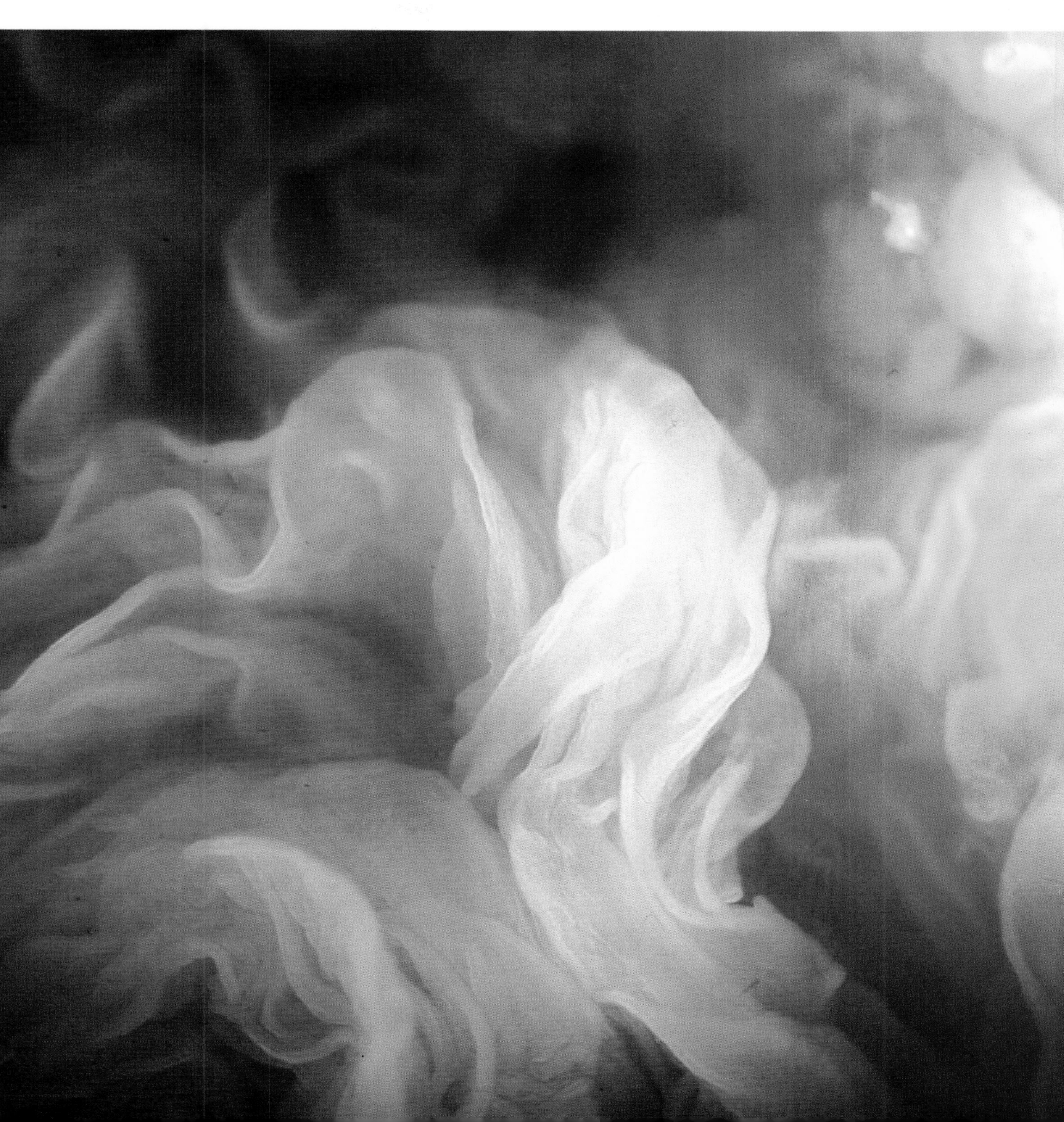

An explosion that frees an egg

At the inner ends of the female genital tract lie the ovaries, two oval sacs an inch or two long, that nestle like twin islands at the sides of the womb. In a woman of child-bearing age, an opportunity to conceive a child occurs once a month, when a ripened egg, ready for its rendezvous with sperm, bursts free of an ovary and enters the nearby Fallopian tube. The remarkable sequence of photographs at right records this process of ovulation as it took place within a woman's body. To capture these scenes on film, the Japanese photographer Junichiro Takeda used an endoscope, a flexible, pencil-thin tube fitted with lights and lenses. Threaded harmlessly through the vagina, uterus and Fallopian tube, the endoscope transmitted images from the body's interior to an external camera.

The egg seen embarking on its journey to the womb was present in the woman's body before she was born, in the form of an undeveloped egg cell called an oocyte. At birth, her ovaries contained about two million of these cells. Most are short-lived; at puberty, about 300,000 remain, and of that number only some 400 will ever mature and break free. They do so according to a strict schedule. Chemical messengers called hormones, released in a cyclical pattern as orderly and measured as the phases of the moon, trigger each ovulation. The same hormones also prepare the mobile end of a Fallopian tube *(opposite)* for the impending event. At ovulation the tube end moves toward the ovary to ensnare the emerging egg. Waving movements of the tube's fringed mouth gently sweep the drifting egg into a five-inch corridor—the tube itself—where muscle contractions and the beating of hairlike cilia move it to the uterus.

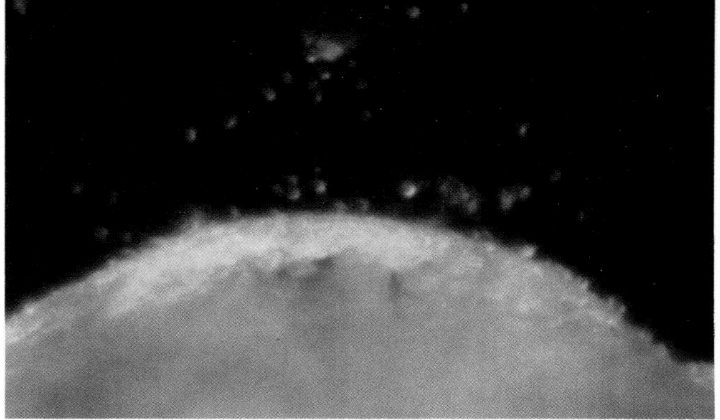

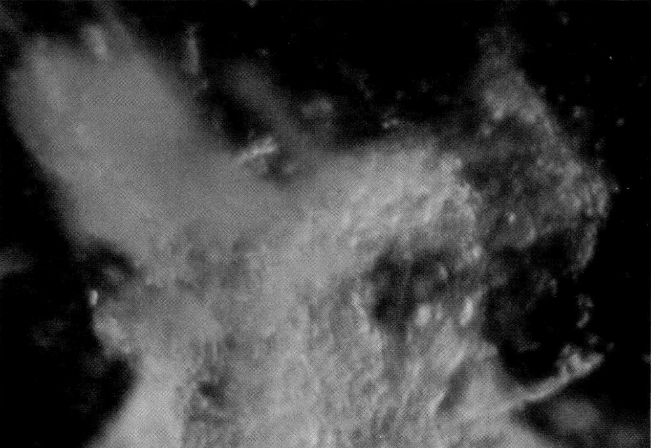

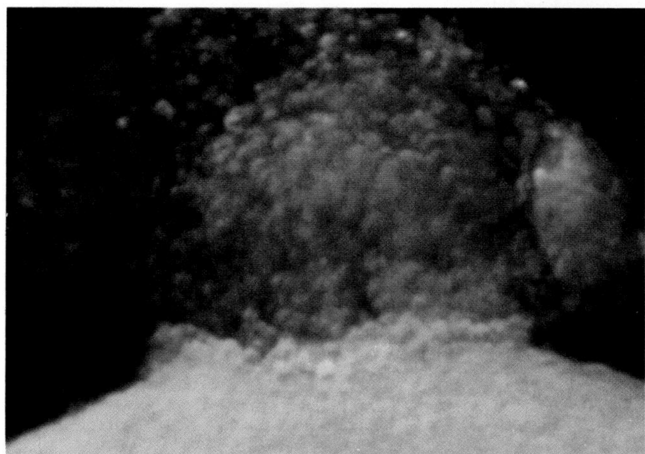

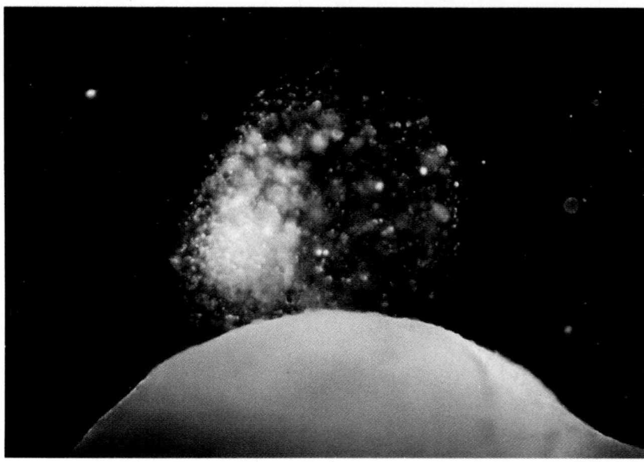

Magnified hundreds of times, the surface of an ovary reveals a blister-like bulge marking the position of a follicle, or capsule, that houses a ripening egg (top). Twelve to 16 days after the follicle begins to swell, its wall ruptures explosively (second from top). For a moment, the contents of the follicle float above the burst ovarian wall in a cloudy greenish globule of hormones and nutrients (third from top); then, seconds later, the mature egg, partly obscured by the thick fluid that surrounds it, drifts free of the ovary (bottom). The fluid will nourish and protect the egg as it travels on the first leg of its journey, from the ovary to the end of a Fallopian tube—as much as an inch away.

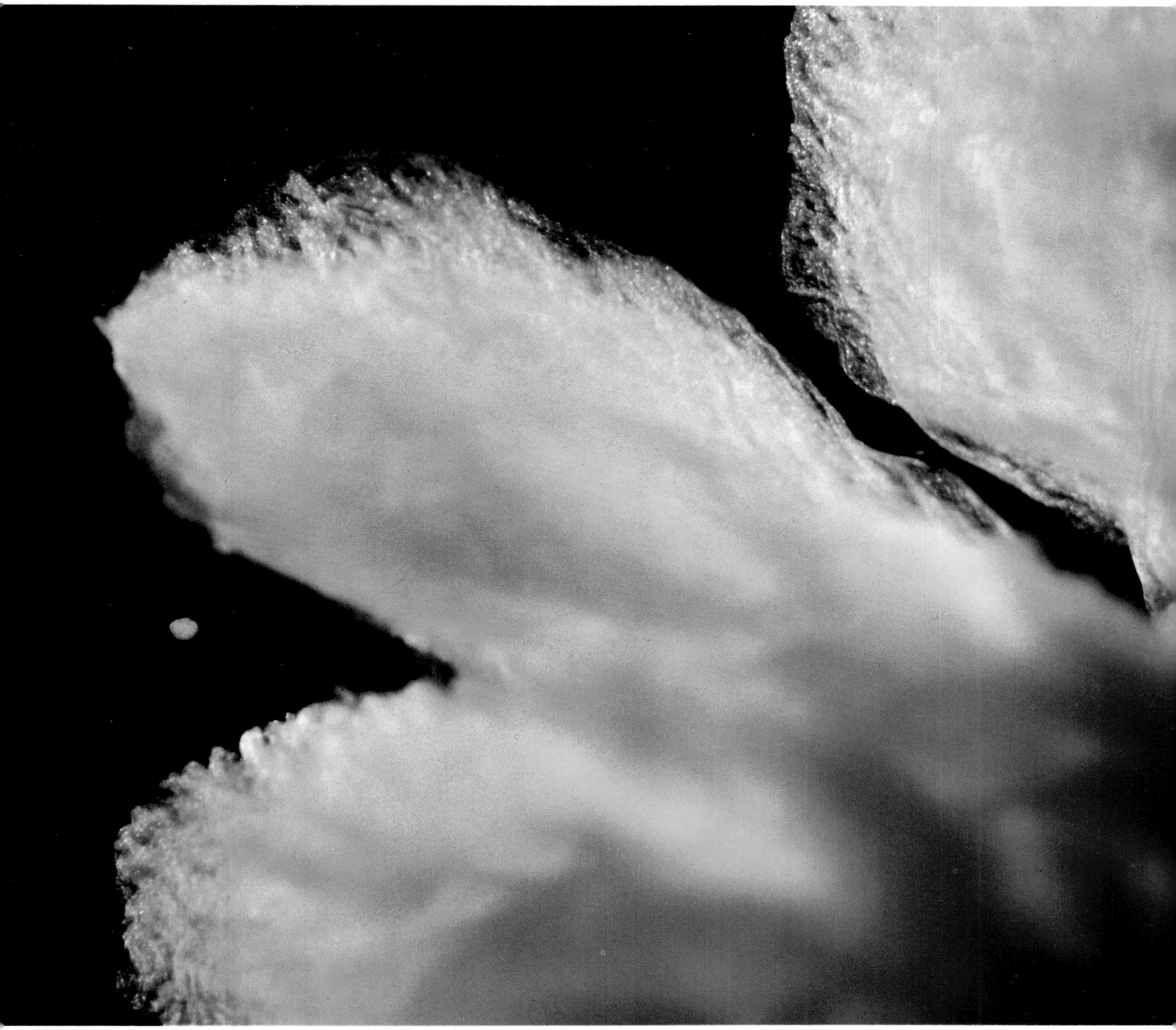

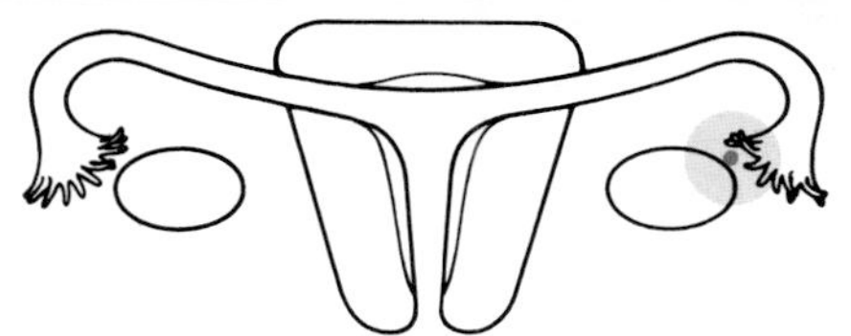

In the gap between the ovary and the Fallopian tube, indicated by a pink circle in the diagram at left, finger-like projections called fimbriae expand from the end of the tube toward the tiny floating egg (above). The egg can neither propel nor steer itself; it is drawn into the tube by sweeping motions of the fimbriae.

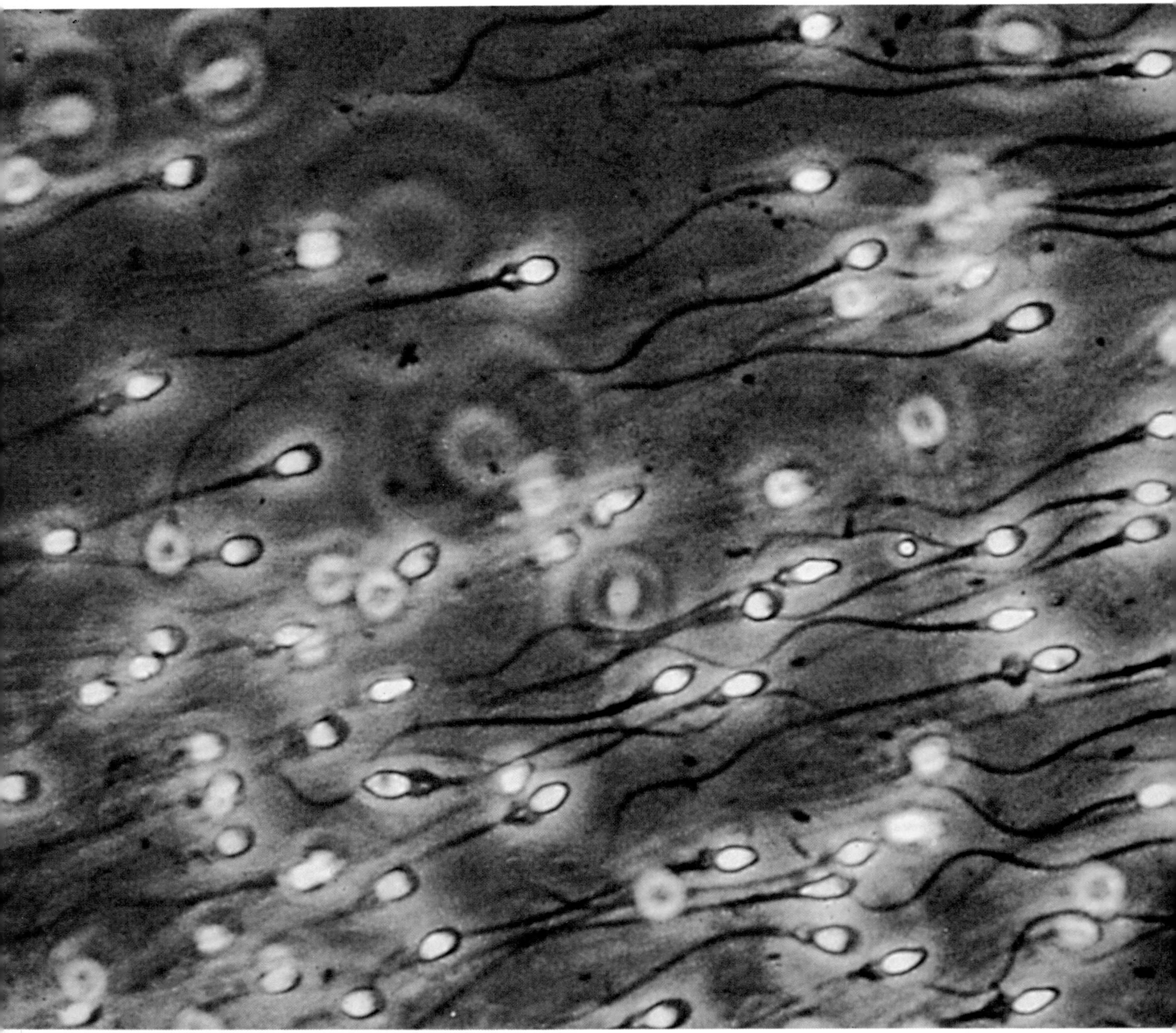

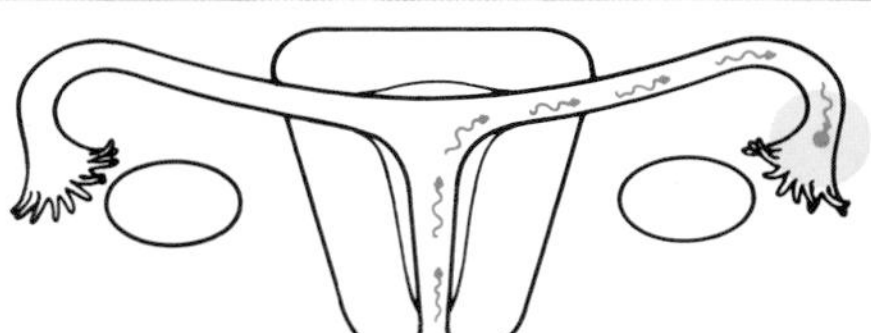

Swimming sperm cells, representing only a tiny fraction of the more than 100 million released in an ejaculation, are seen here on a laboratory slide. Their route in a living body, marked by a stream of sperm in the diagram at left, leads through the uterus and on to a Fallopian tube. Union with an egg typically occurs toward the far end of the tube (pink circle in diagram).

A sperm cell's upstream struggle

By comparison with the egg's short, free flight from ovary to Fallopian tube, the sperm's pilgrimage against the currents of the female reproductive tract is long and difficult. Deposited in the vagina, sperm cells stream through the uterus and up the tube, propelled by their lashing tails at about three inches per hour. The vast majority drop out along the way; of the millions that begin the journey, a few thousand get as far as the uterus, and only a few hundred make their way to the inner section of the Fallopian tube.

There, in the convoluted folds of the tube's lining, conception takes place. The sperm cells that reach the egg surround and besiege it, butting their heads against the surface in a furious attempt to penetrate the interior. The partners in this frenzied dance are grossly mismatched in size: If an egg were enlarged to the diameter of a dime, a correspondingly enlarged sperm would be no bigger than the period at the end of this sentence. Yet both carry equivalent burdens of hereditary information to their union.

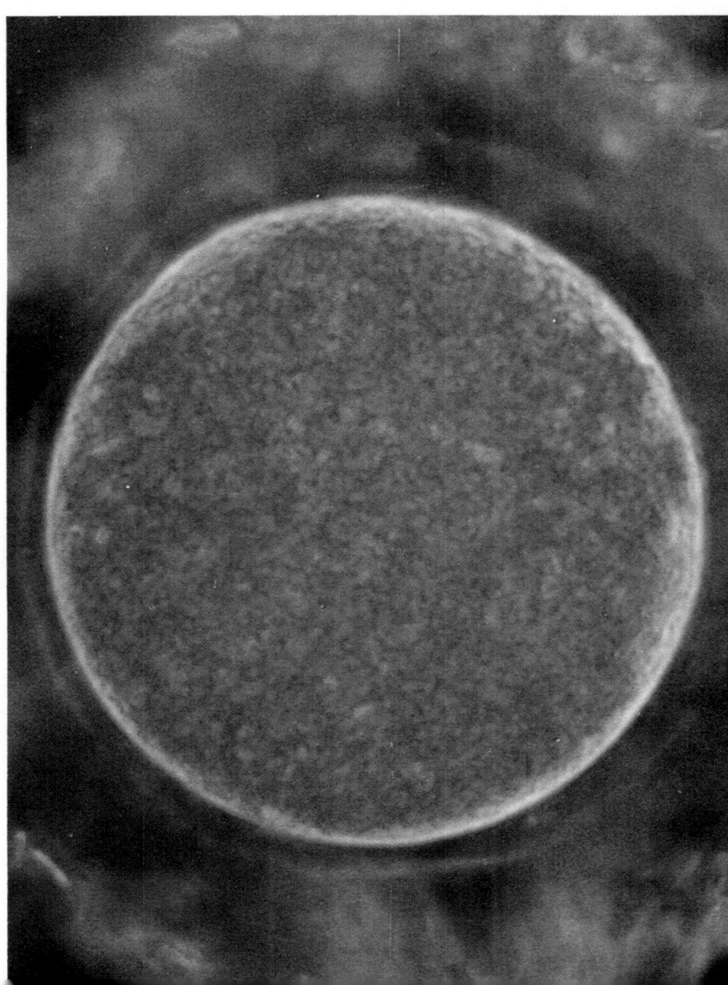

In a photograph taken inside a rabbit's Fallopian tube, an egg is surrounded by a luminous ring of sperm cells. When a single cell penetrates the egg, no others can enter; the rival sperm simply die off, while the fertilized egg begins to multiply.

The snowballing progress of cell division

With fertilization, the sperm cell's work is done; the egg takes over. During the first day after fertilization, the egg undergoes a process called mitosis, or cell division. Its single cell splits in two; the two become four; the four, eight. Eventually, at the end of its journey through the Fallopian tube, the egg reaches the uterus as a knobby, mulberry-like mass of as many as 50 cells, enclosed in a clear protective sac, the *zona pellucida*.

The sequence of pictures on these pages follows the week-long transformations of a fertilized rabbit egg from the Fallopian tube to the uterus. In one respect the pictures are misleading. For clarity, they were made at increasing magnifications, so that the egg appears to grow in size. In fact, both rabbit and human eggs remain the same size; both are barely visible specks throughout their journey in the Fallopian tube. But as embryos lodged in the uterus wall, they do grow—enormously. In humans, the newborn baby that emerges from the uterus 266 days after conception weighs a billion times as much as the original egg, and contains 200 million cells—including the rudiments of sperm or egg cells that can start a new generation of life.

A photograph made 30 hours after fertilization shows an egg that has already divided into two distinct cells. The whitish structures in which the egg rests are part of the ridged wall of a Fallopian tube.

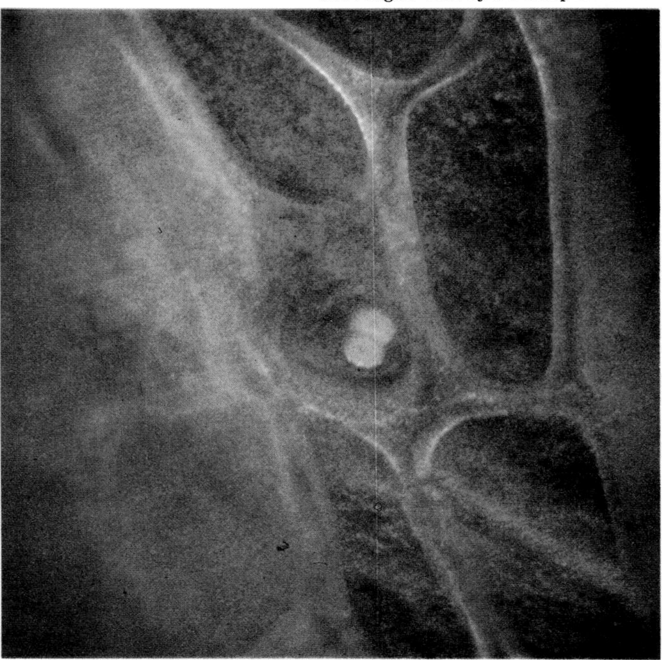

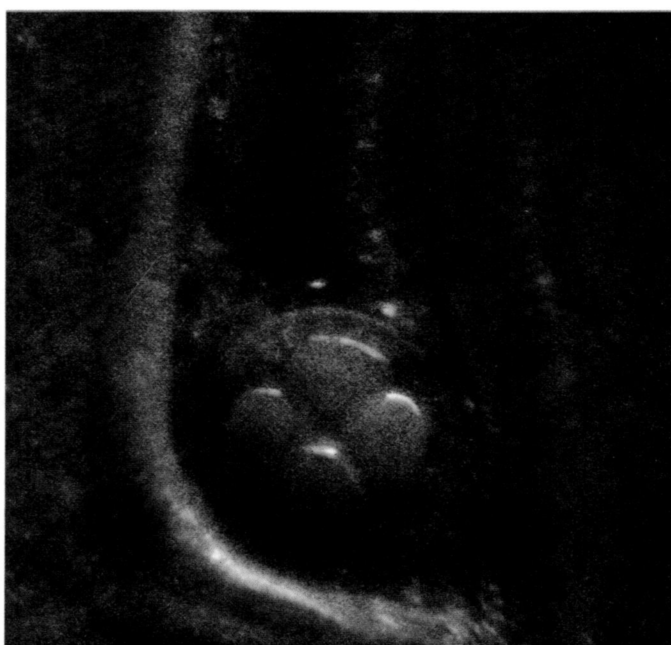

Forty hours after fertilization, the double-celled egg shown at top right has divided again to form a four-celled body, briefly nestled in a curved ridge during its slow progress toward the uterus.

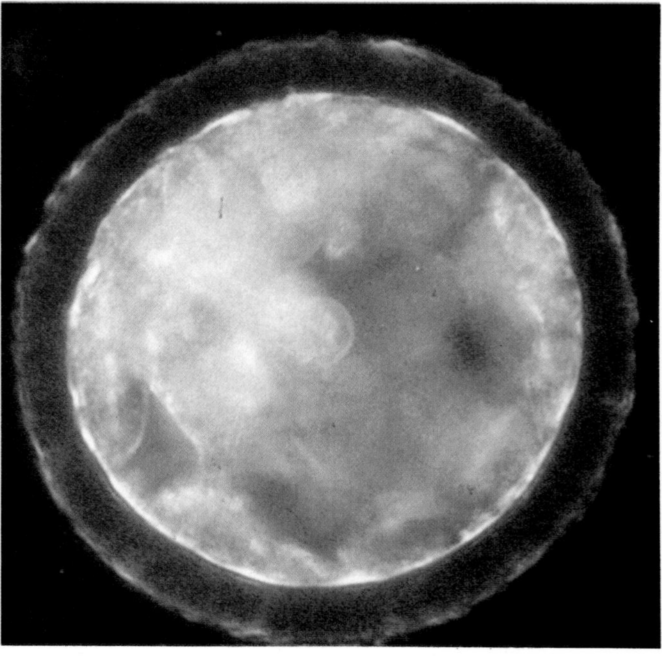

Floating free in the uterine cavity three days after fertilization, the egg has now burgeoned into a mottled, multicelled mass. The sac that envelops and protects it appears as a shimmering, semitransparent halo.

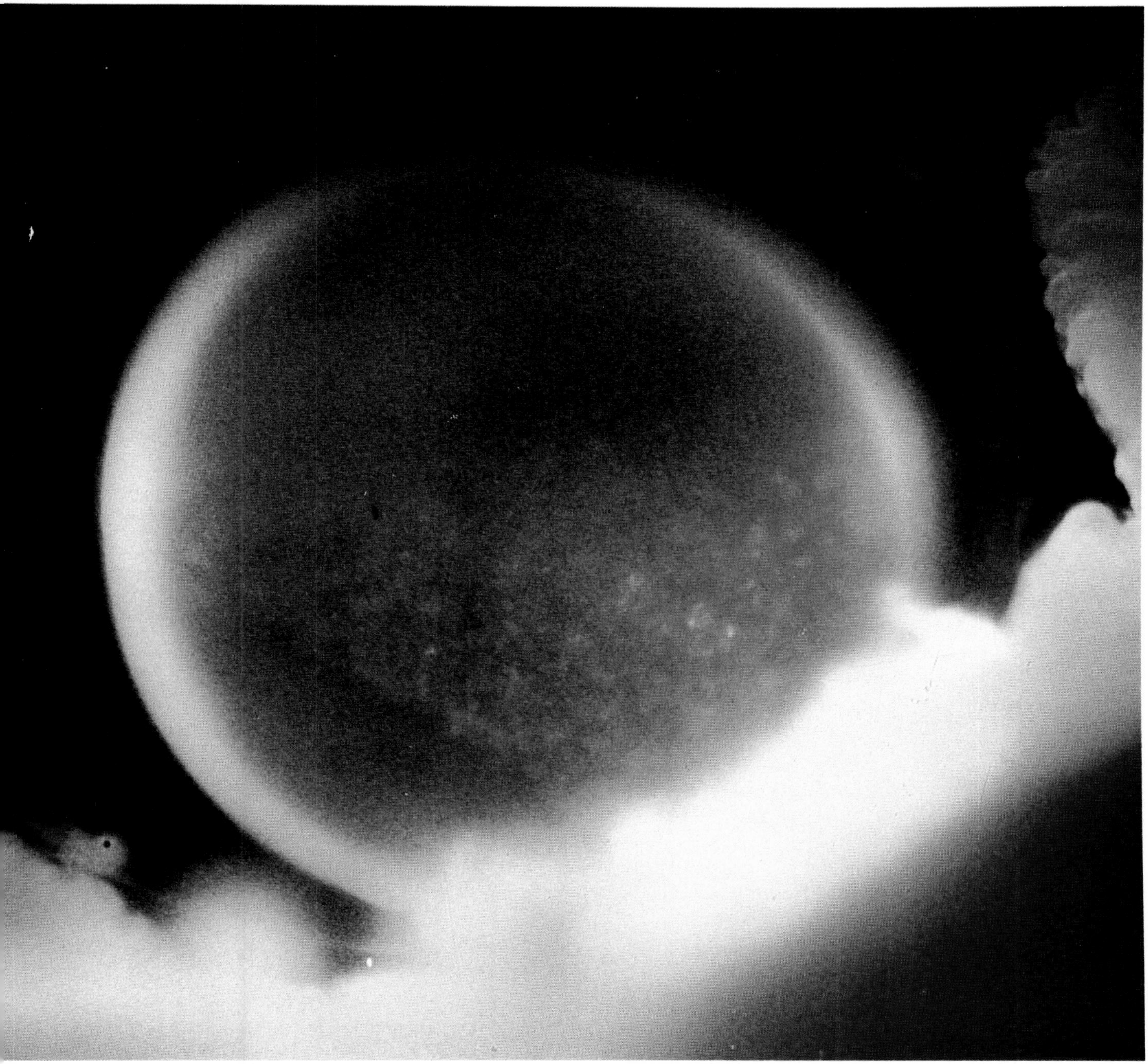

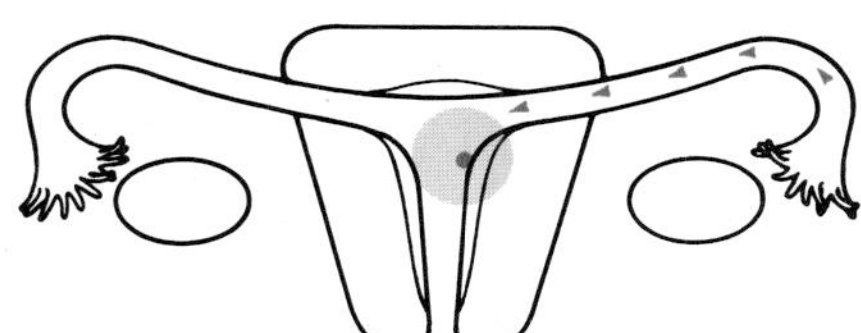

A week after fertilization, the egg reaches its destination—the rear wall of the uterus (pink circle). Nesting in the spongy uterine lining (above), the egg is a fluid-filled capsule with an inner mass of cells—the embryo-to-be—clustered at one pole. The area of attachment will form the placenta, a nourishing organ linking the mother's body with the growing baby's.

Managing a healthy pregnancy

Until quite recently, a woman expecting a baby was likely to be described from time to time as "indisposed." One 19th Century medical manual put it more bluntly: "Child-bearing is a kind of nine-months' sickness." Today, doctors and prospective mothers know better. For the most part, pregnant women are perfectly healthy. Recalled one mother of five, "I always enjoyed being pregnant, especially in the final couple of months. It was like being a ship under full sail."

Minor discomforts and problems there will be, however, even in the easiest of pregnancies, as the mother's body changes to nurture and make room for the baby growing within. Many of these problems are transitory, or disappear after delivery. Others can usually be dealt with effectively, thanks to a host of new diagnostic and therapeutic techniques that pinpoint and resolve difficulties as they arise.

The best way to keep problems to a minimum and ease the entire nine-month experience is to plan early. Ideally, you should start planning as soon as the decision to have a child has been made, but even when planning is deferred until a woman knows she is pregnant, the steps are much the same. Begin in an obvious way, by talking with friends who have recently had children. Their advice may be highly subjective, but their recollections and insights will help you make two key decisions: the choice of a doctor, and the choice of the hospital or other facility where the baby will be born.

In the United States, most women choose a specialist in obstetrics and gynecology to care for them during their pregnancy. In all likelihood the same physician will also deliver the baby, and will do so in a hospital. By contrast, about 80 per cent of all deliveries worldwide are attended by midwives, often in the mother's home. One reason for the difference is a shortage of trained obstetricians elsewhere; but the use of midwives is increasing in the United States as well. The women's and consumers' movements have tended to foster the increase, on the ground that a midwife often permits the mother to exercise greater control over her body. For its part, the American College of Obstetricians and Gynecologists endorsed the practice of midwifery as far back as 1971. There is little doubt that, in the 90 per cent of pregnancies that are normal, a trained nurse-midwife provides competent prenatal and delivery care.

Nevertheless, to ensure the greatest safety for mother and child in case of an emergency, most physicians recommend —and about 90 per cent of American women still seek—the care of an obstetrician-gynecologist. To begin with, such a specialist is proficient in the treatment of the entire female reproductive system. In addition, he or she is trained to deal effectively—by surgery, for example—with any of the numerous complications that may occur during childbirth. And for a pregnancy or delivery that is predictably difficult or complicated, the medical specialist is indispensable.

Finding the right doctor

Look for a physician certified by the American Board of Obstetrics and Gynecology; this means the doctor has completed specialized graduate training and passed written and

A doctor presses the abdomen of a pregnant woman to determine the position of the fetus. Secured to his head is a special stethoscope that enables him to listen for a fetal heartbeat while leaving both his hands free to probe the abdomen.

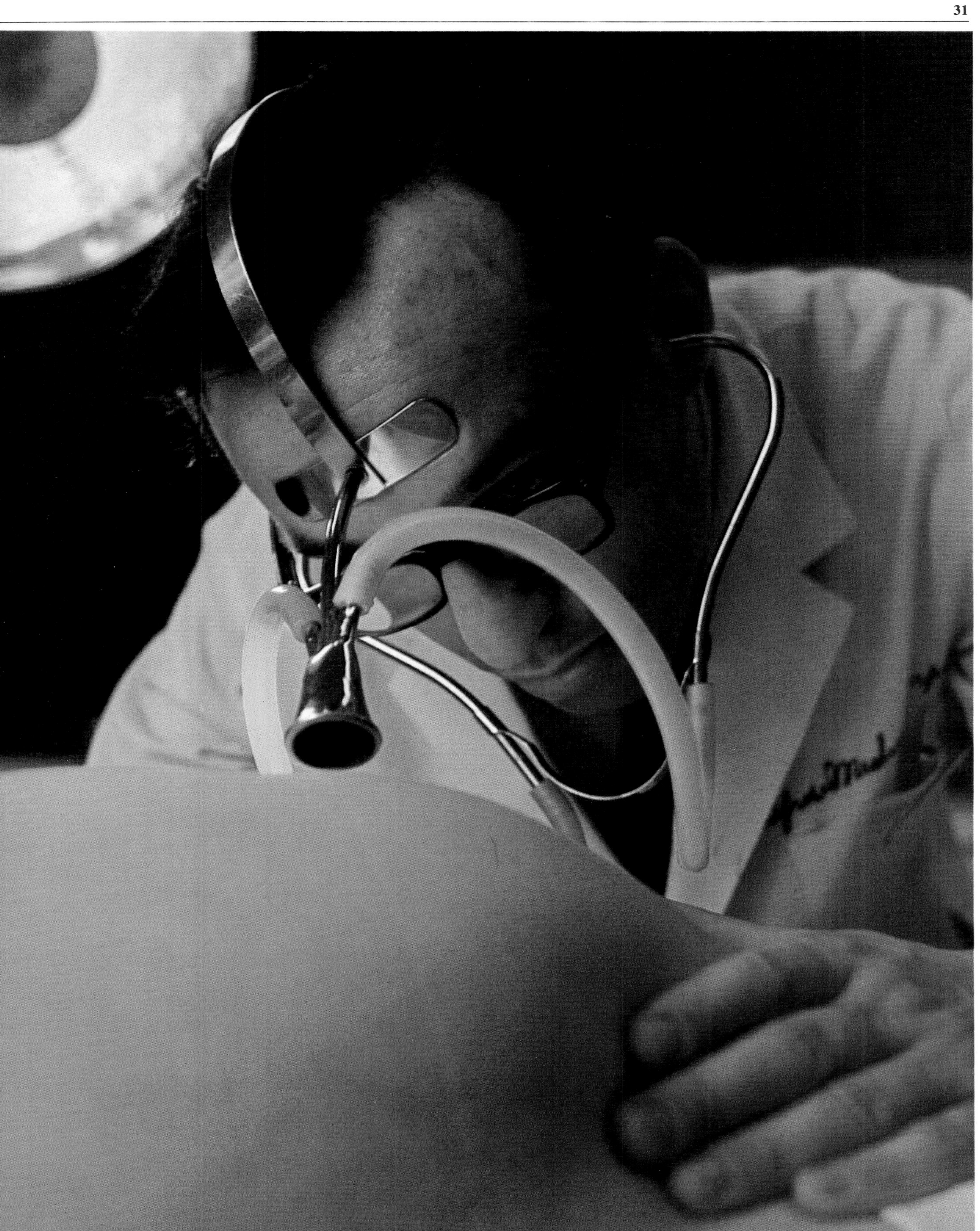

oral tests given by the board. Beyond this criterion, a good source for a doctor is the obstetrics department of a teaching hospital (a hospital associated with a medical school); as in any profession, the insiders know who the best people are. If there is no such hospital in your area, call the local medical society or a major hospital for a recommendation.

Finding a qualified doctor does not, of course, mean that you have found the doctor who is right for you. It is also important to take into account whether the doctor's general approach matches your own attitudes, your opinions and—yes—your prejudices. In conversations with friends and using the information in this book, work out your position on controversial questions in the management of pregnancy and childbirth. Then interview and assess the doctor you are considering. Is he plainly old-fashioned or faddish? It is best to avoid both extremes. Does he explain problems and procedures clearly, and is he both patient and forthcoming when you ask for further clarification? What is his customary procedure during delivery, particularly his attitude toward sedation? A few doctors prefer to anesthetize the mother completely, while others favor little or no sedation. Make sure that you and your physician agree on this question.

The choice of a doctor often determines the hospital you will use; most physicians are affiliated with only one or two institutions. But if you do have an option, find out if the hospital allows fathers in the labor and delivery rooms and how newborn babies are treated. Is the mother permitted to hold the baby immediately after delivery? (Many mothers feel a great desire to establish an immediate bond with their infant; others just want to go to sleep.) Check out the hospital's policy on breast-feeding: Do staff members bring the baby to the mother for a feeding at any hour, or just during the day? Do they allow all family members to visit the new baby (some hospitals bar children from the nursery floor) and do they permit visitors not only to see the baby but to hold him?

A physical exam—and the advice that goes with it

With the doctor chosen, the next step is a complete physical examination. It may and often does take place after pregnancy begins, but the best protection is in a pre-pregnancy examination, ideally made at least three months before conception. It has much in common with a routine physical exam, but focuses on problems of pregnancy and childbirth. In taking a medical history, for example, the physician pays special attention to reproductive or genetic disorders in the families of both the mother- and father-to-be; such information enables him to cope with the possibility that the baby might inherit the disorder. Tests could be administered during a pre-pregnancy exam to indicate whether a woman has been exposed to a venereal disease; if she has, the physician can usually prevent complications for her child by treating her before pregnancy begins. If a woman is anemic, her doctor may start a systematic program of iron supplements.

The doctor will also conduct an internal pelvic examination at this time. Using his hands and such instruments as a speculum, which opens the vagina to view, he will check the birth canal and reproductive organs for abnormalities. In addition, he will determine the size and shape of the pelvis to be sure that it will permit the safe passage of a baby. If the woman's pelvic structure is too narrow or shallow for normal birth, the surgical delivery called a cesarean section may be considered at this point, long before the time it would be performed.

One question the doctor will surely ask is whether the prospective mother has ever had rubella (German measles) or been vaccinated against it. If so, she is immune to it, and her baby will be free of it in the womb. If she is not sure or cannot remember, the doctor will test her for the disease—and with good reason. A woman who contracts rubella during pregnancy, particularly in the first three months, exposes her baby to a high risk of being born with a severe defect, such as heart disease, mental retardation, deafness or blindness. A vaccine at this point would immunize her, but the vaccine itself is dangerous during pregnancy: It contains weakened disease organisms that could infect the developing baby. In a pre-pregnancy examination, the doctor will advise the woman to wait at least three months after immunization before becoming pregnant; if her pregnancy has already begun, he will not risk giving her the vaccine.

The first visit is not devoted to medical procedures alone.

The doctor is likely to discuss precautions and informal rules that apply during all the nine months of a pregnancy. Among the subjects he is certain to cover sooner or later are smoking, drinking, the use of drugs, diet and exercise.

There is no question that smoking can be harmful to a baby in the womb. It depletes essential vitamins and minerals in a pregnant woman, and thus in the offspring she is carrying. What is worse, children born to mothers who smoke generally weigh less than those born to nonsmokers, and underweight infants are especially vulnerable to disease. According to an estimate by the U.S. Public Health Service, more than 4,500 American babies die at birth or soon afterward every year simply because their mothers smoked. Almost universally, doctors urge their patients not to smoke at all during pregnancy.

The consensus is less clear on alcohol. Some obstetricians believe that small amounts of wine or liquor in the evening are probably harmless and may help to relax the prospective mother. But alcohol in excess is clearly damaging. "The equivalent of two drinks a day has a mild effect on birth size," says Dr. David W. Smith of the University of Washington. "At four to six per day, mild to moderate fetal effects become more frequent. At eight, 10 or more drinks per day there is a 30 per cent to 50 per cent risk of multiple effects that have been termed the fetal alcohol syndrome." Some of the syndrome's effects on a newborn baby are mental deficiency and heart defects; at seven years of age about 45 per cent of the victims of this syndrome have subnormal intelligence. For safety, then, go easy on alcohol, preferably with a limit of about an ounce a day—perhaps two glasses of wine or a single drink of hard spirits.

Just as tobacco and alcohol can harm a baby in the womb, so can the improper use of drugs and medicines. Almost any drug in the mother's bloodstream passes eventually into the baby's blood, carrying with it a potential for harm. Even such an apparently benign substance as aspirin may be inadvisable for a pregnant woman. It is best to check with the doctor before taking any medicine that he has not specifically recommended.

Certainly pregnant women should avoid contact with any toxic substances found around the home. Some poisons may be obvious; few women, perhaps, would expose themselves to dangerous fumes by painting a room that is not well ventilated. Yet other hazards are more subtle, and no less dangerous. One that is little known is a microscopic, single-celled parasite called toxoplasma, which grows in some cats and in raw or undercooked meat; it can infect women, causing a disease called toxoplasmosis. A woman who has had the disease before becoming pregnant is immune to further infection, and her baby will be safe. But almost half the pregnant women who contract the disease pass it on to their fetus, with a risk of mental retardation, blindness or epilepsy. In addition to shunning uncooked or very rare meat, it is a good idea to avoid contact with the feces of cats—the husband should empty the cat litter. Some physicians, however, urge expectant mothers to refrain from handling cats in any way.

As to diet, most doctors advise eating somewhat generously. A modest gain in weight is normal; over the nine months of pregnancy most women carrying a single baby will put on 20 to 30 pounds. To achieve the weight gain, the Food and Nutrition Board of the National Research Council recommends increasing the daily intake of calories by 300—the equivalent of two cups of yogurt. Doctors recommend a diet that is rich in protein (meat, eggs, cheese, poultry and fish), is well balanced in other respects and includes a full quart of milk daily. Vitamin and mineral supplements are generally prescribed by the doctor. They should not be chosen by the mother or taken in excess; for example, large amounts of vitamin C, taken by some women in the belief that the regimen will shield them from common colds, can interfere with the absorption of an equally essential vitamin, B_{12}.

Breaking outdated taboos

While a few restrictions on drugs and foods are in order, the doctor will impose almost no limits on daily activities. Gone is the old attitude that pregnant women should be protected like delicate plants. During a normal pregnancy, exercise, work and travel, pursued in moderation, endanger neither the mother nor the fetus. Contact sports and such risky activities as mountain climbing or skiing should be avoided, but tennis, golf or swimming can be continued well into the last three months of pregnancy. Joggers in late pregnancy have run in marathons with no ill effect. These facts should not be surprising. Exercise makes good sense for a pregnant woman: Giving birth is a strenuous physical task, and a mother with well-toned muscles will be all the better prepared for it.

Another taboo now banished is the age-old rule against sexual intercourse. Doctors agree that sexual relations can be continued throughout a normal pregnancy, up to—but not necessarily including—the final month. Intercourse does not bring on premature labor, infections, bleeding or any of the other complications traditionally ascribed to it. Orgasms do not cause miscarriages or even labor, though they may induce some uterine contractions. There are a few exceptions: A woman with a history of spontaneous miscarriages would be better off abstaining, particularly at the stage of pregnancy when she miscarried in the past. And some doctors do advise against coitus in the ninth month; research indicates a slight danger of infection for the baby in the womb.

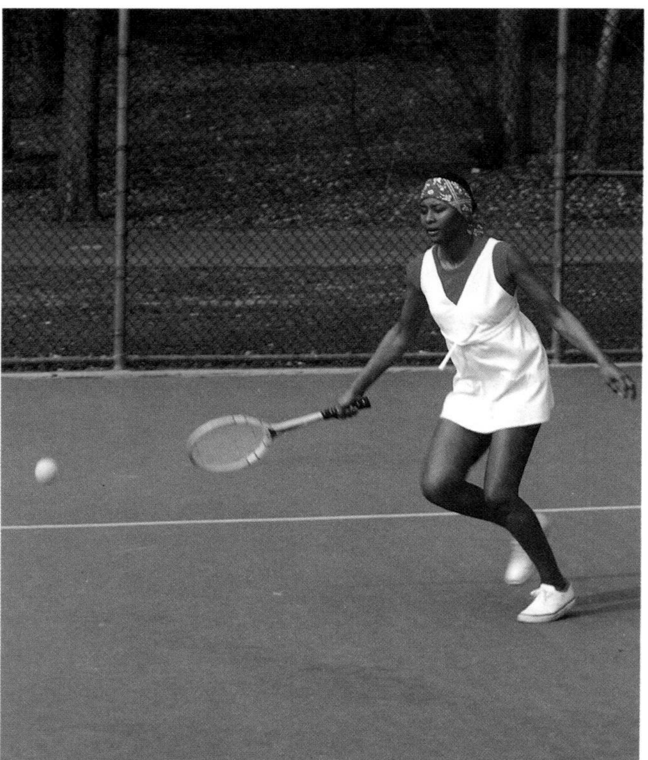

A woman four months pregnant enjoys an energetic game of tennis. Regular exercise improves circulation, minimizes aches and swelling and relieves tension during pregnancy; afterward, good muscle tone promotes an easy delivery and a quick recovery. Expectant mothers should not, however, engage in activities that carry the risk of a heavy fall—horseback riding, for example.

In his discussion with a new patient, a doctor is likely to make one point on a matter that is not physical: Emotional swings and shifts can be expected during pregnancy, and should be taken in stride. A pregnant woman may be frequently depressed, self-absorbed and repeatedly irritated by minor matters that at other times would be taken lightly. Her mercurial emotions are understandable on a number of counts. The fatigue stemming from the demands of another being within her, her own concerns about her appearance and identity, and her apprehensions for the baby's health—all are ample causes for emotional upset. The physician will urge the prospective mother to stay busy, voice her concerns to her husband and family, and, above all, maintain contacts outside the home, which help to smooth her swings of mood.

The mother's stresses may be compounded by the emotions and behavior of the father. Many prospective fathers, finding their wives attracting so much attention and becoming so preoccupied with their pregnancies, suffer feelings of insecurity or even of outright jealousy. Some compensate by absorbing themselves in their work and staying away from home just when their wives most need support and intimacy. Knowing that this may occur, both partners can alleviate the problem with frequent shows of affection.

Occasionally an even stranger phenomenon will occur. The father may actually suffer some of the same pregnancy discomforts that his wife endures, such as weight gain, morning sickness and abdominal complaints. This psychosomatic response, called couvade from the French word meaning "to hatch," reaches its extreme in cultures in which men take to their beds for ritualistic enactments of labor and delivery. Normally, however, most men respond well when they realize that their symptoms stem purely from their emotions.

Whether or not he is afflicted by couvade, the father-to-be will benefit from being brought into the process of pregnancy as much as possible. He should meet the obstetrician, accompany his wife on at least one of her office visits, and attend some or all of the birthing classes that the hospital will offer her. All this will help relieve his anxieties and make the entire nine-month experience more rewarding.

In their conference with the doctor, both parents-to-be may encounter a term that is new to them: *trimester*. Obstetricians divide the 40 weeks of a normal pregnancy into three sections, or trimesters, each lasting a little over 13 weeks. The division is not merely arithmetical or arbitrary; it corresponds to specific phases of the baby's development and of the symptoms felt by the mother in response to that development. Simply put, during the first trimester the baby is essentially being formed, while the mother experiences problems caused by her body's adjustment to its new role as nurturer and bearer. In the second, the baby undergoes rapid growth, while the mother's discomforts arise mainly from the increase in his size. The third trimester is marked principally by a gain in the baby's weight; any annoyances the mother may feel are generally caused by the added weight.

The first trimester: A baby takes form

Because doctors rarely know the exact day on which a baby is conceived, they calculate it from the onset of the mother's last menstrual period: Pregnancy is assumed to have begun about two weeks later. Conception, of course, is not marked by any outward sign; the mother has no way of knowing when her egg cell is fertilized by a sperm cell. Even when the egg divides in a Fallopian tube, moves to her uterus and begins to grow there, she will be unaware of its existence; when the dividing egg, or embryo, is six days old it contains more than a hundred cells but is no bigger than a pinprick. Her first symptom, the absence of the next menstrual flow, is still a week or more away.

In fact she may never know that an egg has been fertilized. Frequently, the gestation process goes awry in the first crucial days. Up to about two weeks after conception, the egg may be sloughed off from the wall of the uterus, and the only sign of the event might be a slight delay in the woman's next menstruation. According to some estimates, as many as 75 per cent of all conceptions are spontaneously aborted as the result of some abnormality in the egg or its surroundings, or some "insult" to the mother's body, such as excessive drinking. After two weeks, however, a spontaneous abortion may be apparent in the form of an especially heavy or clotted menstrual flow.

As the days pass, the embryo's cells continue to divide and grow; some can be identified as the beginnings of vital organs, and one group forms a stalk that will become the umbilical cord, linking mother and child. During the third week after fertilization, the embryo lengthens along an axis that will contain the spinal column; most of this area of growth eventually becomes the baby's head, which develops earlier than the rest of the body.

Meanwhile, thin membranes collectively called the amniotic sac begin to form around the embryo. The sac fills with a clear liquid that serves a variety of functions: It is a cushion for the baby against blows from the outside, a reservoir of vital nutrients and a storehouse for wastes. Outside the sac lies the relatively thick placental membrane, attached to the wall of the uterus and laced with a labyrinth of blood vessels and other tissues vital for maintaining the baby. Its connection with the embryo is the rapidly growing umbilical cord, which now begins to carry a steady exchange of nutrients and wastes between baby and mother.

By the end of the fourth week after conception, the embryo is about as long as the eraser at the end of a pencil and somewhat resembles a tiny caterpillar, with a prominent head and heart, and buds that will later develop into arms and legs. In another two weeks, the fertilized egg has become a complex piece of whitish-gray, almost transparent flesh about an inch long. Fingers and toes have begun to take shape; facial features emerge. By the end of the seventh week a neck separates the head from the torso. The embryo is beginning to look human.

The eighth week is generally taken by doctors to mark the point at which the embryo becomes a fetus; technically, it will remain a fetus until the moment of birth. At this early stage of its development, the fetus measures nearly an inch and a half in length, and most of the major parts have formed:

A pregnant woman demonstrates the correct adjustments for a car safety belt and shoulder harness. Both are buckled snugly, but not tightly, with the belt angled downward against the pelvic bones rather than the abdomen. Pregnant women should sit up straight to prevent the belt from sliding up across the abdomen; on a long trip they should stop and stretch every two hours or so.

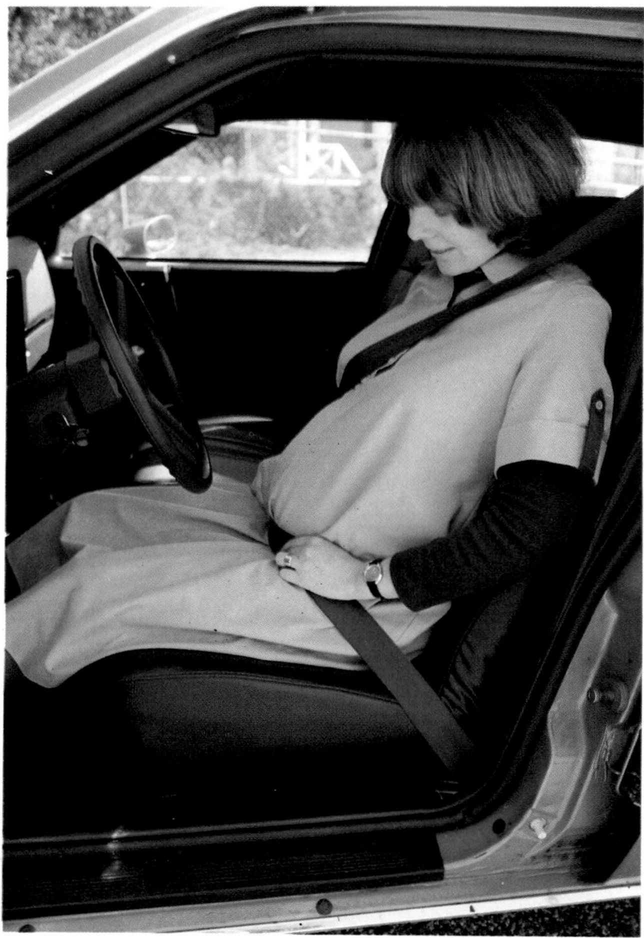

The heart is beating; the eyes, though closed, are in position; and the growing baby has developed sexual characteristics, with a rudimentary penis or clitoris.

Morning sickness and other discomforts

By this point in the first trimester, the mother is well aware that something is occurring within her. For most women the first sign is amenorrhea, or the absence of menstruation, about two weeks after conception. Amenorrhea alone, however, does not necessarily indicate pregnancy. It can also be caused by menopause, by illness or by stress—even the stress of a concern about becoming pregnant. On the other hand, menstruation may continue for a time during a pregnancy, then suddenly stop; such a sequence of events should be discussed with the doctor.

A more certain and familiar sign of pregnancy is nausea, the traditional morning sickness, which often shows up after the first missed period, lasts for six to eight weeks, then ceases spontaneously. Typically, the woman awakes in the morning feeling an urge to vomit, and may do so. Sucking a sweet mint or nibbling dry crackers before rising may forestall the nausea. If it does not, and if the condition persists, more drastic measures may be required.

One remedy for morning sickness, a drug called Bendectin, has proved to be effective and has been widely prescribed, but some recent studies suggest that it can cause fetal malformations. These studies are based solely on animal subjects, and the U.S. Food and Drug Administration has not withdrawn its approval of Bendectin. Nevertheless, in view of the controversy, a pregnant woman should consult her physician and make her own decision.

A complex pattern of other signs, taken together, increases the probability that a pregnancy is under way. If some or all of the following symptoms appear, tests for pregnancy are called for.

- Fatigue and drowsiness. In the course of its rapid growth, the embryo consumes much of the mother's store of glucose, and it may be a drop in her blood-sugar level that makes her feel weary.
- Breast changes. A feeling of fullness in the breasts, normally experienced at the onset of a menstrual period, may be continuous during pregnancy. Heightened sensitivity in the nipples and tenderness and tingling in the breasts, particularly in first-time mothers, may occur and persist for a time, then disappear.
- Frequent urination. The expanding uterus exerts pressure on the bladder, reducing its capacity and its ability to retain liquid.
- Vaginal coloration. The swelling of blood vessels in the pelvic area changes the walls of the vagina from their normal pinkish color to a bluish hue.

Many peoples have used bizarre methods to determine whether a woman has conceived. One practice in ancient Egypt, for example, called for smearing an arcane oil on the woman's body at bedtime; if her skin turned green by morning, she was declared to be pregnant. Today, any woman who misses a menstrual period can make a far more conclusive test in her own home, using a kit that is available over the counter at most drug stores. At least nine days after what would have been the onset of the menstrual period, she pours a few drops of her urine into a small glass tube. A chemical in the tube can indicate the telltale presence of a hormone, human chorionic gonadotropin (hCG), secreted into the mother's blood and urine by the placenta. If, after two hours, a brown ring is visible in the mixture of liquids, the chances are that she is pregnant.

The test is not foolproof. A positive result obtained the first time is about 97 per cent accurate—but a negative result leaves a 20 per cent chance of pregnancy, and the test should be repeated a week later. If either test is positive, the woman should arrange for further, more sophisticated tests at a doctor's office. To confirm pregnancy, the physician will look for the following signs:

- Softening of the cervix. Normally firm, the cervix or neck of the womb generally softens after a month of pregnancy. This sign is not definitive; contraceptive pills can cause a similar softening.
- Changes in the uterus. At about the eighth week of pregnancy, the uterus assumes a globular shape some three inches across. The doctor can manipulate it by inserting two gloved fingers into the vagina while pressing down from the outside with his other hand. A uterus that feels elastic, doughy and soft is a probable sign of pregnancy.
- Hormonal changes. Using precise equipment available only in the laboratory, the doctor repeats the test for hCG.

Later on, the doctor may look for three conclusive indications that his patient is pregnant: the detection of a fetal heartbeat, movement by the fetus, and a picture of the fetus made by a technique called sonography.

Although the fetal heart begins beating after about five weeks, it cannot be detected with a stethoscope until the second trimester. Pulsing 120 to 160 times a minute, the heart sounds like a muffled, ticking watch. The notion that the heart of a male fetus beats slow and that of a female beats fast is false: There is no difference.

The mother's perception of active movement by the baby begins around the 18th to 20th week. Usually the pregnancy has long since been detected by other means, but the first movement is a sure sign of life. Later on, movement becomes more vigorous, and a small bulge in the abdomen may betray the pressure of a tiny arm or leg inside.

Sonography, which uses sound-wave echoes to take pictures of the woman's interior, is basically a diagnostic method *(page 38)*, but can also be used to detect a pregnancy; a sonogram can usually reveal a baby's outlines by the end of the first trimester. X-rays, which can damage the fetus, are never used unless there is no alternative means of examination and the risk is outweighed by other factors, such as a suspicion that the mother has cancer. Sonography is substantially risk-free, and it is painless.

Once the pregnancy is confirmed, the mother and her doctor generally arrange a schedule of regular visits. Typically, she will see the doctor once a month for the first seven months, twice during the eighth month, then once a week until the baby arrives.

The second trimester: a burgeoning growth

Growth is explosive during the second three months of life in the womb. By the end of the second trimester the baby will be about 14 inches long, roughly the length of his mother's fist and forearm, and will weigh about two pounds. What is more, the baby is active and takes on the rudiments of an identity almost from the beginning of the trimester. Sonograms show that at three months his face may assume an expression curiously like a smile whenever one of his fingers accidentally strokes his lips (in fact, he is pursing his lips in a sucking reflex). A month later he begins to move in the womb; his mother can tell when he is still, and therefore asleep, and when he is moving about, and she may offer a guess as to whether he will become an energetic child or a more placid one. A unique and unmistakable individuality is actually forming at the ends of his fingers and toes, where ridges and whorls are assuming patterns that will be his alone throughout his life.

As the baby's trunk and legs lengthen, his head takes on a more normal proportion with the rest of the body. His skin loses its transparency as fat builds up beneath it, and the skin begins to grow a coat of downy hair. Eyelashes and eyebrows appear, though the eyes will remain closed until the end of this second trimester.

Immersed in the amniotic fluid, the baby's skin is now covered by a cheeselike, pasty coating called vernix, a mixture of oil from the skin and dead skin cells. The amniotic fluid itself undergoes continuous recycling; every hour, a third of it is absorbed into the mother's bloodstream and replaced by fresh liquid secreted from the amniotic membrane. Each day the baby swallows about a pint of the fluid, and returns fluid to the sac by urination. He cannot drown, however; his oxygen requirements are fulfilled by blood from the placenta.

By the end of the second trimester, the baby approaches self-sufficiency. If born prematurely at this point, he might live on his own for a few hours, or even a few days. With expert hospital care, one out of five premature babies of this age survives.

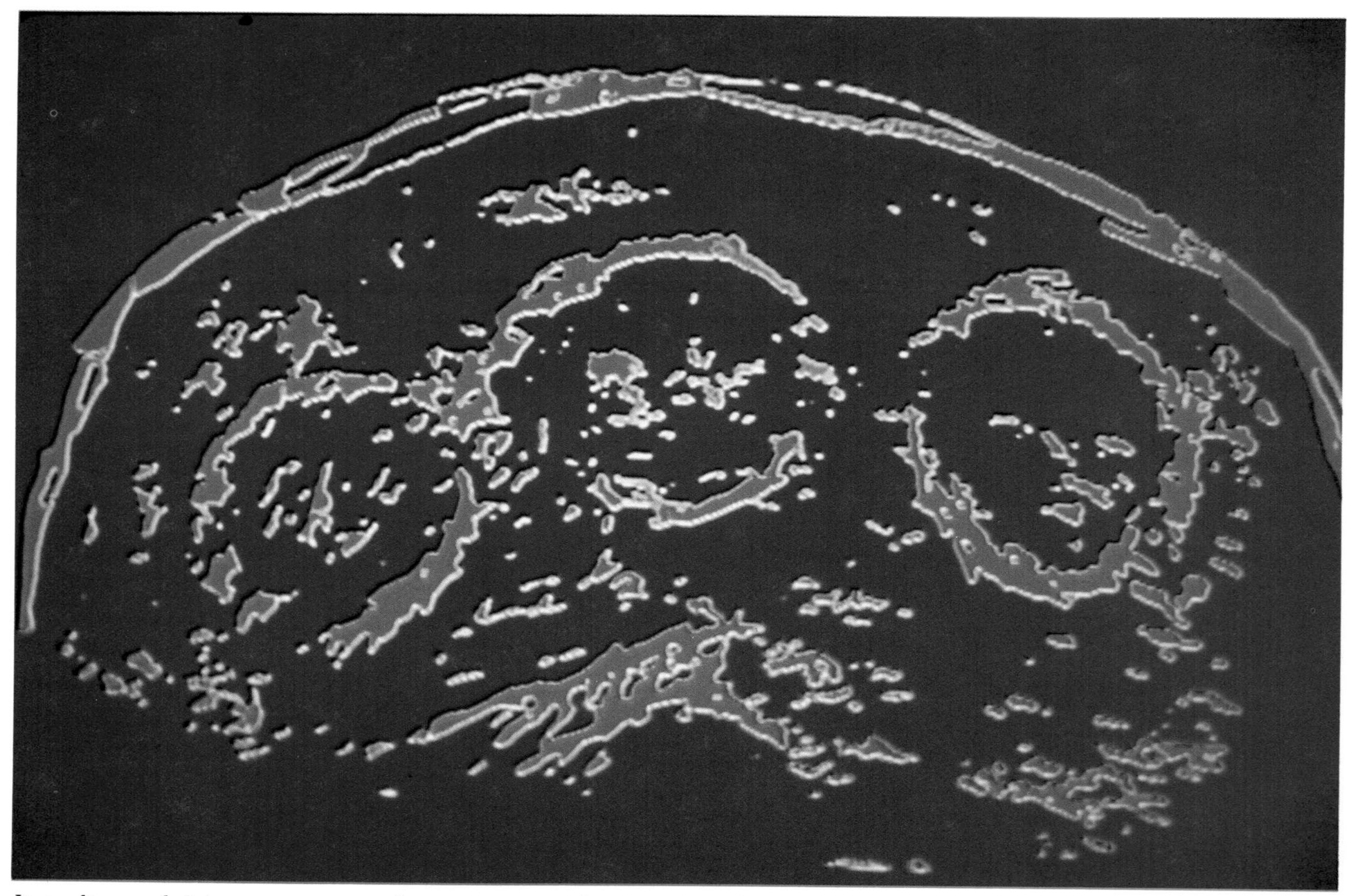

In an ultrasound picture, or sonogram, of a pregnant woman's womb, the heads of a set of triplets are outlined as three colorful rings. Sonography, which records the echoes of high-frequency inaudible sound waves, is a major advance in modern obstetrics: Unlike X-rays, it clearly depicts soft tissues as well as bones, and creates little or no hazard to mother and child.

But the baby's growth is having its effects on the mother. Her uterus enlarges and exerts pressure on her other internal organs, including the large intestine. One frequent and perfectly normal result of this pressure is constipation or flatulence, made more severe by hormonal action that interferes with the functioning of the bowel muscles.

Tried-and-true remedies for these complaints include plentiful fluids, especially upon awakening in the morning; a diet rich in coarse cereals, green vegetables and fruit; and regular exercise. Set a time for going to the bathroom, but do not worry if these visits are without results; your body will eliminate wastes as necessary, and at its own pace. Do not resort to enemas or over-the-counter laxatives, particularly mineral oil, which blocks the intake of nutrients that the baby needs. Reduce flatulence by steering clear of such gas-producing foods as beans, fried foods, cabbage, corn and sweet desserts.

The expanding uterus may also interfere with blood flow in the rectal area and the legs. A common but temporary annoyance is hemorrhoids, tiny varicose veins in the rectum that can itch and bleed. Regular bowel habits help, and so does soaking the area with warm water, but check with the doctor before using any ointment other than cold cream or petroleum jelly.

You can reduce varicose veins in the legs by elevating the legs for 10-minute periods three or four times a day. If the condition persists, wearing support stockings may help. Put them on before rising; otherwise, the veins in your legs will fill with blood when you stand up, and the stockings will be of no use. Do not wear panty girdles or tight stockings, both of which restrict blood flow.

If you experience an increased vaginal discharge, notify the doctor, but do not worry: It is a normal outcome of higher blood and hormone flow to the area. Take daily baths, and use sanitary pads, if necessary, but avoid tampons; they can cause bleeding and foster infection.

Cramps, backache, bleeding gums and insomnia also begin to afflict many women during the second trimester. Generally, the best antidotes are simple ones: extra rest during the daytime, and the cooperation of a sympathetic husband willing to help with chores and give back rubs and leg rubs. But as always, discuss any severe or persistent symptoms with your doctor.

The third trimester: weight gain and finishing touches

For the fetus, the last three months of pregnancy is a time to gain weight. The baby stores up protein to build muscles, calcium for his bones, iron for red blood cells—and a considerable amount of fat. This familiar "baby fat" will insulate him against changes in temperature after he leaves the protection of the womb.

By the end of the seventh month the baby's brain has generally matured enough to control breathing and swallowing, and his feeding instinct may have developed to the point where he regularly sucks his thumb. If born now, he would have a 90 per cent chance of surviving.

Not only his brain but also his senses undergo their greatest development during the last trimester. For some months he has been hearing sounds from the outside world. Now his eyes open, though they are still unable to perceive shapes and colors. His taste buds can distinguish between sweet and bitter substances: If a sugar solution is injected into the amniotic sac, he will swallow more of the amniotic fluid; if a bitter substance is injected, he will swallow less. Finally, at the end of the eighth month, the baby looks much as he will when born. Though his lungs are not yet fully operational, he now has a 95 per cent chance of surviving if born prematurely.

By now, the baby's sheer size has made him more than a mere burden to his mother. The top of her womb reaches nearly to her breastbone, and her abdomen protrudes hugely. Her belly may be laced with reddish "stretch marks" caused by its expansion; the marks will fade to silver after delivery. A streak of dark-brown skin pigment may run down the middle of her abdomen, the effect of a hormone secreted by the pituitary gland during pregnancy; the streak usually disappears completely after the birth. Because the baby is so large, he cannot easily twist and turn—but he can poke and kick, and often does so. The mother may feel at times that her ballooning body is about to burst.

Because the top of the womb now pushes against the mother's diaphragm, she may suffer shortness of breath, particularly at night. An extra pillow or two should ease it. Backache is now a common complaint, as her back muscles strain to balance her unwieldy load; she should avoid bending over to pick up objects and should, if possible, use a firmer mattress. Within the abdomen, ligaments that hold the womb in place may become enlarged and painful; a heating pad, rest and, if necessary, a maternity girdle will ease the pain.

Another common cause of discomfort is heartburn, in which digestive acids back up from the stomach into the esophagus, causing pain that may become so severe as to mimic a heart attack. The condition stems partly from crowding of the stomach, partly from increased levels of the hormone progesterone; the best remedy is to eat smaller meals, chew food thoroughly and refrain from lying down immediately after eating. If heartburn persists, ask the doctor to recommend a mild antacid.

Despite all these difficulties, this is a good time to prepare for life after the baby comes home. You will, of course, buy clothes and baby supplies; more important, you should select the pediatrician who will care for the baby after birth. Be as diligent in choosing him as you were in searching for the obstetrician: Find someone who is board-certified, easily accessible and sympathetic, and who can be trusted implicitly.

If you plan to breast-feed the baby, start to prepare your breasts and nipples. Begin by expressing some of the watery fluid called colostrum to open up the milk ducts. Gently support a breast with one hand while using the thumb and forefinger of the other to squeeze the dark areola area around the nipple until the liquid appears. To forestall tenderness or soreness in the nipples, exercise them once or twice daily by pulling them out firmly until they are slightly uncomfortable; then apply baby oil or cold cream to keep them soft.

Sometime during the last month of pregnancy the baby generally turns head down in the womb. In addition, during

Making room for a growing baby

During pregnancy, virtually every system in a woman's body changes to meet the needs of the developing child and to prepare the mother for childbirth. Hormones step up her respiration, heartbeat, blood volume and total body fluid. Her urine increases as her kidneys filter the wastes of two bodies from her blood; her breasts grow larger as they prepare to produce milk.

But the most striking transformations occur in the abdominal cavity, and are caused by the maturing fetus. Since the spine and the pelvic joint block the uterus, or womb, from growing downward or backward, it expands up into the abdomen. Though stretching of the abdominal wall accommodates much of this growth, the uterus also presses against other organs. Some, such as the liver, are merely pushed slightly upward and to the side; others are compressed and hampered in their functions, causing or contributing to such classic complaints as constipation and shortness of breath. The expanding womb also affects circulation in the legs and pelvis by pressing against veins coming from these areas. Slowed in its return to the heart, blood accumulates in the vessels, sometimes causing swollen legs, varicose veins or hemorrhoids.

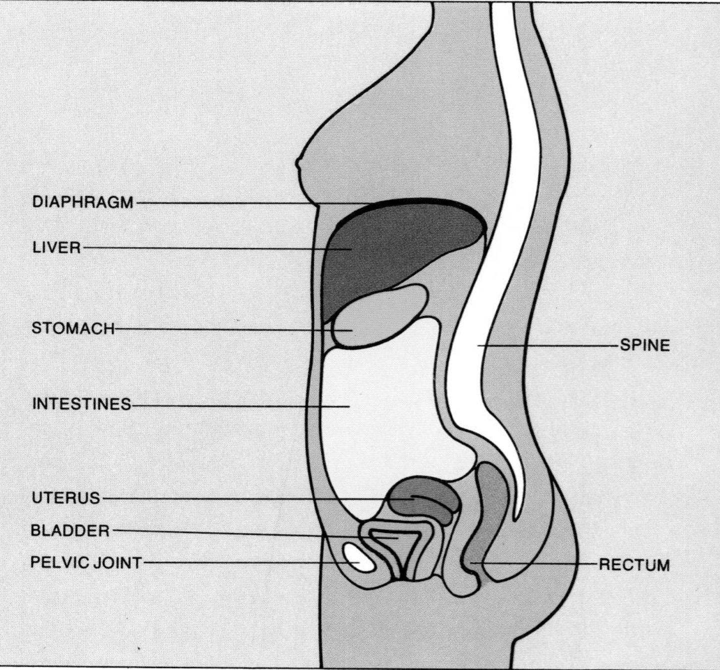

BEFORE PREGNANCY
In its usual state, the uterus is a small organ tucked between the intestines and the bladder. Consisting mainly of thick walls and linings, it has a narrow cavity with a capacity of about ¼ ounce of fluid.

the two weeks before birth, the baby descends about two inches, settling between the mother's pelvic bones. The event is called "lightening," and the mother does indeed feel that her load is lightened; the pressure on her diaphragm and lungs is reduced, and she finds that she can breathe more easily. Barely perceptible and usually painless contractions may begin to shift the baby into the best position for birth and prepare muscles for delivery.

Within the womb, growth slows considerably. The baby receives antibodies from his mother's blood to protect him against infections during the first days of life. He has hair on his head now, and fingernails and toenails. He is ready to emerge from the womb and into the world.

Coping with risks and complications

So goes a normal pregnancy, the predictable lot of the great majority of women. Not all pregnancies, unfortunately, proceed so smoothly. Some carry an inherently higher risk for such reasons as inherited traits, or the advanced age of the mother. Others may be complicated by diseases that attack the mother during pregnancy, and affect both her health and her child's. However, a number of new diagnostic tools can track and even predict the unborn baby's health.

Perhaps the most widely known of these new techniques, and among the most commonly used, is amniocentesis, the removal of a small sample of the amniotic fluid for analysis. Generally carried out after the 16th week of pregnancy, the test can detect such fetal disorders as mongolism, or Down's syndrome, in which the child is mentally retarded; Tay-Sachs, a fatal nerve disease; and spina bifida, a crippling deformation of the spine.

Though it pinpoints some of the gravest and most problematic complications of pregnancy, amniocentesis itself is surprisingly simple. Under a local anesthetic, a needle is inserted into the mother's lower abdomen; the doctor uses a sonogram to avoid striking the fetus. The patient feels little

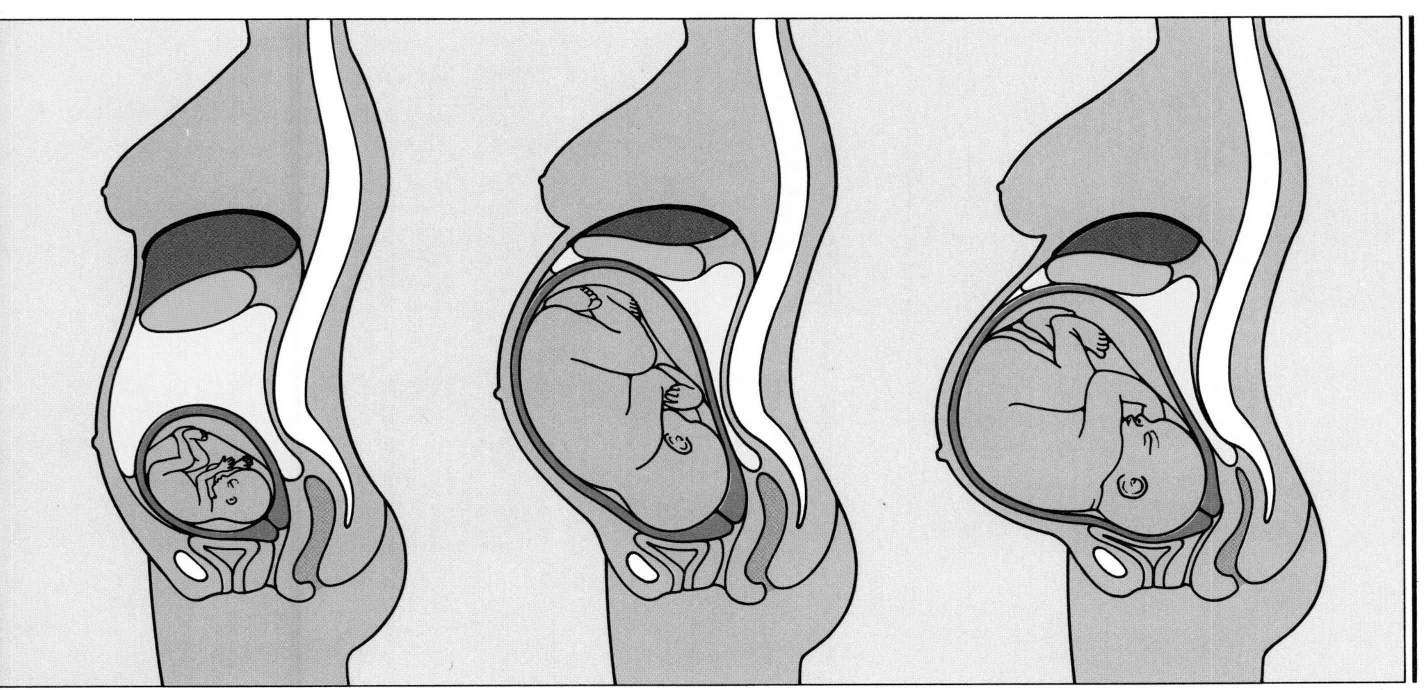

AT 20 WEEKS
Midway through pregnancy, the uterus expands to the level of the navel. One common effect is constipation, as pressure and the effects of a hormone cause the intestines to pass food more slowly.

AT 36 WEEKS
In the last month, the uterus reaches its highest level, greatly crowding other organs. The stomach's displacement may cause heartburn, and pressure on the diaphragm may result in shortness of breath.

THE LAST TWO WEEKS
In the last two weeks, in a shift called "lightening," the baby's head sinks into the pelvis. Breathing is easier, but pressure on the rectum and bladder causes constipation and more frequent urination.

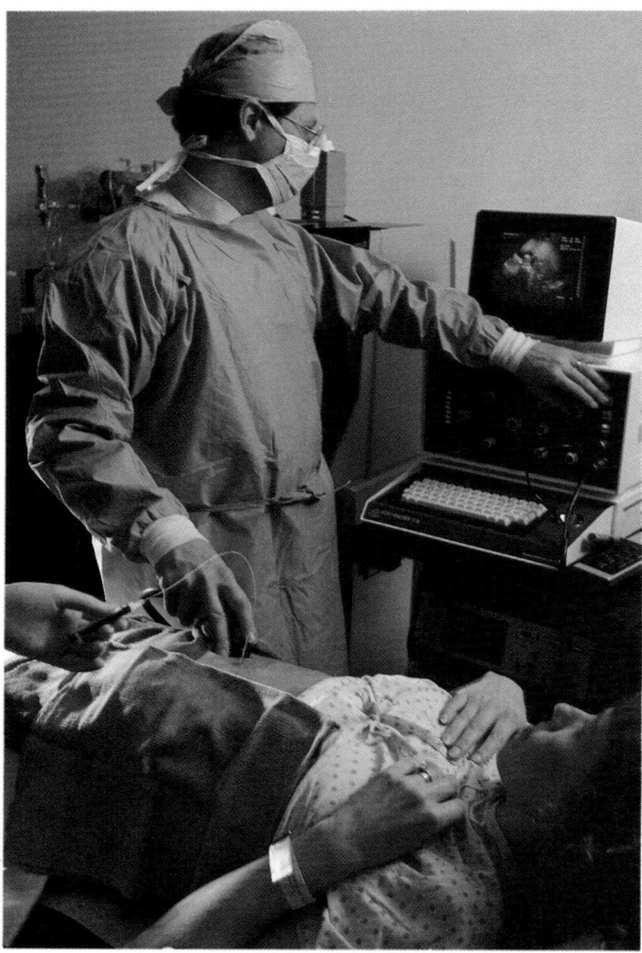

Using an ultrasound projector and screen, Dr. Jason Birnholz of the Harvard Medical School monitors the insertion of a catheter tube into the womb of a pregnant woman for a blood transfusion on her 27-week-old fetus. An assistant (not shown) threads the catheter into the fetus's body, while Dr. Birnholz moves the ultrasound probe over the mother's skin and follows the course of the insertion on the screen. Pioneered in the 1960s, the monitoring technique has since been used during the implantation of drainage tubes in unborn babies, and may someday play a part in the surgical removal or replacement of entire organs.

more than a mild pricking, followed by some temporary soreness. The test does carry risks. A misdirected needle can be fatal to the baby, and infections, premature labor and miscarriages have been accidentally induced. But in the hands of an experienced specialist, and with the help of sonography, the danger is minimal.

Sonography itself is a diagnostic boon. For example, a series of sonograms made over an extended period is a sure way of determining whether fetal growth is normal. Retarded growth is ominous in itself, of course. In addition, it can be an early warning sign of a form of high blood pressure called toxemia. If not controlled, the ailment can be fatal to both mother and baby. Even though an obstetrician routinely checks blood pressure at every visit, such symptoms of toxemia as blurred vision, headaches, sudden weight gain, and swollen eyelids and fingers may appear suddenly, at a time when damage has already been done to the baby. A continuous sonographic record can enable the physician to spot toxemia at an early stage and control it, generally by prescribing rest and low salt intake.

Even more remarkable than sonography is a new fiberoptic device called a fetoscope, which allows doctors to look directly at the baby inside the womb. Made of long, microscopically thin fibers of light-conducting plastic, the fetoscope is inserted directly through the skin and the wall of the uterus, and into the amniotic sac. By its light, the physician can check for such severe abnormalities as nerve trunks that are not adequately protected by the baby's skin; with a modified version of the instrument, he can also retrieve blood and tissue samples. Because fetoscopy is an invasive technique, calling for an incision in the abdomen, it is used only when other procedures have failed to produce a clear-cut diagnosis.

Cures for difficult cases

Armed with information obtained from such sophisticated diagnostic tools, doctors can now perform surgery on a baby in the womb. The techniques are available in only a few highly specialized hospitals, but their successes are astonishing. Relief valves have been implanted to reduce pressure in the heads of fetuses suffering from a build-up of fluids inside the skull. Kidney damage has been averted by draining blocked bladders with an implanted tube. On a few occasions, a complete transfusion of an anemic baby's blood has been performed before birth.

When complications of pregnancy defy all efforts either to prevent them or to resolve them and save the baby, modern techniques can at least minimize the risk to the mother. Diagnosis and prompt treatment, for example, are paramount when a fertilized egg fails to reach the womb but lodges and grows in a Fallopian tube, in an ovary or elsewhere in the abdomen. Called an ectopic pregnancy, from the Greek for "out of place," the condition is generally signaled by abdominal pain and sometimes also by vaginal bleeding. If not discovered early, an ectopic site may rupture, demanding a dangerous emergency operation to remove the damaged parts of the reproductive system and the fetus. But if this doomed pregnancy is detected in time by the standard tests now used to identify pregnancy itself, the fetus can be aborted successfully and the woman stands a good chance of being able to conceive again.

Special considerations apply to prospective mothers who are diabetic. If preventive therapy is not undertaken in time—ideally, before conception—diabetes presents a danger that the baby will be born with heart, bone, kidney or other malformations. Therefore, a diabetic woman should stabilize her condition well in advance of attempting to become pregnant, and must see a doctor at the slightest hint that she has conceived. Two recently developed devices, both still experimental, can help her to sustain a normal pregnancy: a portable glucose meter that monitors her blood-sugar levels, and a portable pump that automatically delivers the correct amounts of the insulin on which she depends. With prompt and proper care, she has an excellent chance of producing a normal baby—and 90 per cent of all diabetic mothers now do so.

Similarly, difficulties once caused by an incompatibility of blood factors between mother and father can now be averted. A small percentage of Americans (about 13 per cent of Caucasians, 8 per cent of blacks, 1 per cent of Orientals) lack a blood component called the Rh factor, named for the Rhesus monkey, the species in which it was first found. Occasionally, the baby of an Rh-negative woman (one who lacks the Rh factor) inherits Rh-positive blood from an Rh-positive father. If so, a chance exists that the mother's blood, intermingled with that of the baby, will produce antibodies that attack the baby's red blood cells at birth or in the womb. Such an attack rarely occurs if the baby is her first, but a second or third baby will be at high risk.

Until recent years, doctors had no choice but to exchange all of a newborn's blood for a type identical with his mother's, a difficult and perilous procedure. But happily, a simple and effective antidote was developed in the 1960s. A serum called Rhogam, it is given to an Rh-negative woman pregnant by an Rh-positive man; the build-up of antibodies is prevented, and what would once have been a dangerous situation becomes a matter of routine therapy.

Despite all the advances in diagnosis and therapy, the primary burden of observation and care rests upon the mother. At best, the obstetrician routinely studies and tests the mother on periodic visits. Between visits, every pregnant woman should be vigilant for any signs and symptoms that may spell trouble for her or her baby. A check list of events to watch for includes the following items:

- Vaginal bleeding of any kind
- Sudden swelling of the face or fingers
- Headaches, either severe or continuous
- Dimming or blurring of vision
- Severe abdominal pain
- Persistent vomiting
- Fever, particularly when accompanied by chills
- Persistent pain or burning sensation during urination
- Discharge of fluids from the vagina
- Absence of fetal movements for a six-hour period during the last trimester

Should any of these symptoms appear, call the doctor immediately, day or night, and discuss it with him. Only by exercising such caution can the mother-to-be—and her developing baby—benefit from the achievements that have so greatly increased the safety of pregnancy. ❋

Exercising away the stresses of pregnancy

Traditionally, a pregnant woman is said to "carry a baby," and the phrase is truly appropriate: Day and night, her physical framework bears an extra load. The most visible change in the mother-to-be is the front-heavy effect of her weight gain—20 pounds or more, concentrated mostly in one place. Under this burden, the pelvis tends to swing forward and the lower back assumes an exaggerated curve; the result is backache and fatigue. The additional load may have other troublesome consequences; varicose veins and swollen legs and feet, for example, can develop when the pressure of the baby interferes with the flow of blood through vessels from the lower limbs.

The program of exercises illustrated here and on the following pages can help an expectant mother cope with the discomforts of her condition by toning and strengthening the appropriate muscles. Some of the exercises actually serve a triple function: They make a woman's pregnancy more comfortable; they help prepare

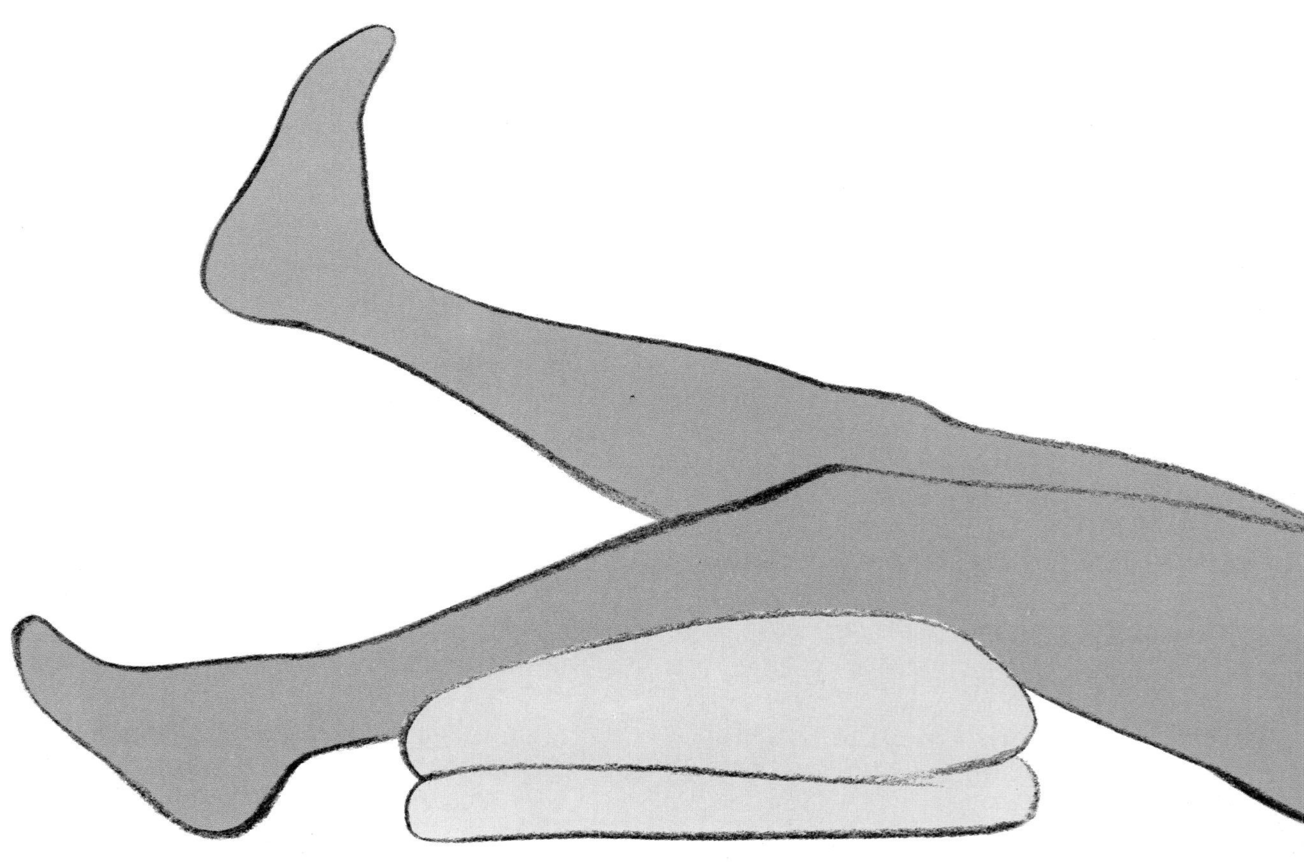

her body for the stresses of labor and delivery; and after delivery, they speed the return of her muscles to their original condition. For example, the exercise shown below, in which the mother practices controlled relaxation, is valuable before, during and after birth. Other exercises are focused upon simple daily movements that become difficult or awkward as the abdomen expands; still others ease minor aches and pains that are characteristic of pregnancy, and a final group helps develop breathing techniques that make the contractions of labor easier for a woman to cope with.

During pregnancy, as at any other time, exercise should be executed with common sense, and only with a doctor's approval. Set aside regular periods in the day for this activity, and introduce new exercises gradually until your body becomes accustomed to them. Two or three short sessions are better than a single long, exhausting one; the point is to make pregnancy easier, not to add another burden to it.

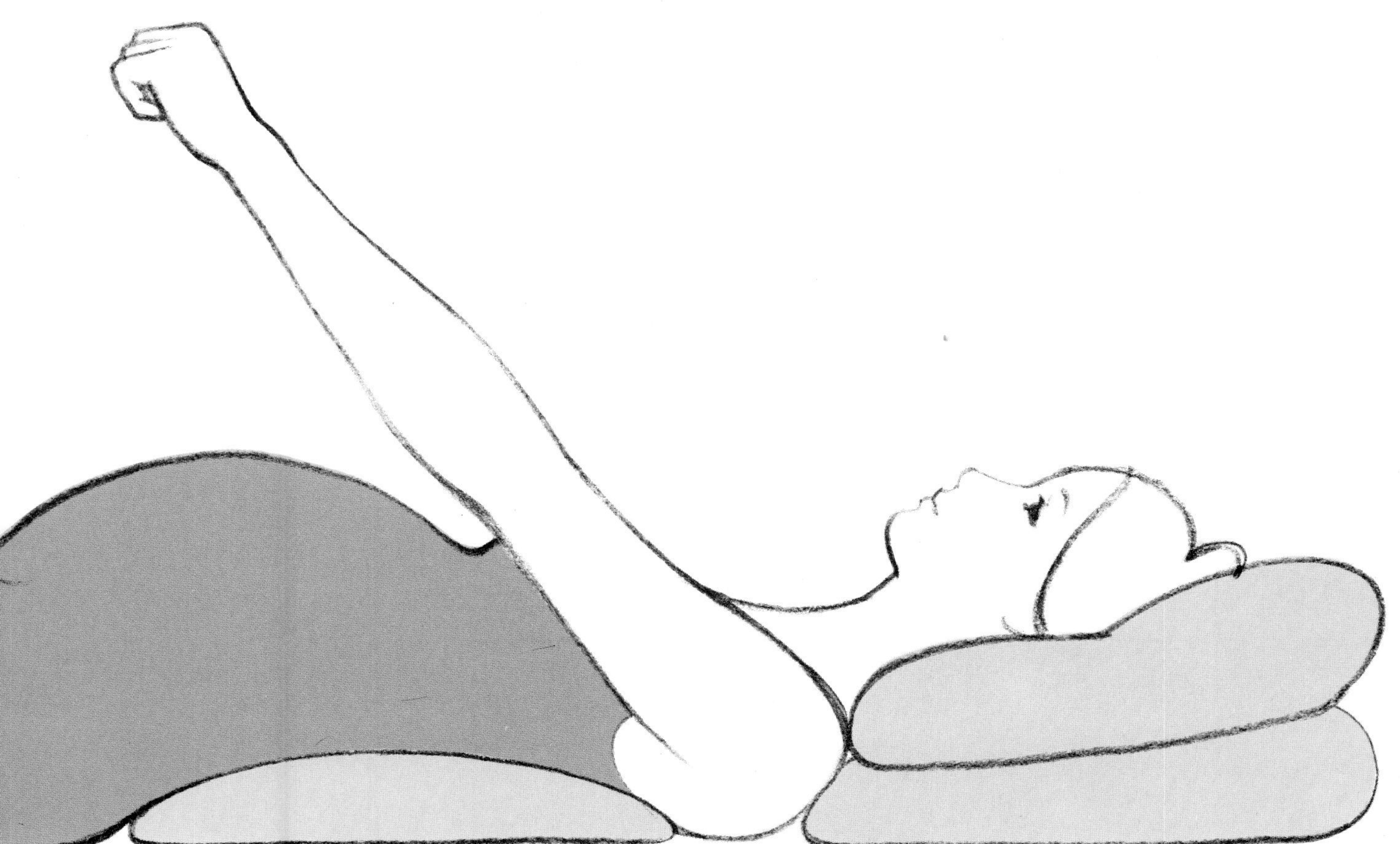

CONTROLLED RELAXATION
Lying on your back, with pillows under your knees, your head and the small of your back, tense sets of muscles—in this example, the muscles of the right leg and left arm—while keeping the rest of the body completely relaxed. The exercise shown here might be preceded by a series of simpler exercises—tightening the muscles of just one limb, then the neck, then the toes and fingers, for example. The ability to relax the body while some muscles are tense is especially valuable during the uterine contractions of labor, but it is also useful in reducing the discomforts of pregnancy and in relieving muscular tensions prompted by emotional stress after the baby has arrived.

Strategies for everyday life

As normally effortless activities and postures such as bending, lifting and lying down become awkward and, at times, even dangerous, a pregnant woman needs different ways of moving during the day and sleeping through the night. For example, a woman in the early stages of pregnancy may rest comfortably while lying on her back; later on, if she lies that way too long, the increased weight of her uterus can constrict blood vessels and cause faintness. In late pregnancy the position shown at the bottom of the opposite page is not only more comfortable, but safer.

In sitting, standing and lifting, good posture helps balance the extra weight and relieve the strain on back and shoulder muscles. Sitting in tailor fashion—with the knees spread wide and the legs crossed loosely enough to permit free circulation *(below)*—carries an extra benefit: It helps condition a woman for labor and delivery by increasing the flexibility of hip joints and strengthening thigh and pelvic muscles.

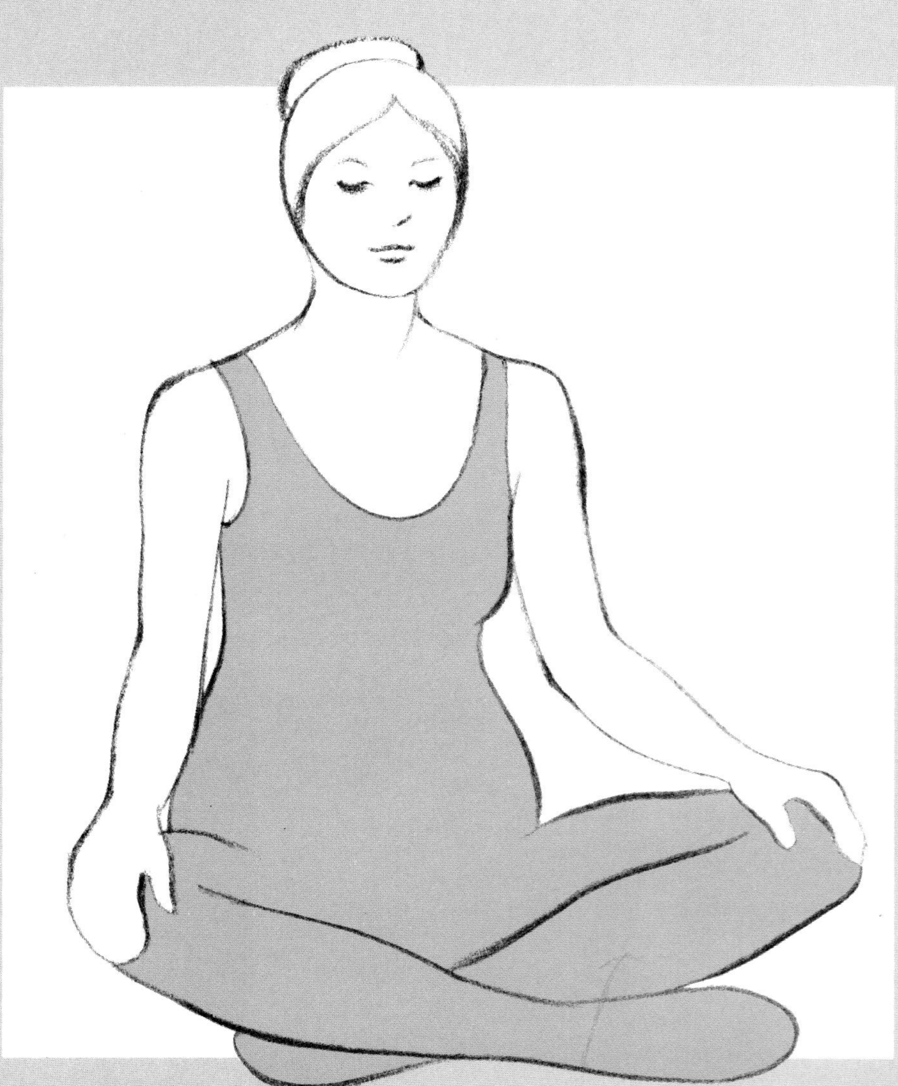

SITTING IN TAILOR FASHION
For such sedentary activities as reading or watching TV, sit on the floor with legs crossed loosely. Intermittently, push gently downward on the knees to stretch the legs apart; release the pressure when you feel a slight strain in your muscles.

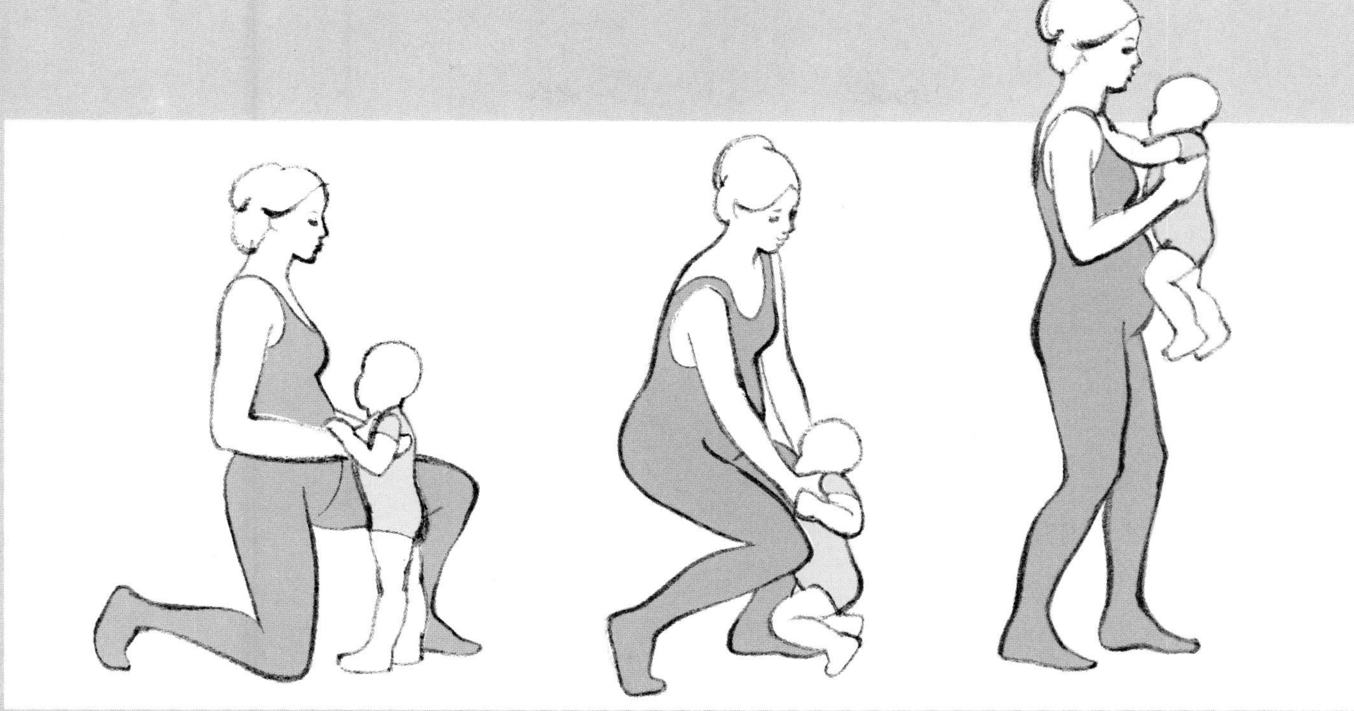

USING KNEES AND LEGS FOR LIFTING
Standing close to a child or object, put one foot forward and drop to the other knee (left), then rise to your feet, keeping your back straight and lifting with the front leg while the back foot balances (center). Carry the weight in front (right), not on the hip.

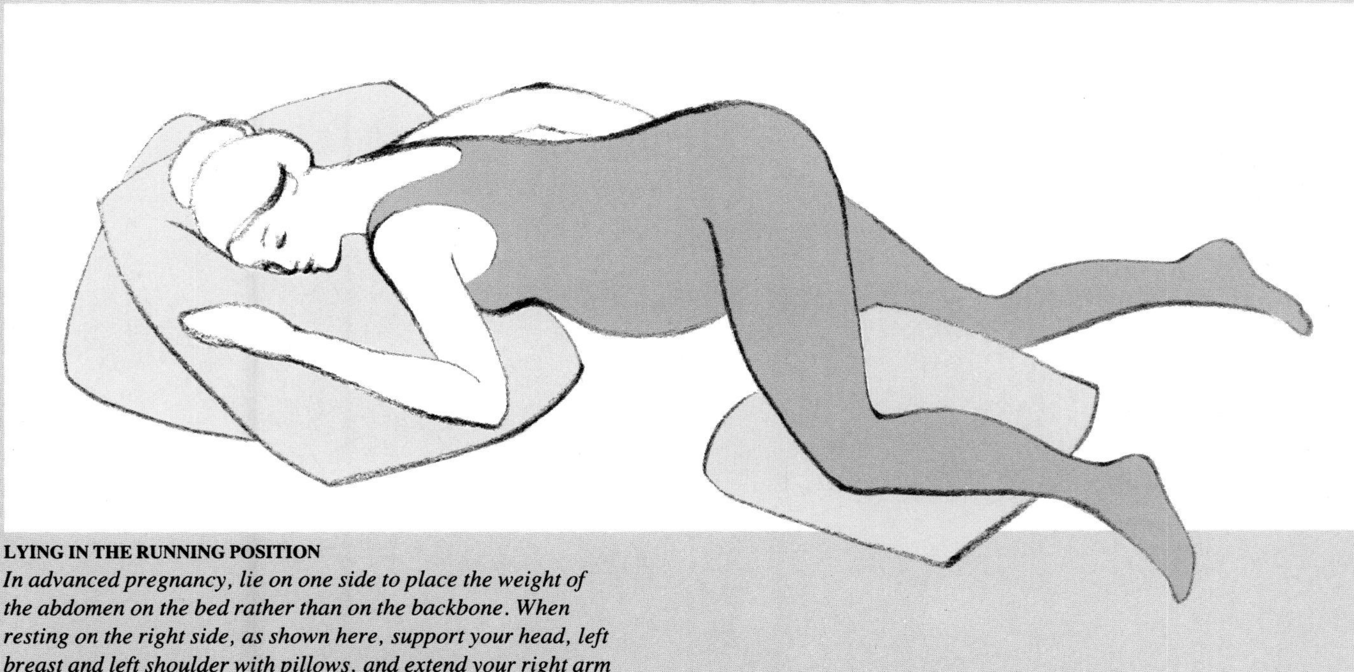

LYING IN THE RUNNING POSITION
In advanced pregnancy, lie on one side to place the weight of the abdomen on the bed rather than on the backbone. When resting on the right side, as shown here, support your head, left breast and left shoulder with pillows, and extend your right arm and leg; an additional pillow may be used under the left leg.

Zeroing in on the common discomforts

Because the minor aches of pregnancy arise largely from localized strains in the muscular, circulatory and respiratory systems, specific exercises have been devised for these trouble spots. Lower-back pain, a frequent complaint caused by the pull of the baby's weight, is relieved by a pelvic-tilt exercise *(bottom)*. Other exercises address problems of the legs and feet, such as varicose veins and swelling, caused by the pressure of the expanding uterus. At the upper end of the torso, the baby crowds the diaphragm, contributing to shortness of breath; here, the appropriate exercise *(opposite, top right)* stretches the torso to ease the strain.

Aside from such formal exercises, some discomfort can be prevented simply by moving around. A woman who insists that she gets plenty of exercise working around the house or office often does not realize how much time she spends standing in one position. Occasional "walk breaks" will improve overall muscle tone, circulation, breathing—and increase her comfort.

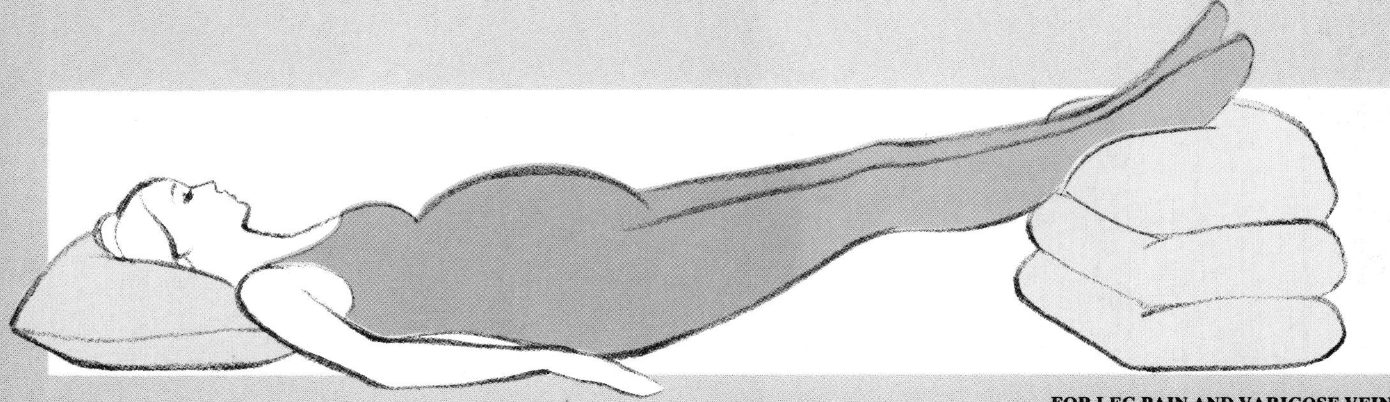

FOR LEG PAIN AND VARICOSE VEINS
Lie on your back with your head supported by a pillow and your feet propped up at about a 30 degree angle—slightly above the level of your heart. No movement is necessary, but the position should be assumed as often as possible during the day.

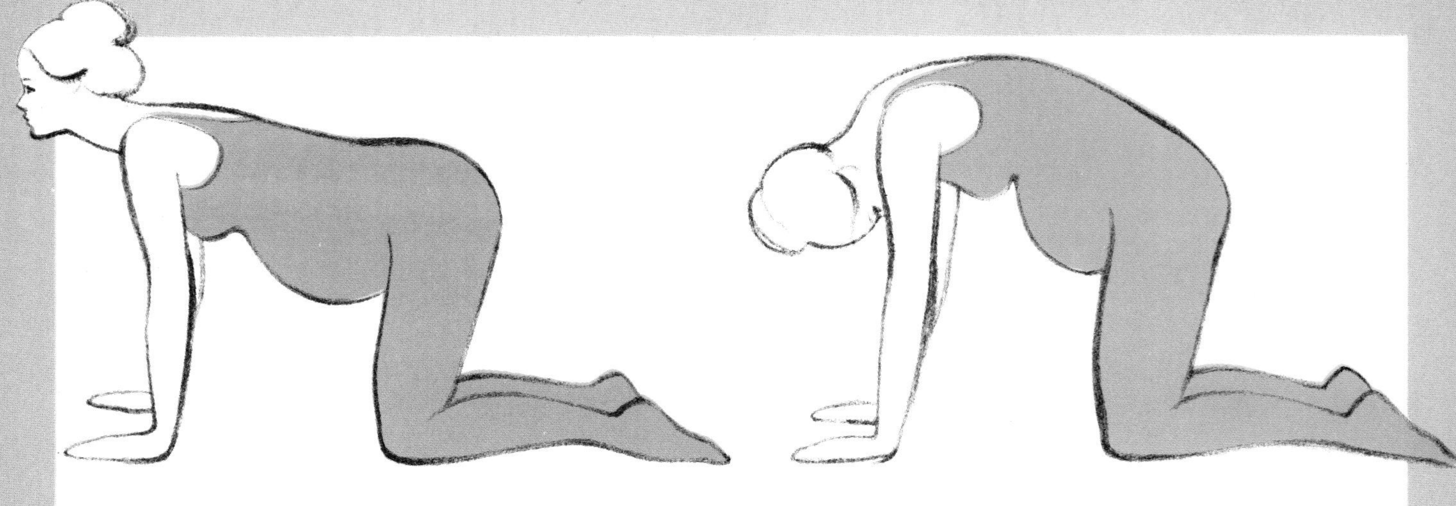

FOR BACKACHE AND FATIGUE
Position yourself as at left, with back horizontal and head lifted; then tuck your chin in, tighten your buttocks and abdomen, and arch your back (right). Hold this position for a few seconds, then relax to the first. Repeat several times, but stop if you feel strain.

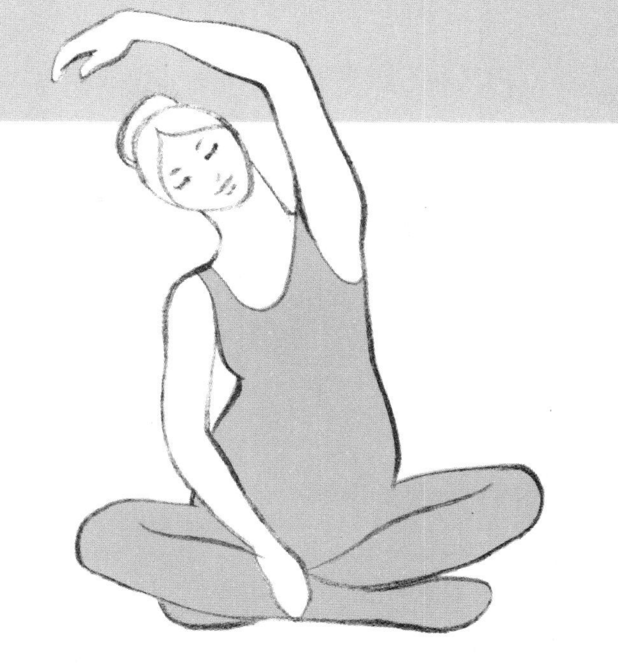

FOR DIFFICULTY IN BREATHING
Sitting with legs crossed loosely, bend the upper torso to the left or right and arch the opposite arm high over your head. Though mainly designed to relieve pressure under the rib cage, this exercise also relaxes shoulder and upper-back muscles.

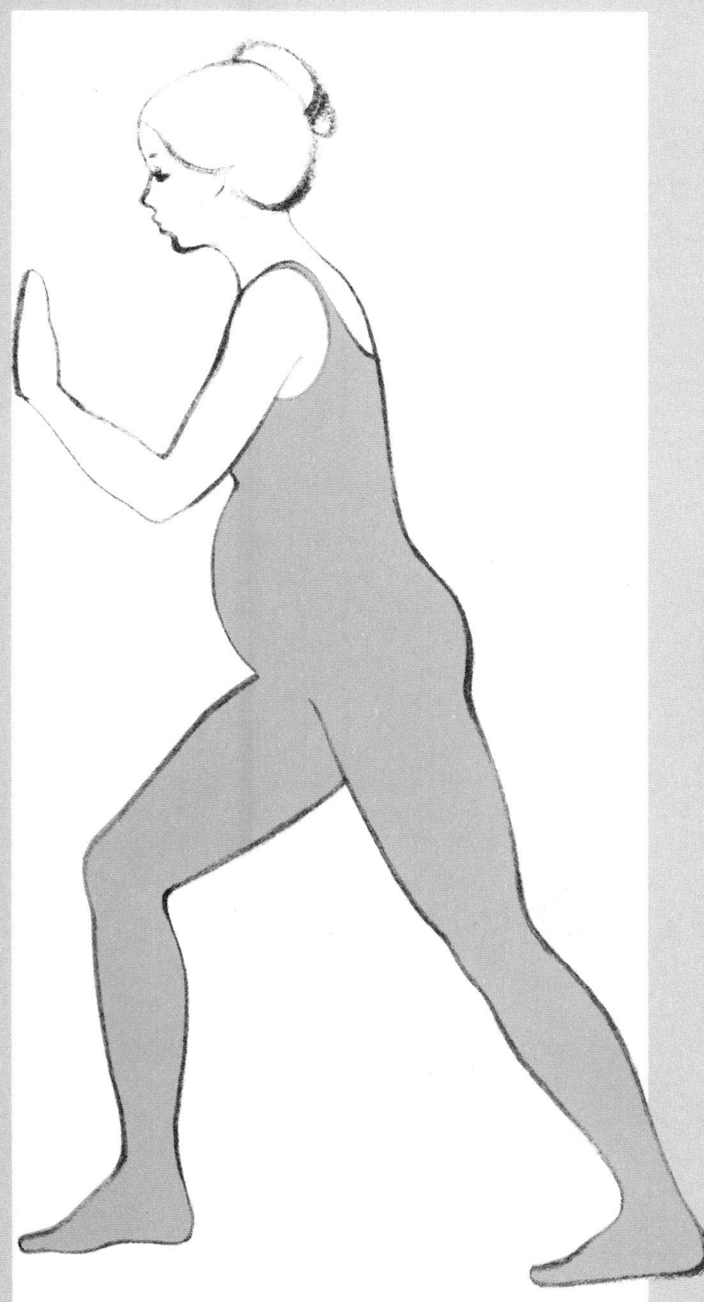

FOR MUSCLE CRAMPS IN THE LOWER LEGS
Stand facing a wall with the more cramped leg behind the other, then lean forward against the wall, bending your front knee but keeping your back foot flat on the floor. This stretching exercise improves circulation as well as muscle tone.

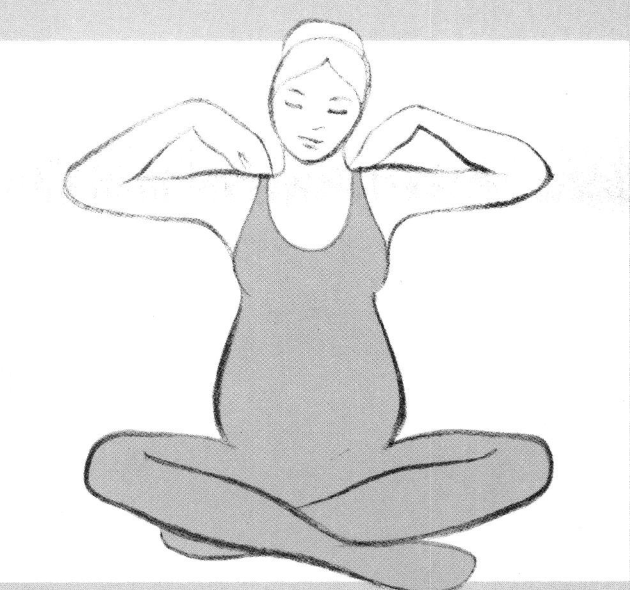

FOR NUMBNESS IN FINGERS
Seated with legs crossed loosely, your back straight, your elbows bent and your fingers on your shoulders, rotate your arms in small backward circles. This exercise not only dispels tingling or numbness in the fingertips but also soothes upper-back pain.

Breathing patterns for the contractions of labor

During labor, breathing the right way can make the difference between a tense, overwhelming experience and one that is calm and manageable. The exercises on these pages, based on prepared-childbirth programs, are designed to teach a pregnant woman how to use breathing to cope with the first stage of labor, in which powerful muscular contractions open the neck of the womb *(page 55)*. This training enables the woman to overcome her natural reaction to pain—tensing muscles and holding the breath. Instead, by breathing with her contractions rather than fighting them, she conserves energy and maintains a good oxygen supply.

In the practice method shown here, the woman sits on the floor with legs crossed loosely while her husband times imaginary contractions and coaches her in the appropriate breathing exercises. The graphs show how her breathing patterns will be synchronized with real contractions at three escalating levels of intensity. Slow chest breathing, in which the diaphragm rises and falls rhythmically, is the basic pattern for the early phases of labor, when contractions begin to feel uncomfortable. As labor progresses, shallower, accelerated breathing, with the diaphragm relatively still, is synchronized with the peaks of strong contractions. Finally, ''pant-blow'' breathing, including a series of blowing or puffing breaths, is used when contractions reach their highest intensity. In all three patterns, a complete ''cleansing'' breath is inhaled and exhaled at the beginning and end of each contraction for maximum oxygen intake.

The goal of the woman is to master these breathing patterns so completely during pregnancy that they will be automatic when labor actually begins. At that time, controlled breathing becomes valuable psychologically as well as physically. It gives a woman something positive to focus on and participate in during contractions, and it sets labor within a time frame, in which each contraction has a beginning, middle and end.

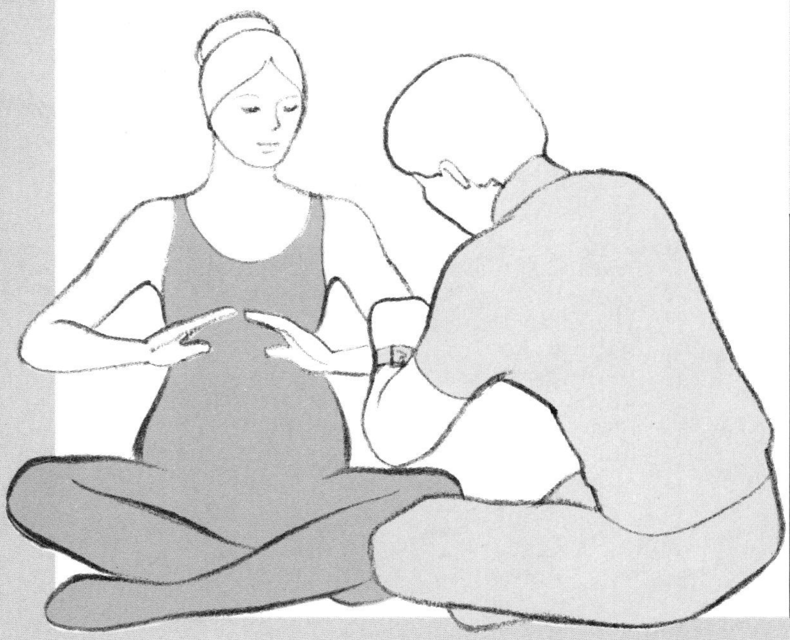

For the moderate, 30- to 45-second contractions of early labor, practice slow chest breathing. As a contraction begins, take a cleansing breath, inhaling deeply through the nose and exhaling slowly through the mouth; breathe deeply throughout the contraction, finishing with another cleansing breath. The woman moves her hands to simulate the rise and fall of her diaphragm.

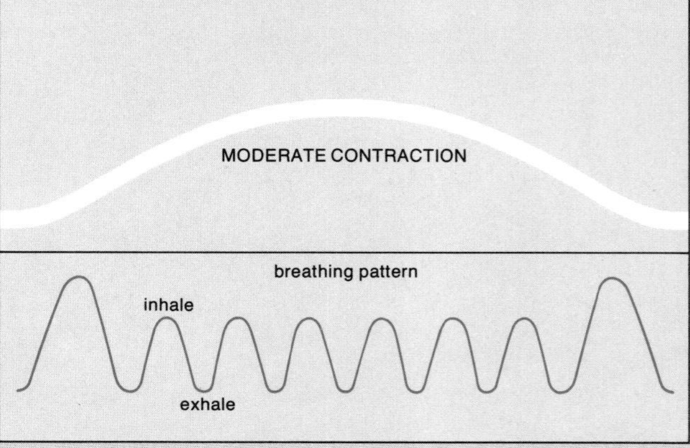

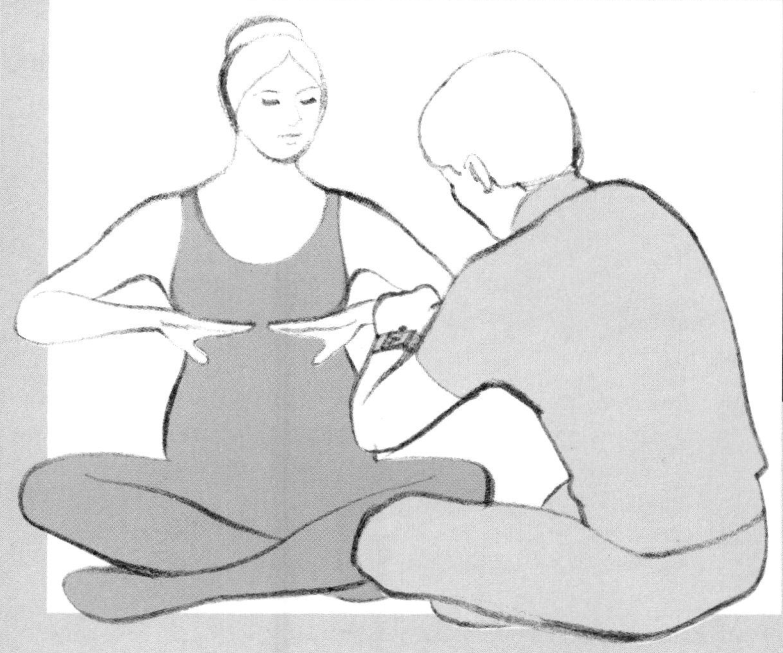

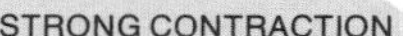

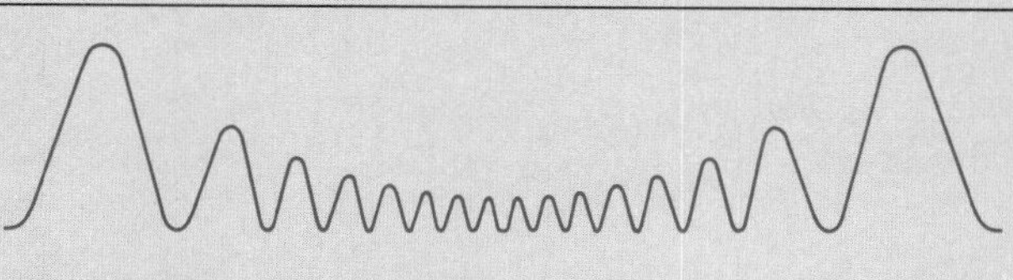

For stronger contractions lasting 60 seconds or longer, change the pace of breathing during each contraction. Begin with a cleansing breath, then breathe progressively faster and more shallowly, in through the nose and out through the mouth, up to the peak; reverse the pacing as the contraction subsides and finish with a cleansing breath. The woman's hands indicate that the diaphragm remains relatively flat.

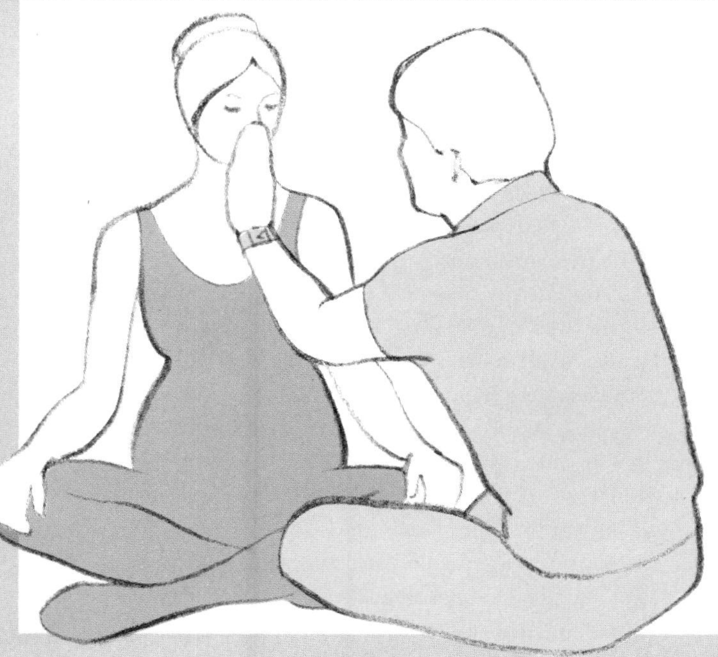

When contractions reach peak intensity, combine shallow breathing with gentle blowing. Begin with a cleansing breath, then proceed with accelerated breathing in and out through the mouth; around the peak of the contraction, exhale every third or fourth breath with a distinct blow or puff. The coach holds his hand before the woman's mouth to check for the puffs.

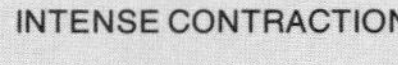

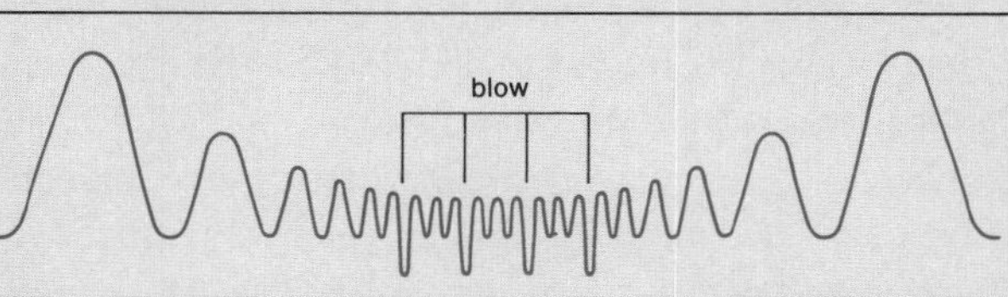

How a baby is born

Of all the predictable pains that afflict human beings, none is awaited with such eagerness as the first contraction of labor. It is a mixed eagerness; the mother-to-be knows that her contractions will be frequent, protracted and intense. Nevertheless, by the end of her ninth month of pregnancy, she hopes that every twinge of her body will be the signal that labor is at last beginning.

For weeks, even months, the expectant mother's muscles may have flexed from time to time in preparation for labor, but these contractions were random and sporadic, in contrast with the rhythmic, escalating pattern of the contractions leading to delivery. As the time of delivery approaches, however, more positive and reliable signs appear. One is lightening—the descent of the baby into the pelvic cavity; as pressure on the mother's diaphragm and upper abdomen is relieved, her breathing becomes easier and her general discomfort lessens. In another sign, the release of the hormone epinephrine sparks a surge of energy that characteristically precedes a birth. One mother summed up this effect with the remark, "It gives you the energy to get through labor." But many a mother has awakened full of zest and, unwittingly, worked off this energy in a frenzy of cooking or house cleaning that culminated with the first contractions of labor. This sequence of events probably gave rise to the old wives' tale that scrubbing the kitchen floor brings on labor.

Whatever the circumstances, the first contraction comes subtly, a slow hardening and tightening of the muscular wall of the uterus. It may not be as easy to recognize as the mother expected, although if she is asleep it will probably wake her up. If she puts her hand against her abdomen at the peak of the contraction, she will find that the muscles are firm as a board. The peak lasts less than half a minute, then the muscles relax. Now the woman is comfortable once more, with time to wonder whether she has felt another false labor pain or the real thing. The best test is to time the contractions and gauge their strength. True contractions often begin as evenly spaced, gentle cramps; as time passes, they become increasingly urgent, longer and more frequent.

As soon as she is certain that her pain is not a false alarm, a mother should stop eating. When labor begins, digestion all but stops, and a stomach containing half-digested food will lead to an uncomfortable delivery at best, and one that could be made dangerous by uncontrolled vomiting. Once labor is under way, intake should be restricted to broth, tea or other clear liquids.

The first signs and contractions

The mechanism that stimulates the first and all other contractions remains a medical mystery. Doctors once believed that the womb simply emptied when full, much like the bladder, but this outdated notion does not account for premature or late labors, nor for the fact that very large babies and twins are born at the nine-month mark just like other babies. Modern theories are generally based upon the role of the chemical messengers called hormones. For example, the level of progesterone, a hormone that prevents muscle contractions,

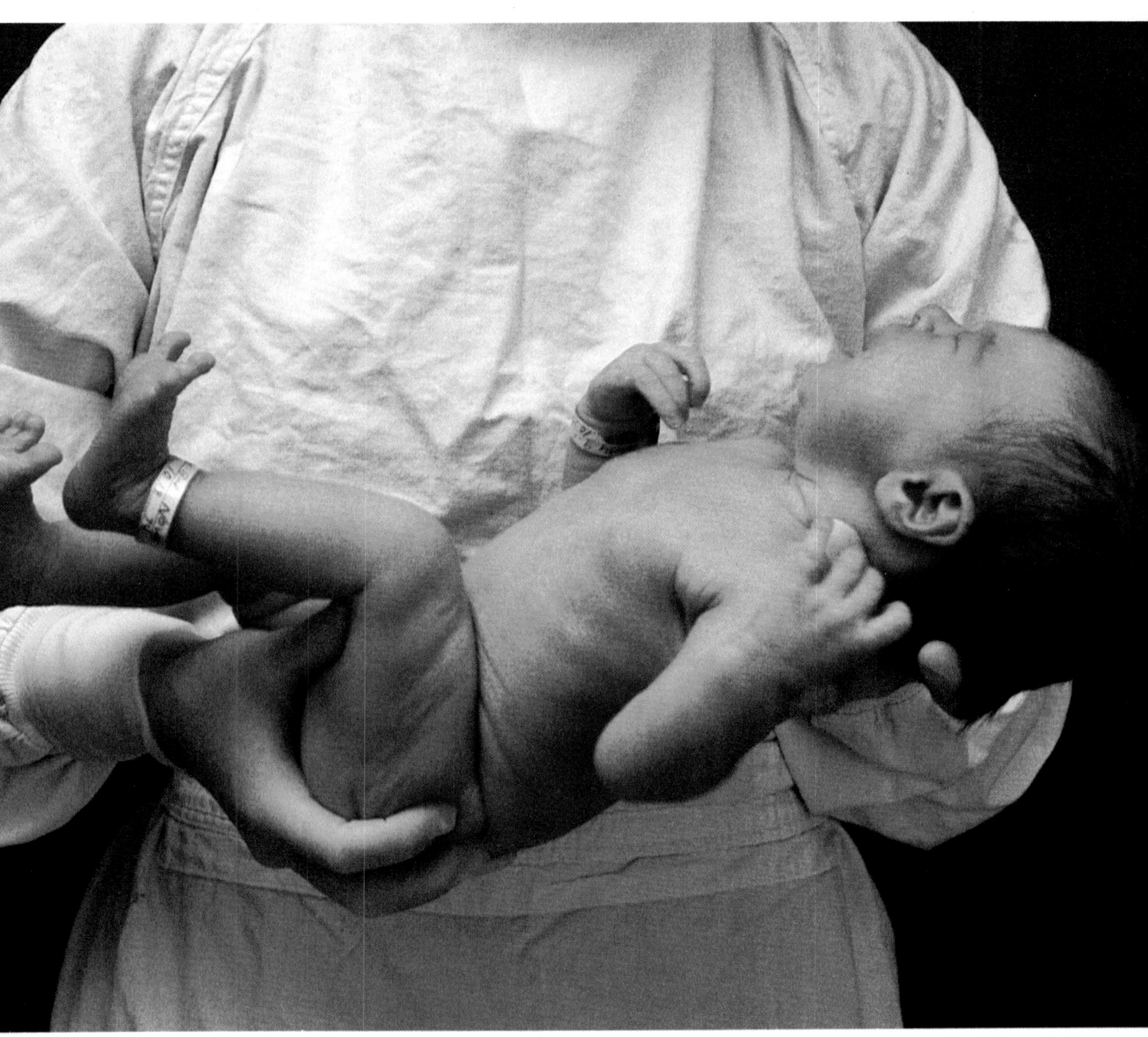

A physician hefts a healthy newborn soon after delivery. In his few minutes of independent life, the infant has already met with a barrage of strenuous experiences, including the suctioning of his nose and mouth, the severing of his umbilical cord, a toweling off, the administration of silver nitrate eye drops, the inking of his footprint and the fitting of identification bracelets.

tends to drop toward the end of a pregnancy. On the other hand, the level of oxytocin, a contraction-stimulating hormone, is above normal during childbirth. Still, the triggering mechanism for such hormonal changes is still unexplained.

Once begun, the contractions of true labor are independent of the mother's control. Breathing and relaxation techniques can make them easier to cope with, just as a sailor's skill can ease a passage over rough seas; but whatever her training, a woman can no more alter the length or strength of a labor pain than a sailor can change the direction of the wind or the size of the waves. What is more, she cannot, of her own volition, speed or slow the labor process as a whole. For a first-time mother experiencing the first contractions of labor, childbirth is still, on the average, 14 hours and 135 contractions away. Subsequent births take less time and labor—an average of 68 contractions over a period of nine hours.

Normally, the time to call the doctor comes at the beginning of the process, when contractions are spaced so regularly that the mother suspects her labor has begun. But even in the absence of contractions, she should call him immediately if her vagina releases either an ooze of slightly bloody mucus or a trickle or sudden gush of watery liquid.

The first of these events, called "show" or "bloody show" by obstetricians, is a relatively quiet signal of the imminence of birth. This is the discharge from the vagina of the brownish, blood-streaked plug of mucus that seals the outer opening of the womb during pregnancy; it often pops loose two or three days before the onset of labor. The "breaking of the waters" is a more dramatic sign that birth is imminent. It shows that the pressure of the baby's body in its descent toward the birth canal has broken the membranes lining the amniotic sac. This reservoir of fluid, which has cushioned the fetus for many months, must break at some point in the course of labor; when the moment comes early, the event apparently helps to trigger labor contractions.

Though the mother cannot consciously induce her own labor, a doctor can and sometimes does make it begin for medical reasons. In a mother with high blood pressure, for example, the blood supply may not meet a baby's needs; the result could be an abnormally small and vulnerable newborn. If such a mother is at her due date or beyond it, she and her doctor may elect to induce the birth. In one method of provoking contractions, the obstetrician snips through the membranes of the amniotic sac; in effect, he breaks the waters by hand. Alternatively, he may use the contraction-stimulating hormone oxytocin, administered intravenously.

Even in a relatively normal situation, inducing labor has certain advantages: The mother arrives at the hospital by appointment, well rested, unfed, and with her household arrangements already worked out at leisure. But contractions artificially induced by oxytocin may be more intense and frequent than normal labor pains, and can place dangerous stress upon both mother and infant. What is worse, there is always the chance that the baby's due date was miscalculated at the outset of pregnancy, and that an induced labor may produce a premature baby who should have been left alone. For these reasons, the U.S. Food and Drug Administration has forbidden the use of oxytocin to induce labor purely for a mother's or a doctor's convenience. There must always be a good medical reason for rushing a baby out of the womb.

When to go to the hospital

For the great majority of mothers whose labor begins spontaneously, the first contractions normally recur at 15- to 20-minute intervals. Mothers who have previously given birth, and can therefore expect a relatively short labor, are generally advised to go to the hospital fairly soon after contractions begin. A first-time mother, by contrast, tends to have time on her hands—time that she can spend more comfortably at home than in a hospital room, where there is little to focus upon but each impending contraction. For her, this early stage of labor is a good chance for a cat nap, a repacking of her overnight case or even a visit with friends. Meanwhile, of course, labor is continuing at its own pace. When the interval between the beginnings of contractions is down to five minutes, it is time for her to depart for the hospital.

Normally, an obstetrician has the mother register in advance, so that the admission procedures can be taken care of in minutes. The trip to the maternity area may be made in a wheelchair if contractions are advanced and severe. Once there, the newcomer will be greeted warmly by nurses trained in the art of reassurance. After a preliminary examination and a change into a sterile hospital gown, most women go into a labor room, for a number of routine hospital procedures. Early in labor, a nurse may give her an enema—unwelcome, but generally necessary, to avoid contamination from feces during the delivery. (The mother will also be encouraged to empty her bladder regularly during the hours to come; if she cannot do so, a nurse may empty it through a catheter tube.) Pubic hair will usually be sheared off or shaved, and the area bathed with a sterile solution.

When the obstetrician arrives, he will check the baby's heart rate and the progress of labor. Ideally, the baby's head is pressing against the cervix, the ring of fibro-muscular tissue that forms the neck of the womb; with each contraction, the head exerts more pressure against the ring, spreading its edges and expanding the opening. Before labor begins, this doorway from the womb is about two millimeters, or 1/12 inch, across. By the time the baby is ready to leave the womb, at the end of the first stage of labor, contractions and pressure will greatly thin the cervix and spread it to a fully dilated width of 10 centimeters, or four inches *(page 55)*.

Doctors and nurses measure the stages of dilation in centimeters, and the numbers from one to 10 become important milestones for a woman in labor. On her arrival at the hospital, with her contractions about five minutes apart, she is likely to be at two or three centimeters of dilation. Later, as her contractions grow stronger and more frequent, the mother will welcome the doctor's announcements of her progress to six, eight, and finally 10—the point at which the baby begins the passage through the birth canal *(pages 58-59)*.

Easing the pain of labor

This first stage of labor is not only the most difficult but the longest, averaging 12 hours for a first baby, two to eight hours for subsequent children. At some point during these hours, most women receive at least some mild medication to take the edge off the contractions.

Mothers expecting medication from the moment they reach the labor room should know that drugs will not be

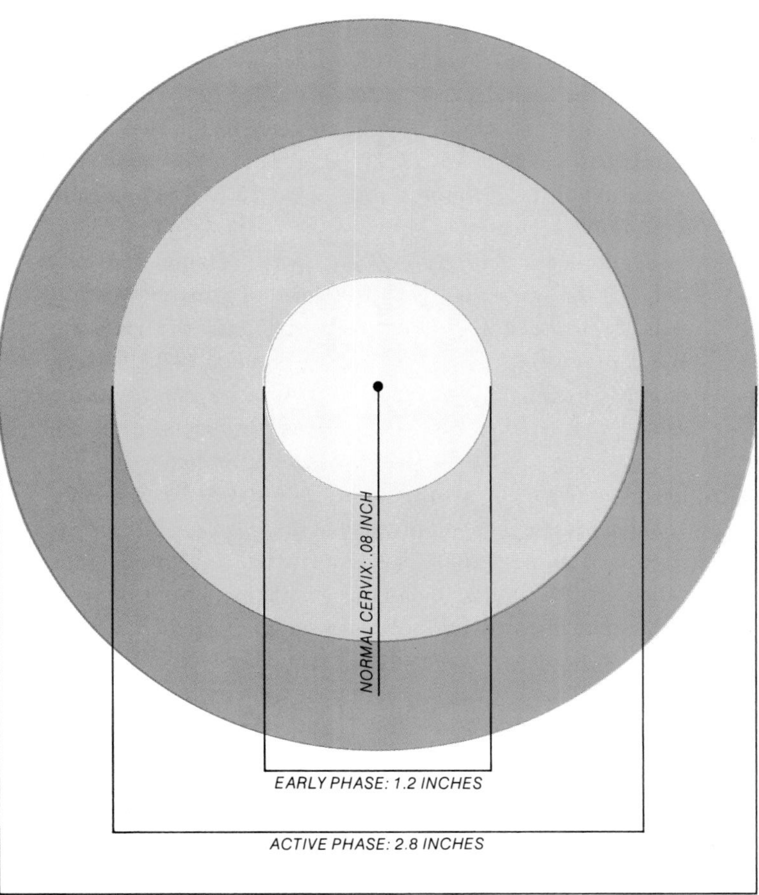

WIDENING THE PASSAGE FROM THE WOMB
During the first stage of labor, in a process called dilation, the cervix, or neck of the womb, widens more than 40-fold to permit a baby to pass out of the womb (pages 58-59). Dilation takes place with increasing speed as labor contractions grow stronger and more frequent, but is often divided into three phases, shown above approximately life-sized. The first, or early, phase, which ends when the cervix is about 3 centimeters (1.2 inches) wide, takes about 70 per cent of the total period. During the active, or accelerated, phase, width increases to 7 centimeters (2.8 inches) in about 20 per cent of the total period. The final, or transition, phase is the briefest: In 10 per cent or less of the dilation period, the cervical opening widens to the 10 centimeters (4 inches) required for delivery.

administered until labor is well under way, usually midway through the first stage. The delay is in the best interests of both mother and child. Given too early or too copiously, painkillers can slow or even stop the progress of labor. The effects on the child are less obvious, and have only recently been fully understood.

Beginning in the early 1900s, mothers in labor were customarily drugged in a "twilight sleep" of groggy forgetfulness, from which they would awaken to greet the newborn. But the powerful narcotics used to produce twilight sleep crossed through the placenta to the baby in the womb with the same sleep-inducing effect; what is worse, they affected the respiratory center in the baby's brain, often hampering his first attempts to breathe. And because the drugged mother could not participate in the effort of delivery, doctors resorted to deep and sometimes damaging insertions of metal tongs called forceps to draw the infant from the mother's body.

Modern research has yielded a range of medicines that, when properly administered, can reduce or block the mother's pain without greatly affecting the baby or the progress of labor and delivery. Ironically, many women now prefer to experience the full strength of every contraction. A first-time mother should keep an open mind on the subject. Until she is actually in labor, she really cannot know how her body reacts to its pain. She may wish to avoid medication as long as the contractions remain manageable—and for some women, that means right through delivery. But if the pains become intolerable, she should by all means ask for relief—preferably through a type of medication she and her obstetrician have agreed upon beforehand—without feeling that she is a coward or a failure.

Four methods of pain relief are now generally used in labor and delivery. Three—analgesics, amnesics and anesthetics—are drugs. The fourth, prepared childbirth, is designed for a woman who prefers to forgo medication either completely or as long as possible; this method copes with pain mainly by psychological means.

Analgesics, such as aspirin, diminish the sensation of pain; the analgesic most commonly used for labor and delivery is Demerol. An amnesic—scopolamine, for example—removes the memory of pain; it is usually given in combination with an analgesic. A woman who receives an amnesic drifts off to sleep, moans and writhes in a half-alert state during contractions, but finally awakens after the delivery to ask when the birth will occur.

Anesthetics, which completely suppress sensation in all or part of the body, fall into two broad categories. A general anesthetic, given as an injection or a gas, renders the mother temporarily unconscious. Because of the risk of complications for mother and baby, general anesthesia is rarely used in normal deliveries. Far more common are local and regional anesthetics, which act directly through the nerves rather than the bloodstream, leave the mother awake and alert, and have little or no effect on the baby. They are now the medication of choice in 70 per cent of all births.

Some local anesthetics are injected into tissues around the vagina to block pain in a small area; a paracervical block, for example, numbs the region of the lower womb. Others, called conduction or regional anesthetics, are injected into cavities in the spinal column to interrupt nerve pathways that serve a larger area of the body. A so-called saddle block, for example, injected directly into the spinal fluid just before delivery, numbs the upper thighs and the outlet of the birth canal—the parts of the body that would be in contact with a saddle if the woman were astride a horse.

One of the most common of the conduction anesthetics is an epidural, which blocks pain from navel to toes. Administering an epidural takes care and special skill, but the effects can be invaluable in the long labor of a first-time mother. To begin with, the anesthesiologist may numb the woman's lower back with a local anesthetic. Then he painlessly threads a plastic tube into the space between two vertebrae and tapes the tube securely to the skin. Using the tube, the anesthesiologist can administer a controlled flow of anesthetic.

The fourth, or psychological, form of pain relief is built upon a training program that teaches parents-to-be exactly what to expect during labor and delivery. In itself, dispelling the mysteries of childbirth does much to relieve fear and tension; in addition, the mother learns to relax and to breathe with her contractions rather than fighting them. Throughout the program the father plays an active role, first as his wife's classmate during pregnancy, later as her coach and timekeeper during delivery.

The ideas underlying this technique are not new. In 1944, Dr. Grantly Dick-Read, an English obstetrician, wrote a book, *Childbirth Without Fear,* on what he called natural childbirth. Dr. Dick-Read argued that women who understood the process of childbirth would be more relaxed and suffer less pain during the event; he insisted, for example, that so-called labor pains be called by their rightful name, contractions. In the 1950s a Frenchman, Dr. Fernand Lamaze, took the idea of drug-free childbirth a step further. According to Lamaze, a mother who learns to focus her attention on something other than the contractions will find that pain assumes a minor role. His technique, called prepared childbirth, teaches women in six to eight weeks of classes to concentrate on specific breathing and relaxation patterns that they will later use while contractions occur.

The patterns vary *(pages 44-51)* during successive stages of labor and delivery, but there is one constant: The mother is never alone. A coach is always near to give her emotional support, help time her contractions, guide her in breathing and relaxation, and massage such painful areas as her lower back. If the mother has difficulty withstanding the pain, no stigma is attached to requesting relief. In fact, about one third of all women who choose prepared childbirth do ask for pain medication, but most obstetricians agree that these women fare better on lower dosages than those who have not been to preparatory classes and do not have the support of a coach.

From labor room to delivery room

For the mother who is doing without pain-relieving drugs, the most difficult moments come near the end of the first stage of labor, in the so-called transition phase. Contractions then last as long as a minute and a half and many recur within a minute, leaving little chance for relaxation. The cervix is now three-quarters dilated, and the contractions that stretch the final inch are the most powerful of all. This time of stress has been appropriately nicknamed the "Hurricane Hour"; during it, a woman may feel confused, irritable or anxious, and suddenly uncertain whether she can endure her travail. But the transition phase is soon over, usually in 20 minutes to an hour. With the cervix completely dilated to four inches, it is time for the second stage of labor, in which the baby moves out of the uterus and down through the birth canal. The mother may feel an urge to push when the baby begins his descent, but she is generally asked to wait until he reaches the halfway point of the canal, in order to save her strength. Sometimes the nurse will instruct her to "pant like a puppy," to help her resist that compelling urge to push.

When the long-awaited permission to push is given, many mothers feel a surge of relief and renewal, as if their bodies were telling them that the hardest work is over and the end is in view. The contractions of the second stage are far less severe than those of transition, and the mother finally has an active role to perform. At each contraction she is encouraged to take a deep breath, hold it, and bear down steadily with her abdominal muscles, as if straining for a bowel movement. Each push inches the baby farther down the birth canal; when the head becomes visible at the opening of the vagina, it is time to move the entire cast of characters from the labor room into the delivery area for the final act.

The delivery room somewhat resembles an operating room. Considerably larger than the labor room, it accommodates a variety of medical paraphernalia, an additional nurse and, before long, another individual—the newborn. Sterility is all-important here; the doctors, nurses and coach wear scrub suits, paper shoe covers, hair coverings, and masks that cover the nose and mouth. At center stage is the delivery table, equipped with leg supports and stirrups to hold the mother's legs bent and spread wide. A large adjustable mirror, set at an angle that permits the mother to watch the birth, may hang over the table. Off to one side an area is ready, with a heated crib or table, blankets, a resuscitator and supplies for the baby's immediate care and identification.

A chronicle of one child's birth

The time required for delivery varies widely. A veteran may expel her child in a few minutes with three or four pushes; a first-time mother needs an average of an hour and a half, and a dozen or more pushing contractions. Generalizations are elusive, but perhaps the best way to convey the quality of a birth is to trace one actual delivery. Here, then, is the experience of a young mother who gave birth to her first child at a hospital in northern Virginia on a Saturday evening in May.

At about six o'clock that evening, after a sluggish, all-day labor and half an hour of bearing down with contractions, the mother was wheeled into the delivery room. Propped up at a comfortable 45-degree angle by a triangular pillow on the delivery table, she was positioned in the stirrups and draped with sterile sheets. Two nurses stood by to help coach her through the delivery. As he swabbed the exterior of the birth area with a brown sterile solution, the obstetrician noted with satisfaction that the baby's head was well positioned for exit. "You could have your baby with the next contraction," he told the mother.

At this point, moments before the baby would squeeze out of the cramped opening, the obstetrician performed an episiotomy. Using a pair of blunt surgical scissors, he cut a slit an inch or so downward from the base of the vagina toward the anus. The simple surgical procedure, sometimes performed under a local anesthetic, is now employed in the overwhelming majority of deliveries, and with good reason. If it is not deliberately cut, this bit of skin, stretched beyond endurance in childbearing, usually tears, and a ragged tear requires more stitches to repair and heals with more difficulty than a clean incision. An episiotomy may also save the mother strain by widening the birth passage, and it dramatically eases pressure on the baby's head in the final squeeze out of the birth canal.

Despite her episiotomy, however, the young mother's baby did not arrive with the next contraction, nor the next after that. "Oh, come on!" she cried in exasperation. When the next contraction came, at 6:06, she caught it well and pushed long, strong and steadily to a chorus of coaching: "Keep it coming . . . Right on through . . . You're nearly there!" Another contraction started at 6:08. "Two-yard line and goal to go!" exclaimed a nurse. "Push her down . . . Good . . . Great!" But the contraction subsided, with the baby still within the canal.

Another contraction, at 6:11, brought the baby almost, but not quite, out into the doctor's waiting hands. "It hurts," the

Three stages of delivery

The passage of a baby from a mother's womb to the outside world occurs in three successively shorter stages, shown in the four pictures at right. During the first, generally lasting about 12 hours in first-time mothers, eight in women who have previously borne a child, the muscular contractions of labor open the cervix, or neck of the womb. In the second stage, which typically takes between 30 minutes and an hour and a half, the baby passes out of the womb and through the birth canal, twisting and turning to slip through with the least resistance. During the final stage, which takes about 10 minutes, additional contractions expel the placenta.

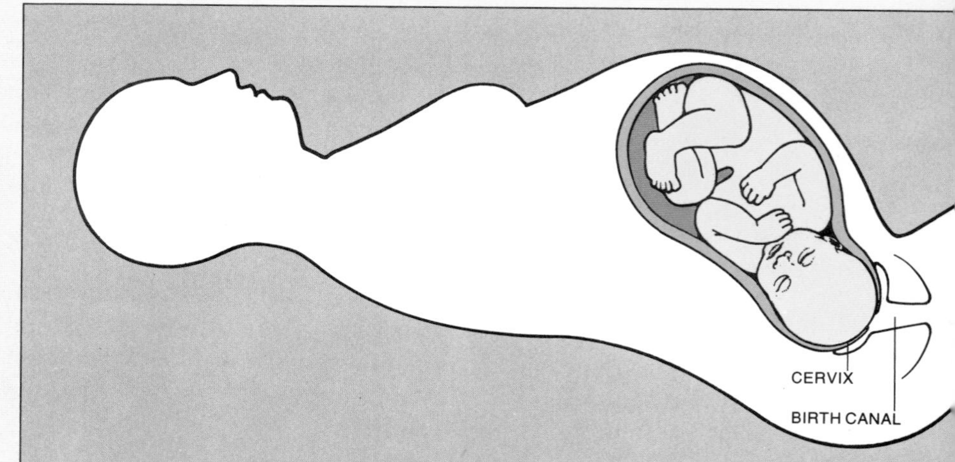

As rhythmic contractions signal the onset of the first stage of labor, the baby's head settles deep in the pelvis, near the birth canal. The pressure of the head and the pull of contracting muscles stretch the cervix; its walls, normally as much as 4/5 inch thick, become almost paper-thin, and the cervical opening eventually dilates to a diameter of about 4 inches.

mother whispered, in an extraordinary understatement after 16 hours of labor.

But the very next contraction was the magic one. With the mother's heaving, red-faced push, her baby's head and neck made their way out of the vaginal opening. Immediately, the doctor drew mucus from the baby's nose and mouth with a rubber suction bulb, while the mother panted at rest. Her main work was done, for the head is the most difficult part to deliver. With one more strong push, the rest of the baby's body emerged. The eight-pound-five-ounce boy was very white for an instant, then turned bright pink, like a tightly squeezed finger. A nurse made a note of the time—6:14 p.m.

The obstetrician clamped the umbilical cord in two places and cut it between them, then raised the child for his mother to see. She asked, "Why isn't he crying?"—and at that moment her son produced a lusty bellow. However eagerly it is anticipated, and however often it is heard, that cry produces a shock of recognition and carries a semimystical meaning. The poet Carl Sandburg described it in this way: "The first cry of a newborn baby in Chicago or Zamboango, in Amsterdam or Rangoon, has the same pitch and key, each saying, 'I am! I have come through! I belong! I am a member of the Family.' "

From this point in childbirth, the hospital has two patients to care for, each with individual needs. As the delivery room nurses carry the infant to one side, the obstetrician focuses on the third and easiest stage of birth: the delivery of the placenta, or afterbirth. The expulsion of the tissues that linked the circulatory systems of mother and child is usually accomplished within 10 minutes, with one final contraction and, if necessary, gentle external pressure on the abdomen by the doctor's hand. Separating from the walls of the newly slack uterus, the placenta slides down the birth canal and is simply lifted out of the vagina. Finally, the doctor sews the episiotomy incision, using catgut thread that will be absorbed by the mother's body as the wound heals.

Meanwhile, a nurse takes charge of the newborn's first busy moments of life. She wipes the baby's skin clean of excess vernix, the cheesy, protective covering on his skin, and covers his head with a cap to prevent heat loss from his scalp. Then, after a series of quick checks to evaluate such

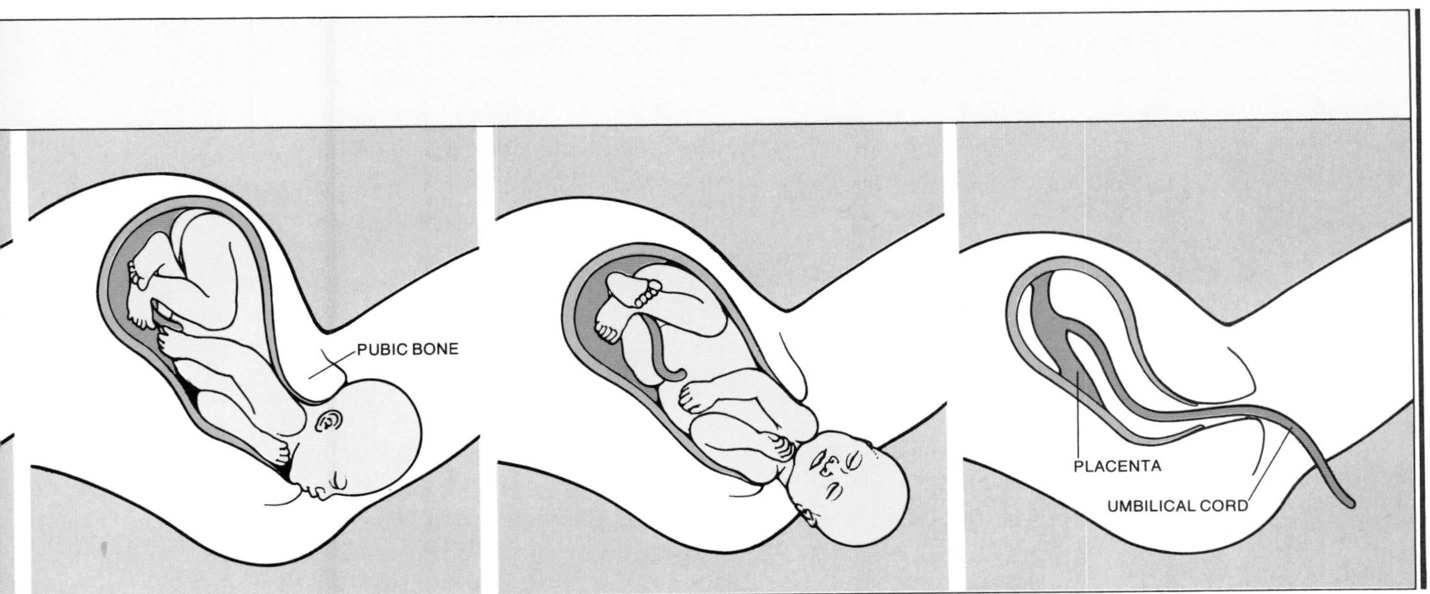

Stronger contractions at the start of the second stage push the head, now face downward, into the birth canal. Though the chin is tucked in at first for compactness, the head soon bends back and up (above) to pass under the pubic bone.

After the head emerges from the mother's body, the baby turns sideways again to ease the shoulders through the canal, top shoulder first. One or two more contractions expel the rest of the body quickly and smoothly, ending the second stage.

In stage three, the placenta separates from the wall of the womb; the womb shrinks and resumes contractions, which soon force the placenta down the birth canal. Outside the mother's body, the umbilical cord has already been cut and clamped.

vital signs as respiration, heartbeat and muscle tone *(pages 68-69),* she swaddles the infant in light blankets and bundles him into the arms of his mother. That exhilarated, if exhausted, woman may now spend an hour or two in a recovery room, visiting with the baby and her husband.

For problem births: cesarean delivery

More than 95 per cent of all babies approach the hour of their birth in the classic style of the boy in northern Virginia—head first, with the rugged but malleable skull forging a path through the mother's tissues and the rest of the small body slipping out easily in its wake. But about one in 25 are nonconformists who present themselves for birth in other positions—sometimes rear-end first, with legs straight up and toes near the shoulders; sometimes cross-legged, or with one leg descending into the birth canal before the other. All of these positions are known as "breech," and all of them call for special methods of delivery.

An obstetrician may decide to go through with a vaginal delivery of a breech baby. If so, he will probably begin by manipulating the exterior of the mother's abdomen in an attempt to turn the baby's body head down. If this maneuver is not successful, the doctor may first use a regional or general anesthetic to block the mother's pain, then reach into the birth canal and assist the final exit of the baby with a gloved hand and, if necessary, the rounded tongs called forceps.

Breech delivery, no matter how difficult, is still a form of natural birth. In two thirds of the cases, however, a breech presentation is so stubborn as to rule out the normal birth-canal route. Instead, the child must be delivered by the operation called a cesarean section.

Breech presentations account for only a fraction of cesarean sections done today. The most common cause, by far, is a pelvic problem—more specifically, a pelvis so small, malformed or blocked by a tumor that a baby cannot squeeze through the opening formed by the pelvic bones. A baby who begins to arrive prematurely may require a cesarean because he is too small and weak to withstand the rigors of natural childbirth. And a whole class of disorders generically called fetal distress account for still other cesarean sections: If, for example, the heart rate of a baby in the womb suddenly declines, or if there is evidence of bleeding or infection within the womb, a cesarean offers a rapid form of lifesaving action.

Whatever its cause, a cesarean section is full-fledged surgery, performed under regional or general anesthesia. The obstetrician cuts an opening in the abdomen, then makes an incision into the uterus and quickly lifts out the baby and placenta. The delivery itself usually takes only five to 10 minutes, but another 50 minutes or so is needed to stitch together the layers of severed tissues.

Unlike the vaginal-delivery mother, who may deliver in the morning and be up and about in the afternoon, a cesarean mother emerges from the operation with serious wounds that take time to heal and cause considerable discomfort. Gas pains are common for several days, and movement may be painful for a week or more; later, because she tires easily, the cesarean mother is likely to have some difficulty in feeding and caring for her new baby for a few weeks. Nevertheless, the number of cesarean sections is on the increase, partly because they are safer than ever. Before the turn of the century, the operation was resorted to only as a desperate last-ditch measure, when there seemed no other way to save the life of mother or baby. Today, cesareans constitute 17 per cent of all births in the United States, with a mortality rate of only one per thousand operations.

A third of these operations are performed on women who have already undergone a cesarean section for a previous child. Years ago, in fact, there was little or no alternative to repeating the operation for subsequent births, and doctors and mothers used to say, "Once a cesarean, always a cesarean." The adage held true for old-style cesareans, in which the abdomen was slit vertically from navel to pubic hair, leaving a large scar that was liable to rupture under the stress of normal labor. Today, only 3 per cent of cesareans are performed in that way. Modern obstetricians make a transverse cut—a horizontal incision so low on the abdomen that even a bikini bottom will cover the scar. Unless the problem that dictated a cesarean for the first baby persists or recurs, a

The newborn's rich repertory of reflexes

The brand-new baby shown here and on the following pages is displaying reflexes—automatic physical responses to specific stimuli, comparable to the knee-jerk response that doctors produce with rubber hammers when examining grown-ups. In the picture below, for example, the stimulus is a light stroke on a corner of the infant's mouth; the reflexive response, called rooting, is a turn of the infant's head in search of a nipple.

Rooting is one of many reflexes a normal baby comes equipped with at birth. All can be stimulated during the first months of life, then all of them disappear. As the nervous system matures and voluntary control of the muscles takes over, the primitive responses fade away in a predictable order. Meanwhile, they form a valuable diagnostic tool for pediatricians. In the words of one authority, Dr. M. D. Sheridan: "It is as if Nature had put them there so that we could test if the circuits are properly laid, and expect that things would work satisfactorily when the current is subsequently switched on."

A word of caution is in order. Many parents who wish to assess or diagnose their own children with respect to the reflexes worry needlessly because, at one time or another, an attempt to elicit a specific reflex is ineffective. In fact, the responses vary widely from child to child; moreover, minor neurological disorders that may suppress a response often resolve themselves spontaneously. A wrong diagnosis can easily be made by an inexperienced examiner or in an examination made at an inappropriate time, when the infant is sleepy, full or crying.

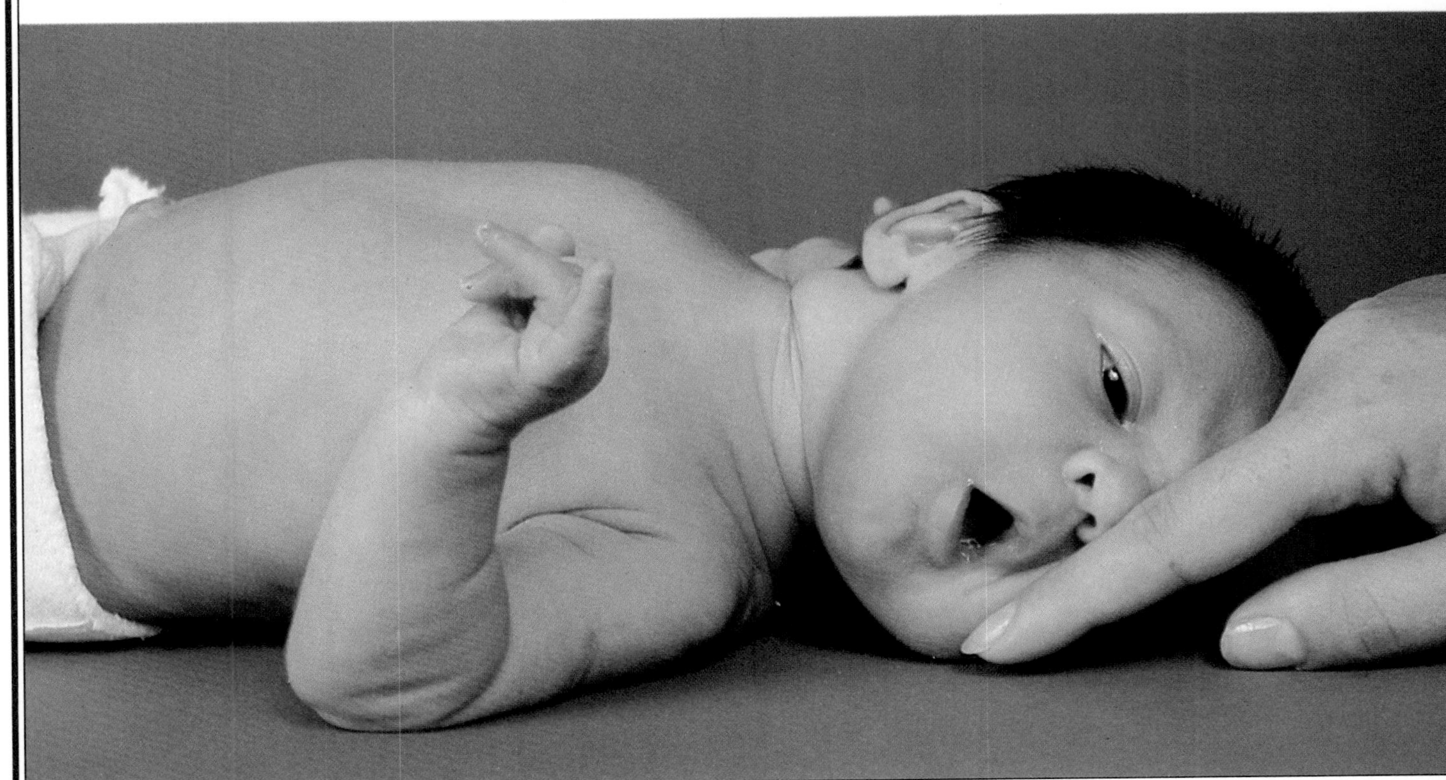

A newborn exhibits the rooting reflex: As the skin near the corner of the mouth is stroked, the baby turns his head to that side and tries to suck the stimulating finger as if it were a nipple. Though it is increasingly efficient during the first six weeks of life, the rooting reflex eventually loses its survival value; by the age of six months it has generally disappeared.

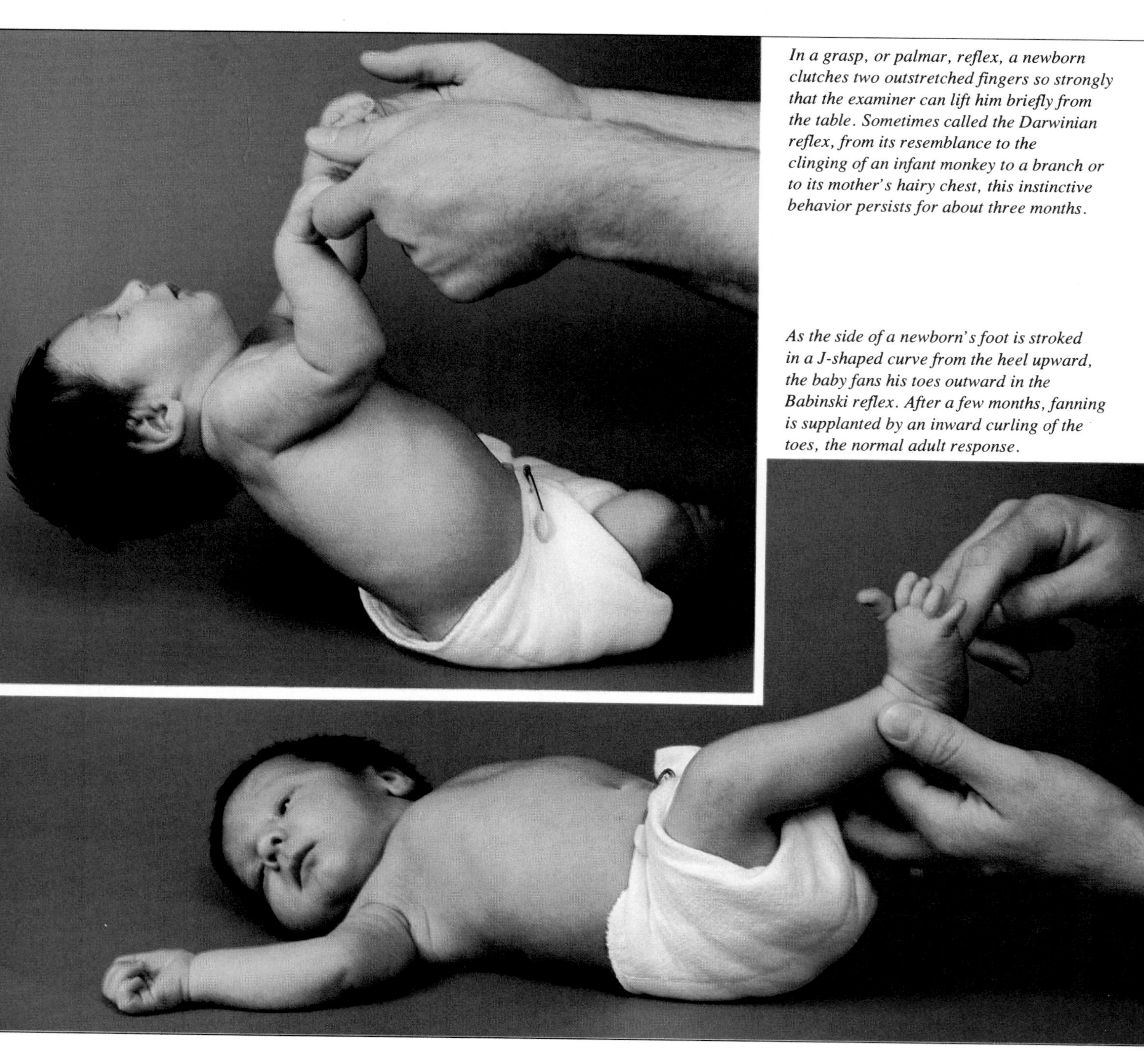

In a grasp, or palmar, reflex, a newborn clutches two outstretched fingers so strongly that the examiner can lift him briefly from the table. Sometimes called the Darwinian reflex, from its resemblance to the clinging of an infant monkey to a branch or to its mother's hairy chest, this instinctive behavior persists for about three months.

As the side of a newborn's foot is stroked in a J-shaped curve from the heel upward, the baby fans his toes outward in the Babinski reflex. After a few months, fanning is supplanted by an inward curling of the toes, the normal adult response.

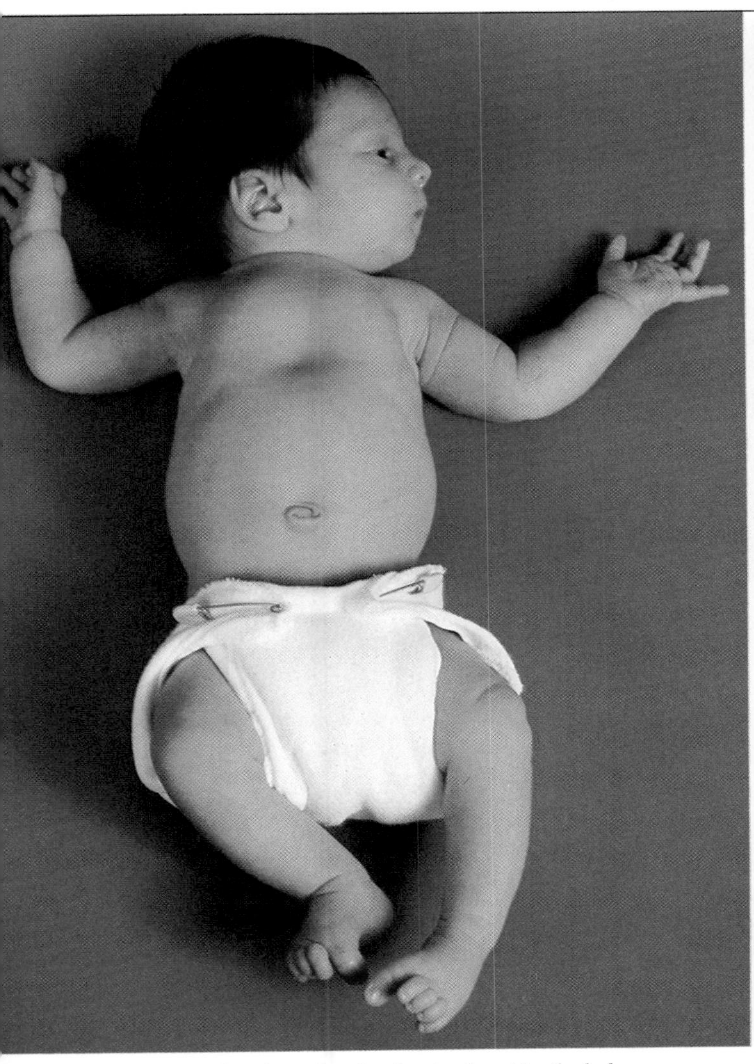

An asymmetrical tonic neck reflex is stimulated by the baby himself: As he turns his head to one side, the arm and leg on that side are extended, and the limbs on the opposite side are flexed. This so-called fencing posture may persist for nine months.

Held erect with the feet touching a hard surface, an infant takes a few quick steps. This step-in-place reflex, which usually disappears by the age of three months, has nothing in common with true walking, which does not begin until a year or so later.

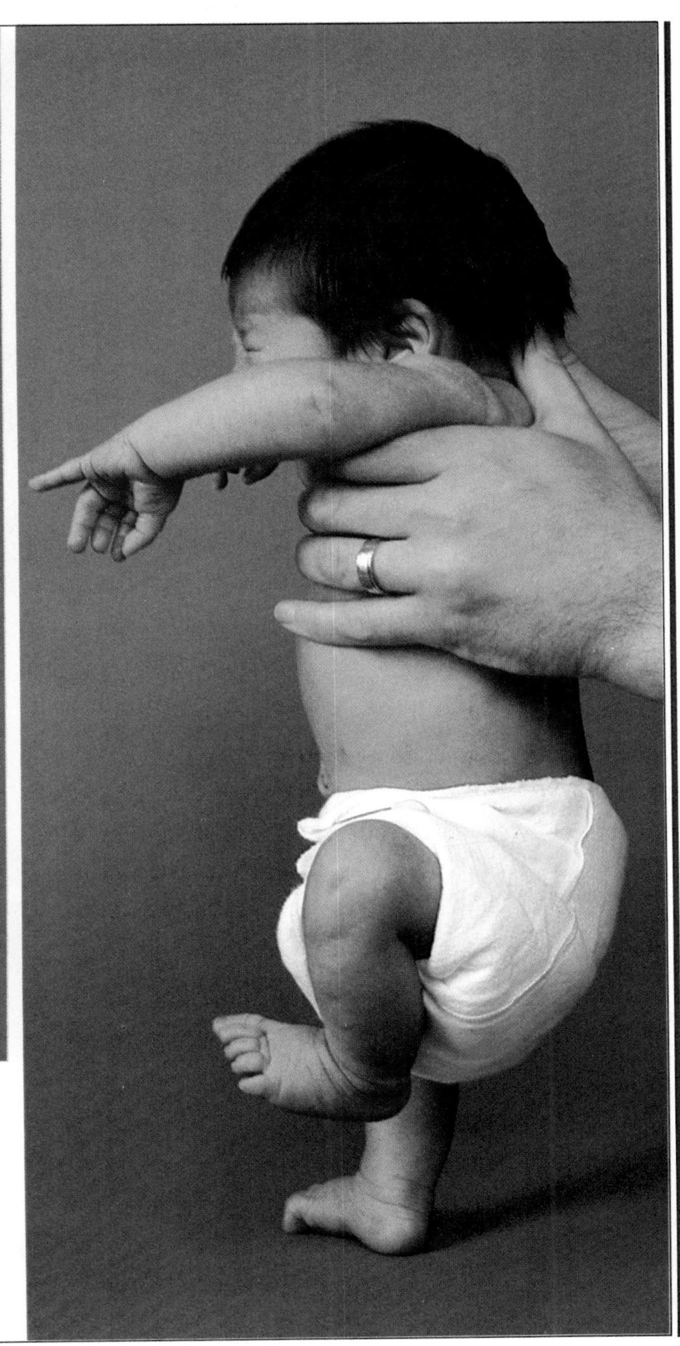

normal delivery is generally feasible for the next birth and is often given a trial.

On the other hand, doctors now often recommend cesareans to mothers who, in an earlier generation, might have attempted natural delivery. A cesarean section can be performed at a prearranged time, chosen for the convenience of both the mother and the doctor; a cesarean baby, delivered without the bruising pressures and risks of a difficult vaginal birth, is pink and perfect. With the development of fetal monitoring and other techniques that permit the early detection of potential birth problems, many physicians apparently prefer to schedule a cesarean in advance rather than chance a lengthy and stressful vaginal delivery.

With the growing popularity of cesarean sections for difficult births, the number of deliveries aided by forceps has been drastically reduced. In earlier days, these metal tongs were inserted deep into the birth canal to pull the baby out, and were used routinely in nearly half of all births; understandably, mothers dreaded them as instruments of torture. Today forceps figure in only 12 per cent of deliveries, and their use is limited to the final inches of the birth canal. Typically, they are employed when pain-relieving medication has interfered with the mother's own efforts to push the baby out, and even then their use is generally deferred until the baby's head is visible at the opening of the vagina. The doctor positions the halves of the forceps separately, sliding one and then the other into place around the infant's head, then links them together at the handle and gently eases the head through the opening.

The first days of a new life

Difficult deliveries impose an extra measure of fatigue upon the mother in the hours just after the birth, but even the smoothest birth leaves a new mother thoroughly exhausted. Well-meaning friends and relatives may bombard her with flowers and felicitations, but what she needs the most is rest. There will be ample opportunity for visiting later; this is the time for sleep, for quiet feeding periods with her son or daughter, for lessons in breast-feeding and care of the breasts if she so chooses.

The hospital stay provides time for the mother to rest, and skilled nurses will guide her first mothering efforts and explain the physical readjustments her body is undergoing. Some light bleeding will occur as the uterus sheds excess tissue from the area that supported the placenta; sanitary pads will be needed for a week or two. For a few days, many mothers may also experience afterpains similar to strong menstrual cramps. Other early discomforts include irritation from stitches if skin was cut in an episiotomy or torn in delivery. Constipation or hemorrhoids may occur as a related problem. If so, ask for help promptly; stool softener taken early can spare you an enema later on.

At birth the mother's breasts are filled with colostrum, a colorless fluid rich in protective antibodies. On the second or third day after childbirth, milk enters and swells the breasts, sometimes making them hard, hot and painful. If a mother has decided not to breast-feed, she may be given a support brassière, hormones to suppress milk build-up, and pain relievers, but her milk supply will soon dwindle for lack of demand. A breast-feeding mother, of course, will be relieved when her nursing baby eases the pressure of the milk; her engorged condition generally passes completely as her breasts soften and grow accustomed to their new role.

Meanwhile, during all these changes, the mother has been getting acquainted with the newborn. He may be somewhat unprepossessing at first—perhaps a bit pointy-headed, flat-nosed and mottled after the rough journey of birth—but he soon fills out and adapts to his new surroundings. The cartilage of the nose and soft bones of the skull regain their shape with surprising speed, and if the baby was born with downy hair on his body, it soon disappears on its own. Almost half of all newborns have a touch of jaundice, a disorder that yellows the skin and the whites of the eyes. The cause is simple and temporary: an immature liver, which fails to eliminate some of the wastes that accumulate as the infant switches over from the mother's placenta to his own breathing and digestion systems. Jaundice, too, usually clears up on its own; if necessary, the doctor can correct it by exposing the baby to fluorescent light that duplicates the effects of sunlight *(page 65)*.

For three out of four baby boys, there is the special discomfort of circumcision. In this quick surgery, performed at the option of the parents, the fold of skin that covers the head of the penis is snipped away. One of the oldest forms of surgery, circumcision figures in religious rites dating back thousands of years, but its effect is quite practical: It makes washing the penis easier and reduces the risk of infection in the area.

As she handles her baby, the new mother will notice inborn muscular and postural reflexes that all newborns have in common *(pages 61-63)*. But her most remarkable discovery is likely to be the individuality, the uniqueness of her child. Even in these early days, a distinct personality is in the making. One baby will thrash and howl, taking the world on as if it were a prize fight, while in the next bed or room a mild-mannered child peers peacefully into space with an infant's typically blurred sight, which distinguishes little more than light and vague shapes.

This initial get-acquainted period for parents and child will be delayed if a baby is born so prematurely or so ill that he must remain for a time in a special nursery under constant care. In most hospitals, the mother and father are welcome there, and are encouraged to touch and hold and help care for their child from time to time. But anxiety is inevitable. All parents, of course, want a perfect baby and dread the small chance that their newborn may be seriously flawed. They should know that the odds favoring the baby's ultimate health improve every year.

Fewer than 3 per cent of all babies are born with defects, and half of those defects are minor or can be readily corrected. If the baby's lungs are not fully developed, they may require immediate help from a resuscitation machine called a respirator. Congenital heart problems demand attention and sometimes delicate surgery. Bone fractures can occur in difficult births, but they heal rapidly. One common problem is the release of the baby's intestinal waste matter, called meconium, into the womb before birth. Because meconium can choke or sicken a newborn, the nursing staff will monitor with care the first hours of those babies affected.

If your baby is kept apart from you during this early period, it can be helpful to know that the emergency is usually brief. If any physical problem is present, the first few hours of a baby's life are generally the most difficult. They contain the hurdle of transition—the massive change from life in the womb to a life of breathing air, digesting food, and circulating nutrients throughout the body. Most babies who make it through the first day do well thereafter.

The mother, too, has undergone a dramatic metamorphosis in the space of a few days. She arrived at the hospital in the temporary condition of a pregnant woman; she leaves it with the permanent status of parent. Throughout the hospital experience, her most constant support has come from a nurse. It is the nurse who holds her hand during the hardest moments in labor, who helps unravel the first mysteries of child care, who reassures her when post-partum tears well up for no apparent reason. By the time she arrives home, the mother has had a sort of cram course in modern nursing techniques—the array of regimens and emergency measures that sustain a helpless, vulnerable human being. Now she begins to understand, in a new and different way, why a baby's room is called a nursery. Practically overnight, she has become her child's nurse. ❋

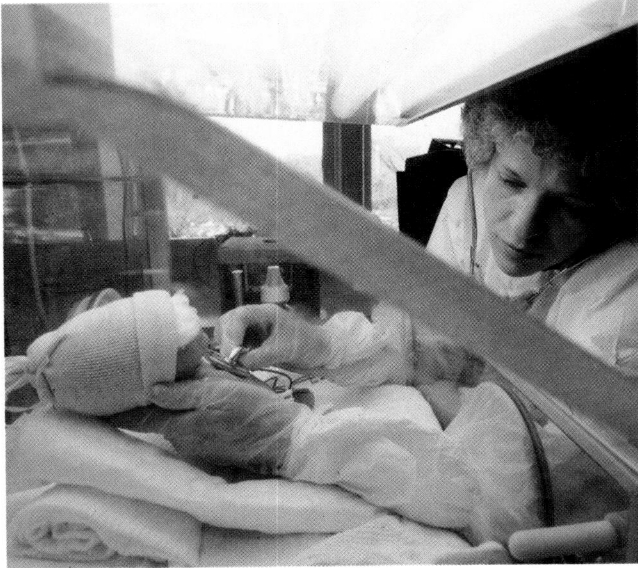

A nurse checks the heartbeat of an incubator baby undergoing treatment for jaundice—a yellowish discoloration of the skin and whites of the eyes that affects about half of all newborns and is caused by the failure of the liver to remove excess amounts of a pigment called bilirubin. A blindfold protects the infant's eyes from the glare of the fluorescent lights that correct the jaundice.

A tumultuous launch into life

For a mother, the moment of birth brings an arduous labor to a joyous end. For the baby, it is the beginning of another kind of labor—the struggle to sustain life outside the haven of the womb. Severed from the umbilical lifeline that linked his body to his mother's, the newborn suddenly switches over to his own tiny systems. Like stubborn balloons being blown up for the first time, the air sacs in his lungs expand and fill with his first breaths of air. His heart takes on the full job of pumping blood to all the tissues of his body. Within hours, for the first time, he will digest food to get the nourishment once delivered automatically from his mother's bloodstream.

A baby born in a modern hospital has help in plenty for this critical switchover. When he emerges from the birth canal, he becomes the object of the most intense five-minute barrage of care and attention he may ever receive. An obstetrician and nurses ease his breathing, protect him against disease, and assess his heartbeat, color, muscular reflexes and other vital signs, searching for subtle abnormalities that demand quick action. Backed up by equipment that can duplicate almost every bodily function, the team is ready for an unexpected emergency as well as the usual trouble-free birth.

The first day in the life of Brian Richard Becker, chronicled here and on the following pages, began with a not-quite-normal delivery; it was brought to a normal, healthy ending by a good doctor in an up-to-date facility—Fairfax Hospital in Falls Church, Virginia. Brian's parents, Fran and Rich Becker, had taken prepared-childbirth classes and also had the benefit of prior experience with their first child, Jenny, two and a half years old. Brian was exceptionally heavy—10 pounds 2 ounces—but the delivery was swift and drug-free.

His arrival, however, was preceded by a potentially dangerous event. During labor, he released his first bowel movement, called meconium, into the amniotic fluid cushioning him in the womb. If a newborn breathes this sticky waste into his lungs, he may get pneumonia. Therefore, the obstetrician began clearing fluid from Brian's nose and mouth as soon as the baby's head emerged from the birth canal; he also placed the baby under observation in the hospital nursery instead of having him join his parents right away.

Unlike Jenny, who nursed at Fran Becker's breast on the delivery table, Brian waited more than five hours for his first breast feeding. They were anxious hours, but the baby suffered no harm from the meconium. Equally important, he recovered beautifully from the first—and perhaps the greatest—trauma of his life: leaving the warm, dark, quiet, soft sanctuary of his mother's body for a world that is cold, dazzlingly bright, noisy and hard.

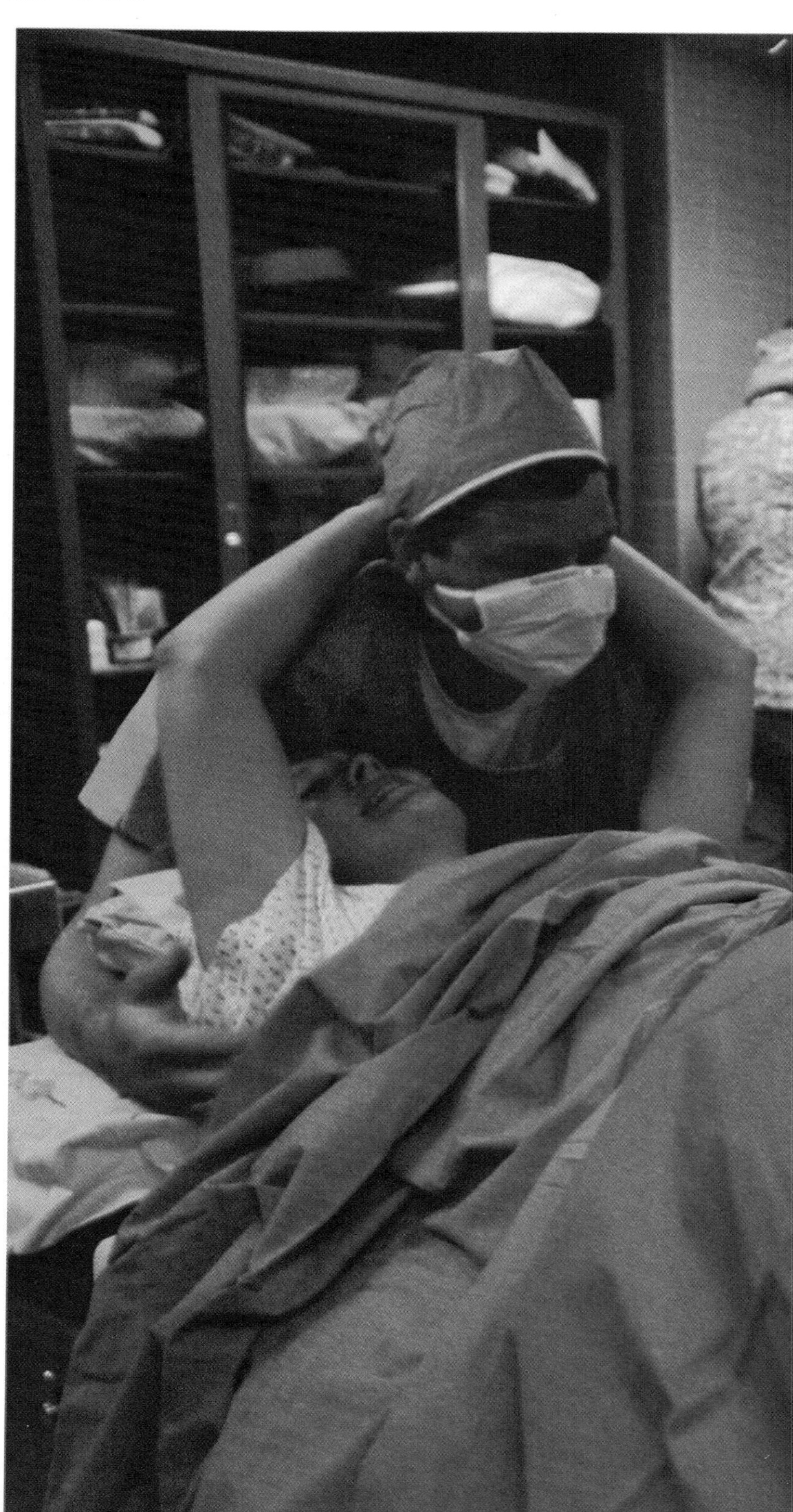

PHOTOGRAPHS BY LINDA BARTLETT

With a staff pediatrician standing by, the obstetrician suctions fluid from newborn Brian Becker's nose, using a plastic tube fitted with a trap to catch fluids. Watching at left, father Rich Becker is still in the position he used to brace his wife for the last hard push of the delivery. Two nurses (rear) prepare to receive the infant in a special warming area of the delivery room.

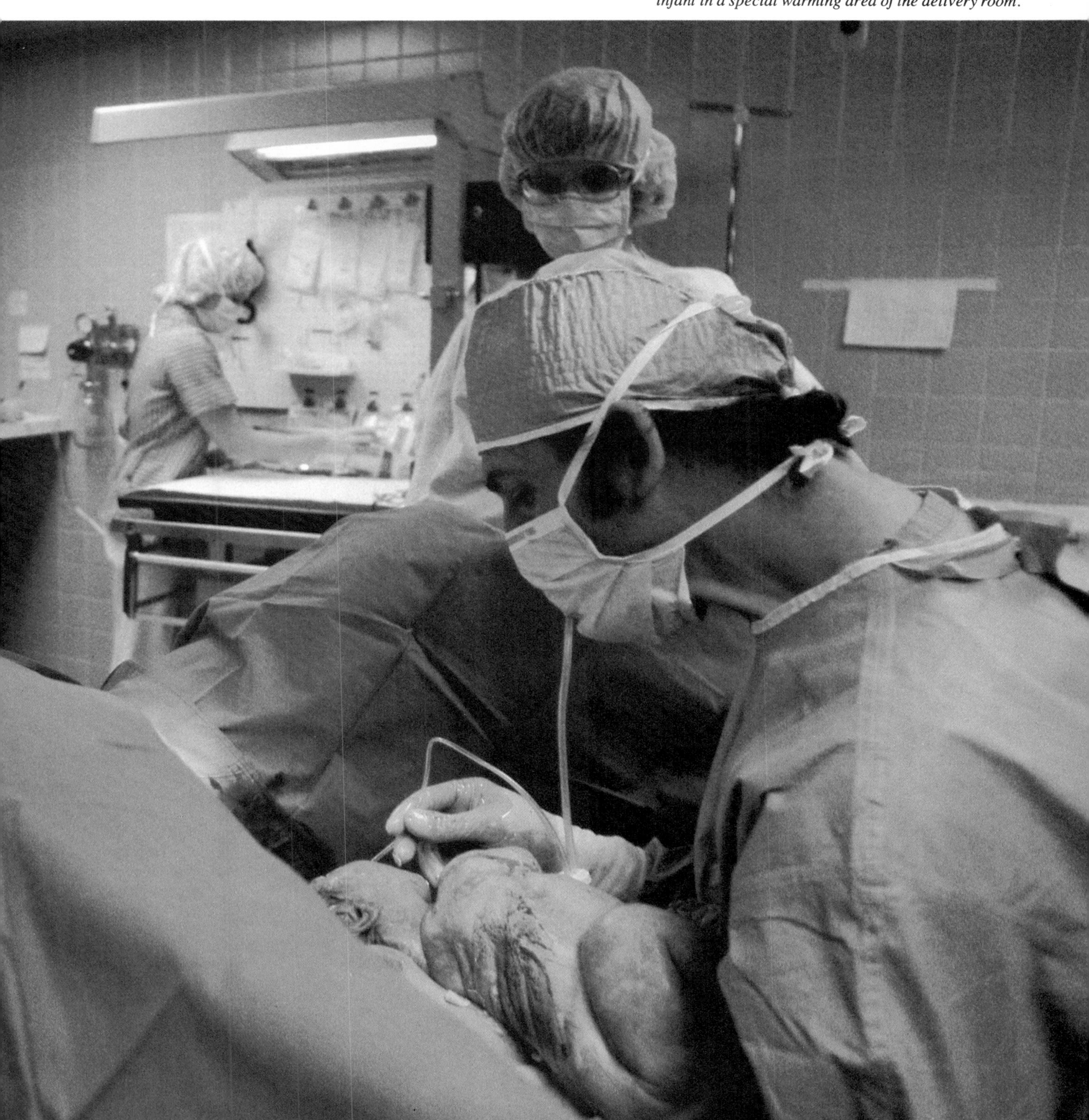

The first tests—and a report card

Upon emerging from the moist, warm womb into a dry, air-conditioned delivery room, Brian Becker was set under a heat lamp that maintained his temperature at around 98° F. Nurses dried his body, then immediately began to check his condition. Like most hospitals, Fairfax evaluates every baby at one minute and again at five minutes after birth, using a five-item checklist called the Apgar Scoring System. Heart rate, breathing, muscle tone, muscular reflexes and skin color (typically blue at birth, but soon changing to a rosy pink) are each rated at zero, one or two points, against a maximum possible score of 10.

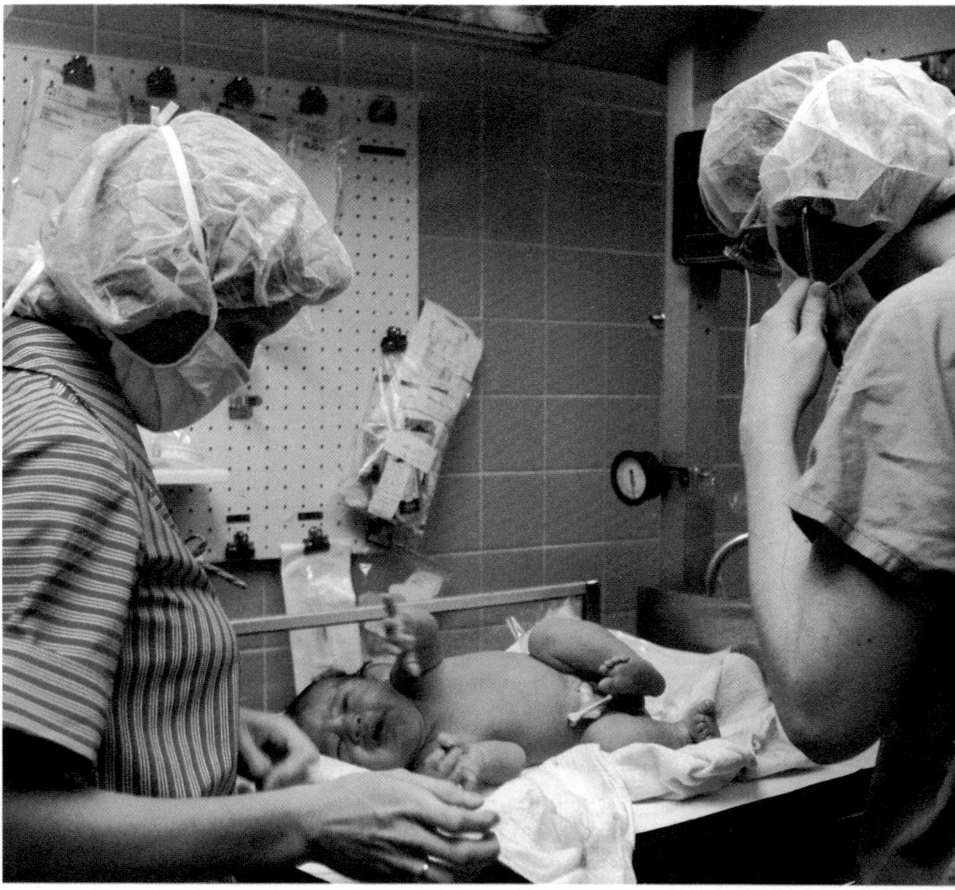

The hospital pediatrician dons a stethoscope so she can check Brian's heartbeat for an Apgar evaluation. At five minutes of age, he scored a healthy nine on the scale of 10, losing one point for a lingering blueness in his head, hands and feet. The condition cleared up in a few hours.

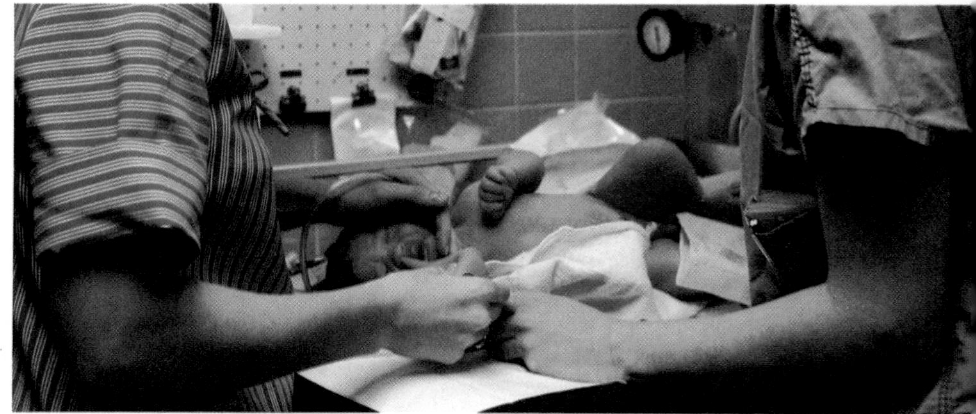

Using a blue suction bulb, a nurse removes mucus and amniotic fluid that can clog the baby's nose and hinder breathing. Brian's grimace is a healthy reaction to the pressure of the bulb; his flexed knees and clenched fists indicate good muscle tone.

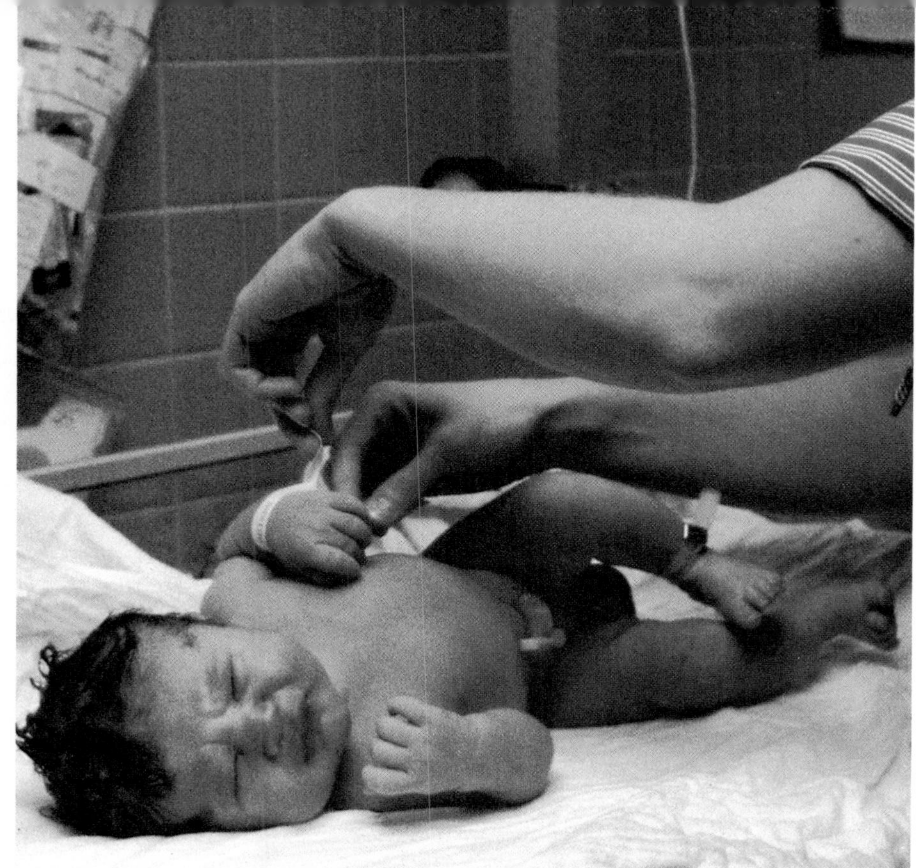

The nurse fits Brian's ankle and wrist with plastic bands bearing an identification number; the same number is imprinted on a bracelet that Fran Becker will wear. To prevent mix-ups, a nursery attendant double-checks the matching numbers each time babies are taken to their mothers.

Moments after the Apgar test, Fran and Rich Becker embrace their son and each other. Both parents were filled with what Fran called ''total joy, total relief'' that Brian had come through the delivery without harm. For this first meeting, the baby was kept warm in a blanket and a cap.

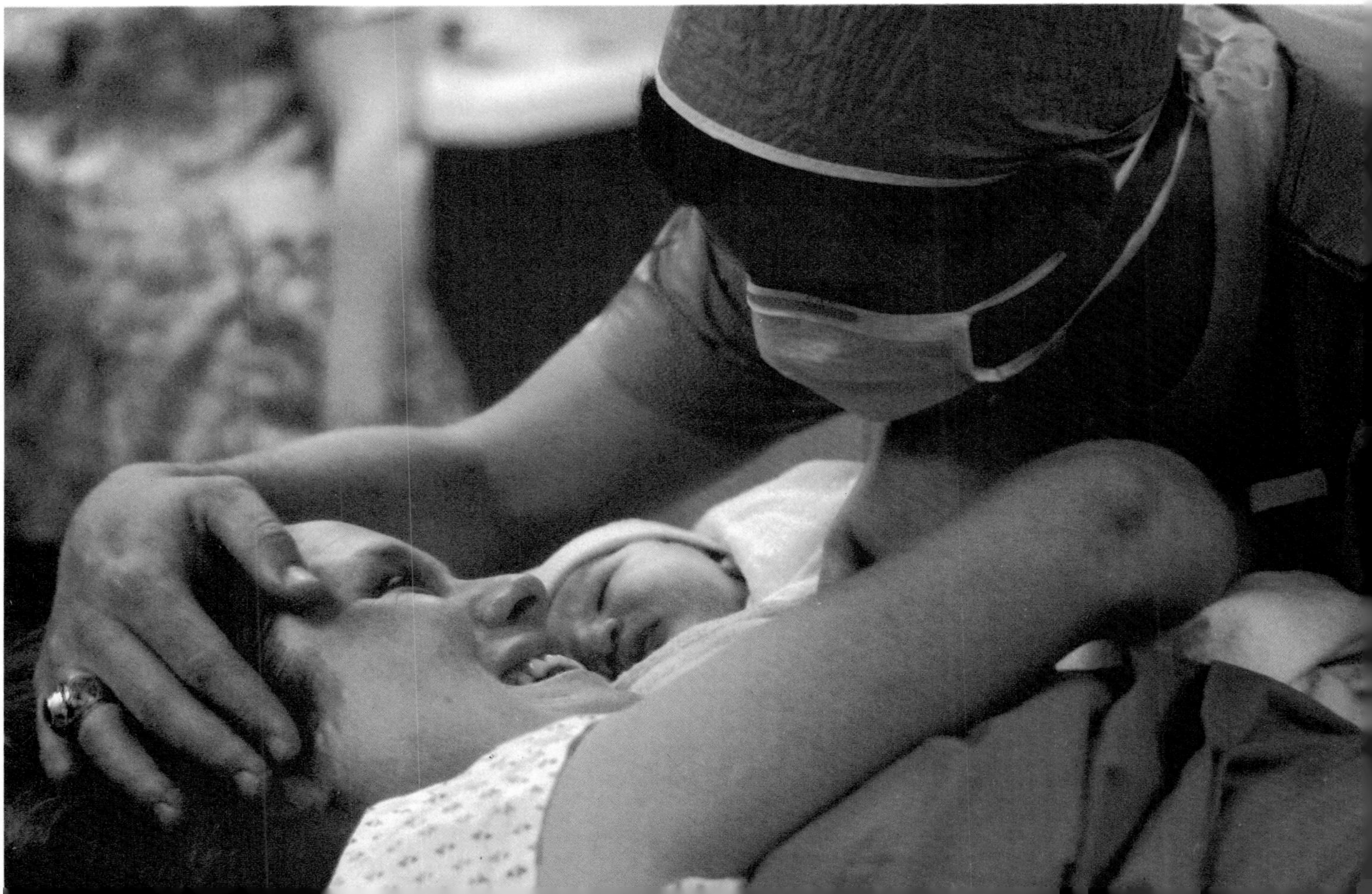

Hours of special care

In the hospital's nursery for the newborn, Brian passed through another crucial transition from the womb to the world. Like a new engine that sputters at the start, an infant needs time to stabilize heartbeat and breathing, and to recover body heat lost at birth. Infants cannot warm themselves by shivering or curling up in a ball; in the nursery, they lie in portable cribs that can be rolled beneath heat lamps. Nothing is taken for granted: Nurses note every physical function, from crying to bowel movements. Routine health measures taken at this point include a shot of vitamin K to prevent bleeding, and silver nitrate eye drops to guard against infection.

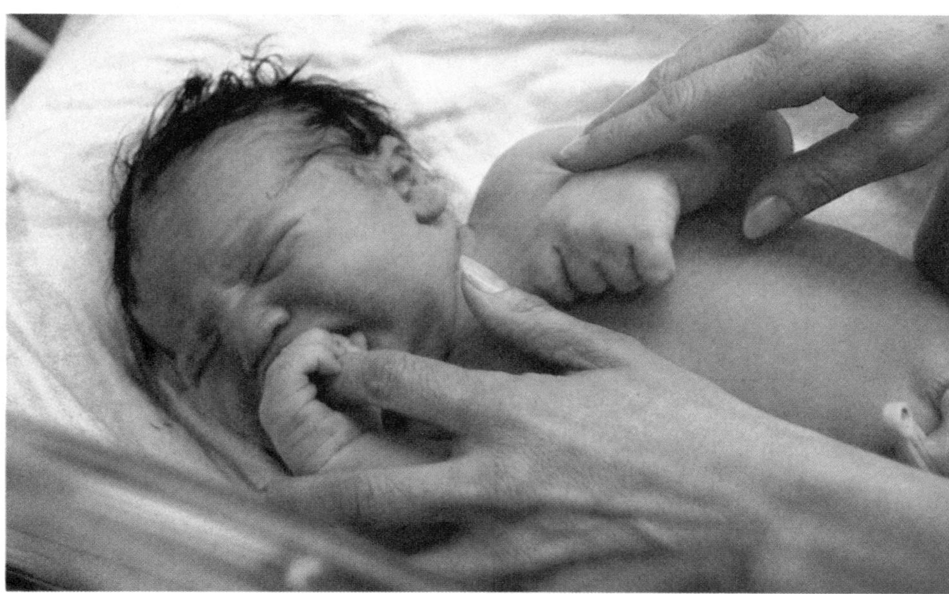

A nurse gently inserts a fingertip into Brian's mouth to check his sucking reflex and tell whether his palate is completely formed. Both reflex and palate were fine.

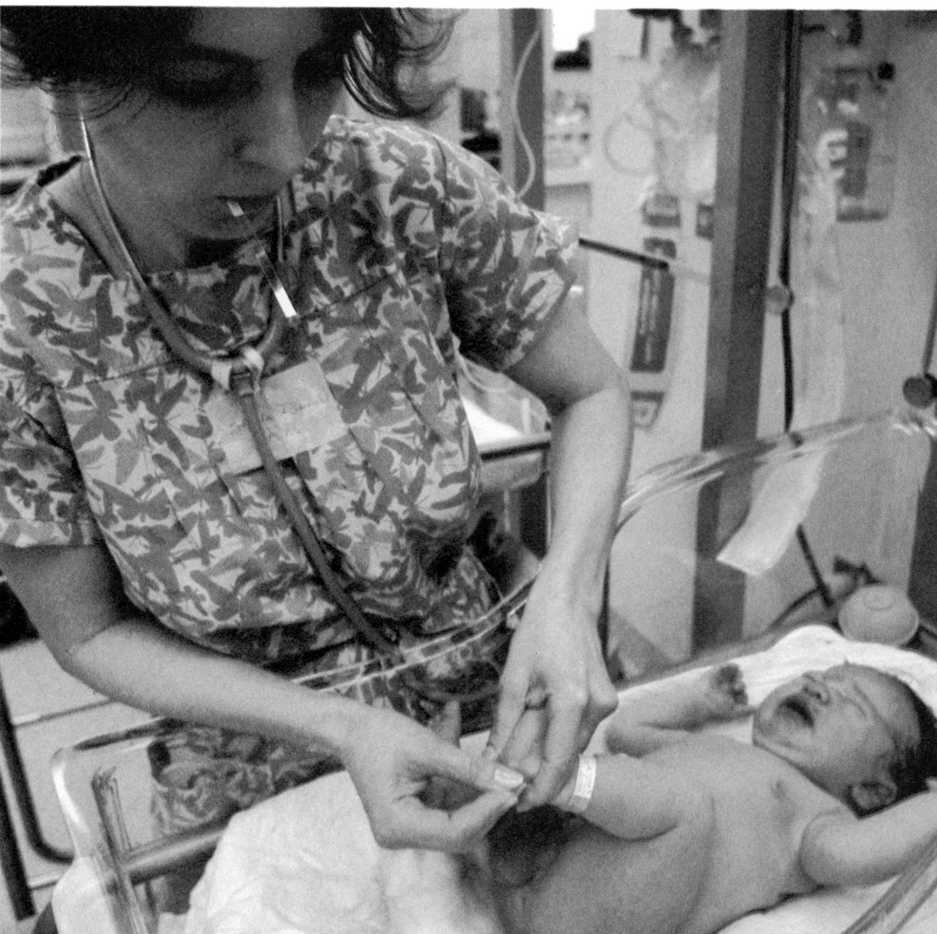

Brian howls as a nurse pricks his heel to bring a drop of blood to the skin. The plastic stick held ready in her mouth is coated with a compound that, when touched to the blood, turns blue in proportion to the level of blood sugar—the higher the level, the darker the color. Low blood sugar indicates a need for immediate feeding.

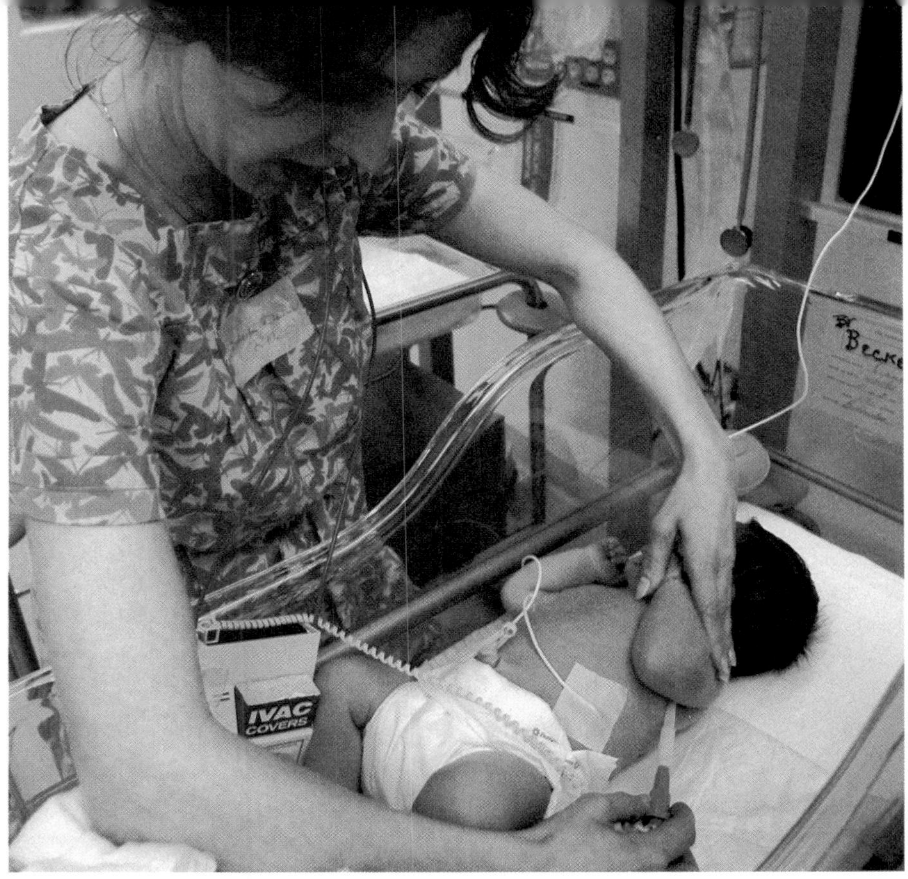

The nurse takes Brian's temperature with an electronic thermometer; she will take hourly readings until his temperature is stable. The wire taped to Brian's side is a sensor for the warmer over his crib. In effect, it lets the baby serve as his own thermostat: When his skin temperature drops below 98° F., the heat lamp goes on.

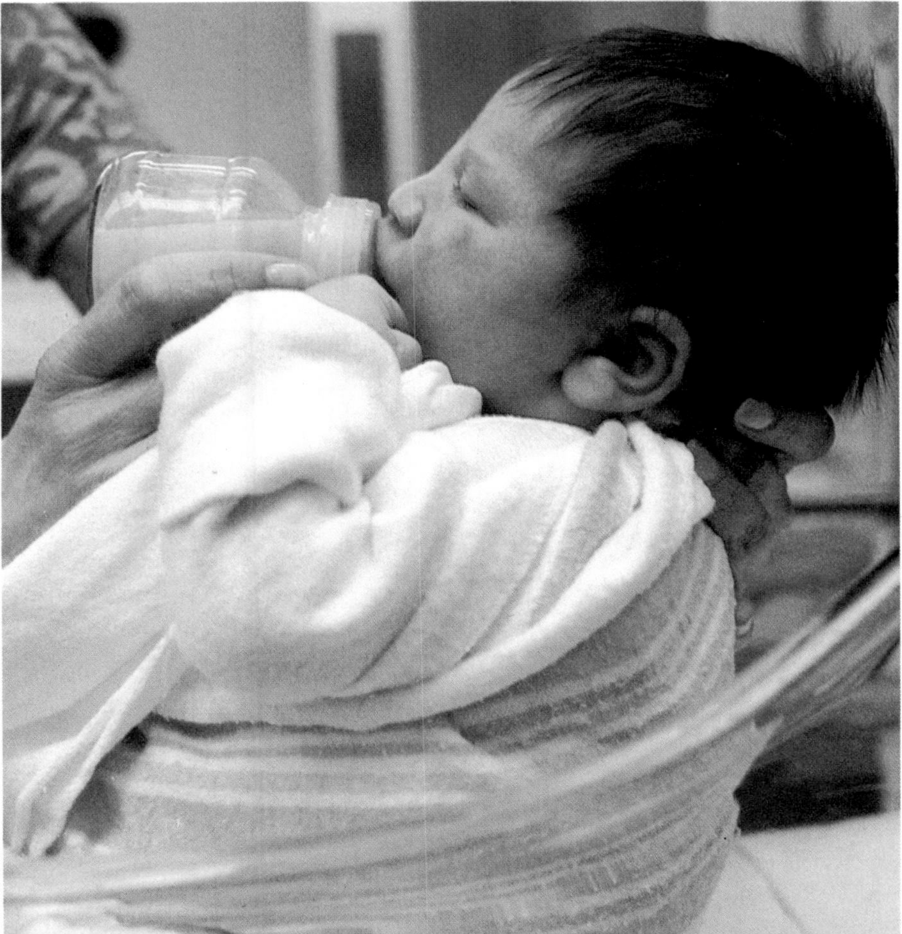

Bathed, dressed and wrapped in a blanket, Brian enjoys his first bottle in the nursery. With his breathing, heartbeat and temperature stable, he can now move into his mother's room for breast feeding.

A time for getting acquainted

Just as Brian's physical condition was monitored and sustained in the nursery, vital emotional needs were met during his first contacts with his mother. Many hospitals now permit babies to stay in their mothers' rooms for extended periods during the day, and Fran Becker took full advantage of the opportunity. Except for the hospital's regular visiting hours, when the risk of infection was high, she kept Brian with her from nine in the morning until nine at night.

For her, as for all other mothers of newborns, these hours transformed the hospital stay into a time when mother and baby get accustomed to each other, free from the distractions of family, friends and the regular household routine. For a first-time mother, particularly, this experience in the hospital, supplemented by guidance from the nursing staff, provides a chance to master the mysteries of a baby's feeding, crying, burping and sleeping patterns.

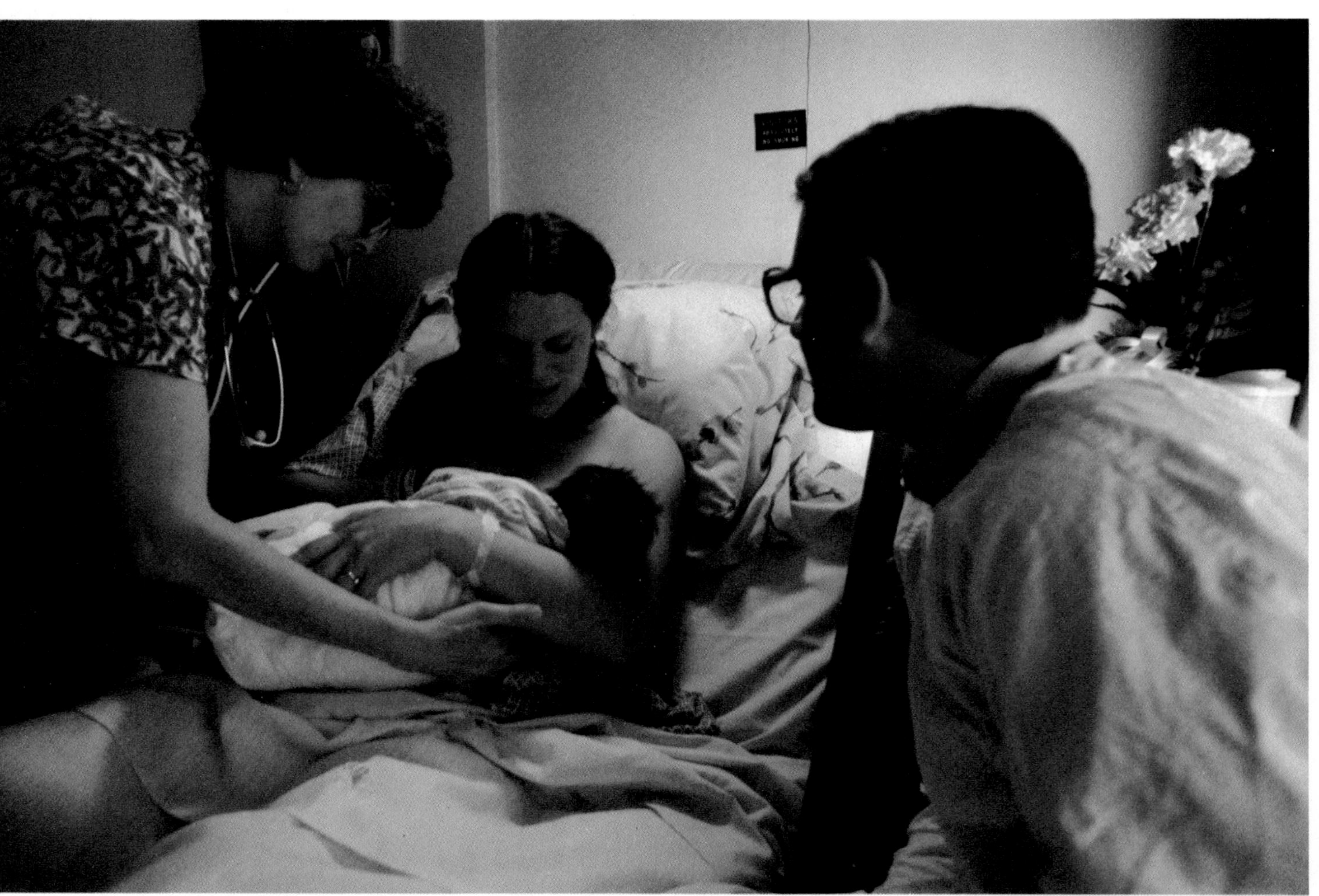

Five hours after Brian's birth, a nurse helps position him for his first breast feeding, while Rich Becker, dressed in a sterile hospital gown, lends moral support from the sidelines. This special moment in a breast-fed infant's life usually takes place within the first half hour after birth; it was delayed in Brian's case because of the time he spent under observation in the nursery.

Fran and Brian settle into their own nursing schedule—one benefit of the rooming-in plan that let Brian stay with Fran all day. For the first 48 hours, a mother's breasts produce colostrum, a fluid that precedes true milk.

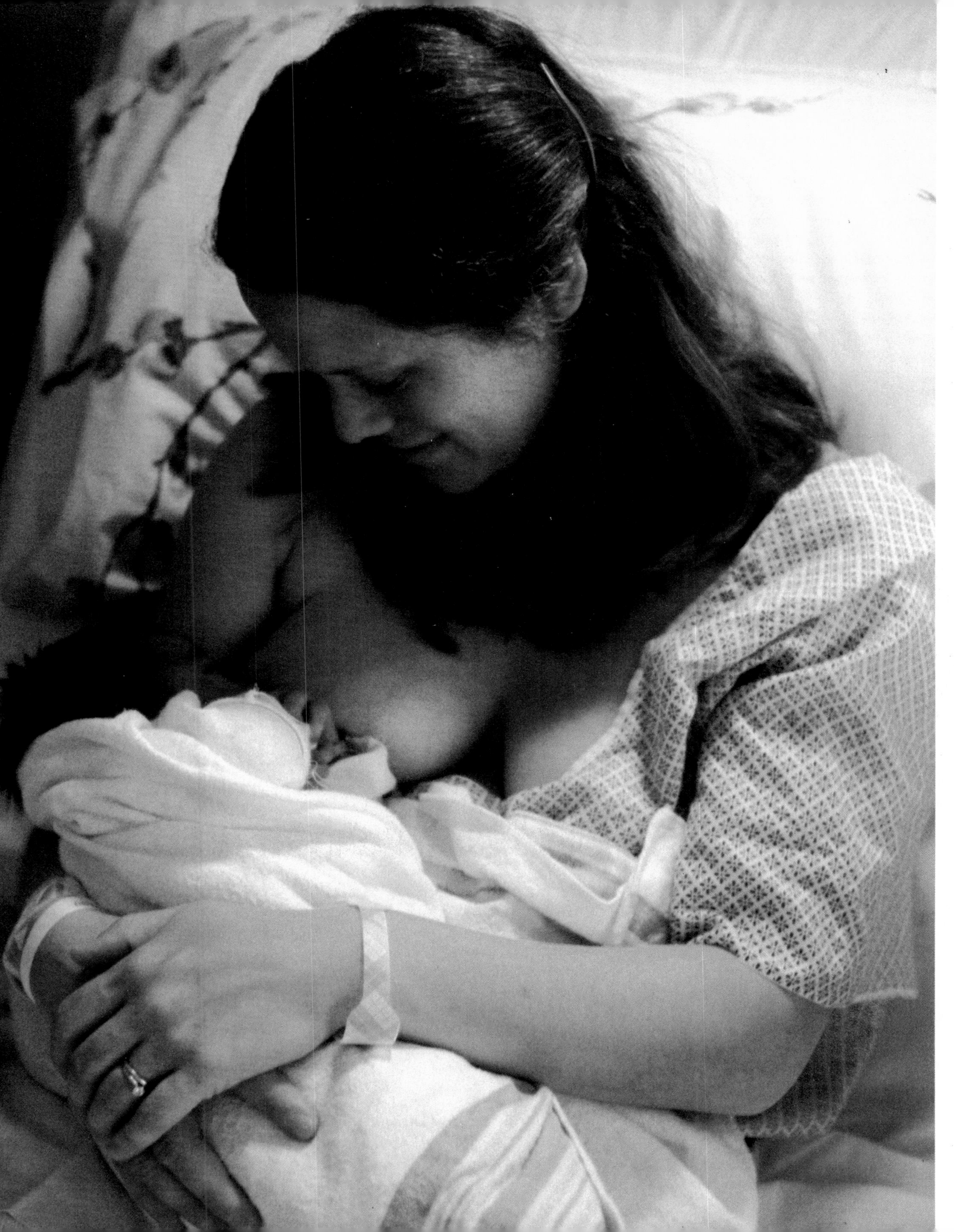

The final tests: making sure that all systems are "go"

At some point during the hospital stay, a pediatrician, generally chosen by the parents, gives the newborn a full physical examination. This assessment rarely uncovers a congenital defect or birth injury not already detected by the hospital staff; the doctor's main concern is to check over the infant's fledgling systems and senses for smooth, trouble-free operation.

The pediatrician's tests are simple but revealing. As the examination gets under way, for example, he will welcome and even provoke a loud, vigorous yell as a sign that the infant is expanding his lungs properly. By the baby's reaction to new postures and positions, the doctor can evaluate reflexes, alertness and muscle tone. Bones and joints, still flexible and relatively soft, are tested for proper alignment; loose or dislocated hip joints, a common problem at birth, may be corrected by simply triple-diapering the infant to fix his hips at the correct angle.

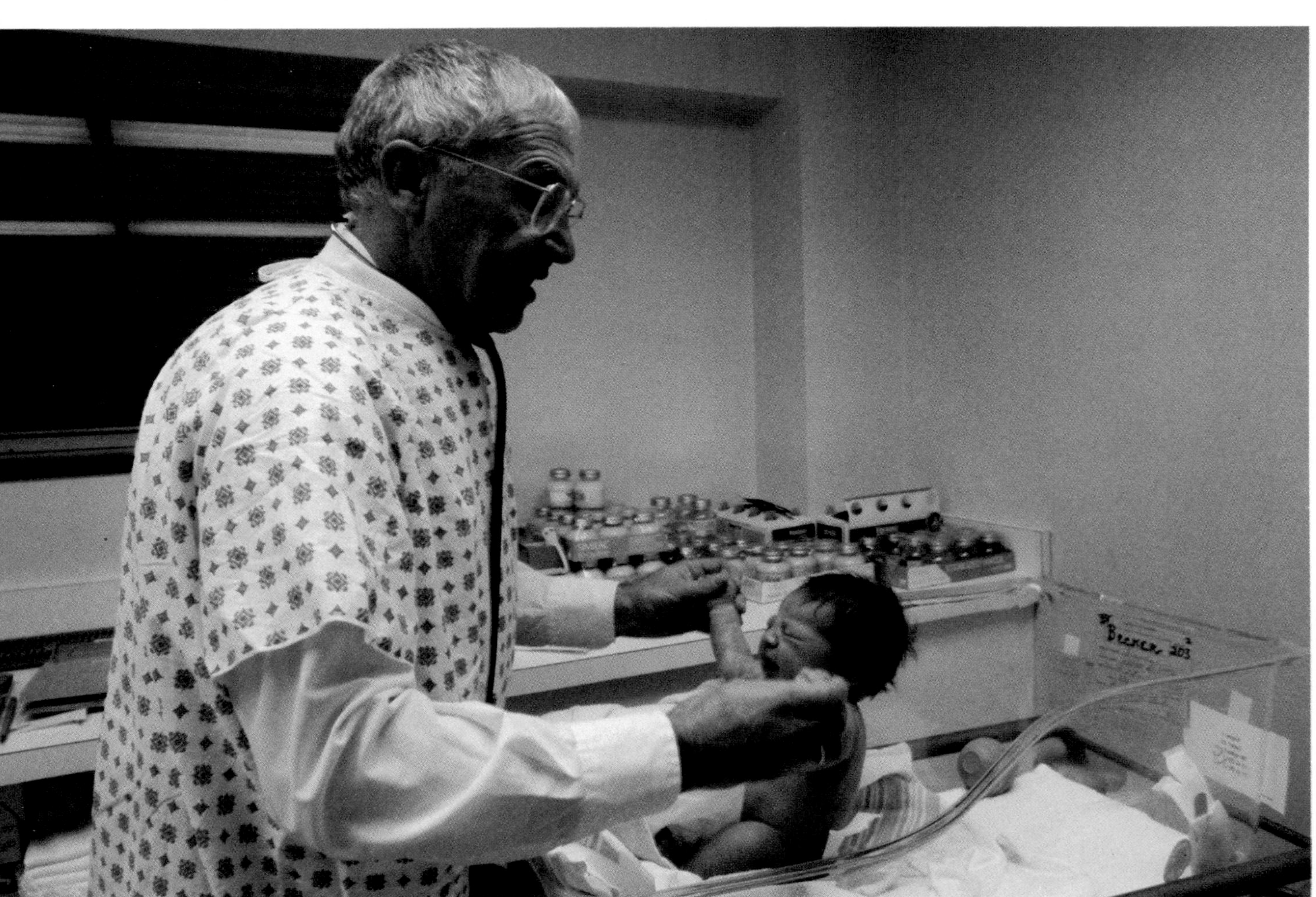

The pediatrician begins Brian's checkup by pulling the infant to a sitting position. This maneuver tests nerve response and muscle tone; it will also reveal any damage to the collarbone suffered during delivery, a special danger for large babies. Throughout the test Brian's tiny fingers tightly grasped the doctor's thumbs, in one of the reflexes common to newborns (pages 61-63).

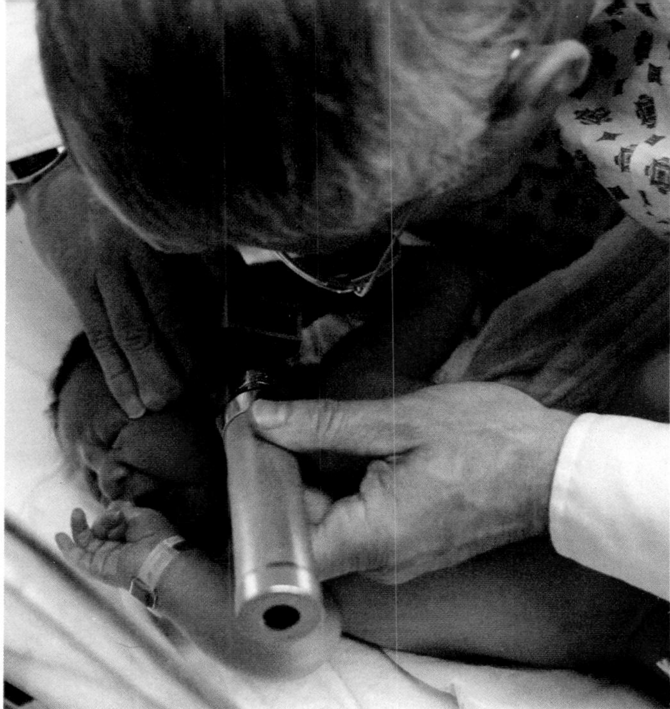

Using an otoscope, which combines a tightly focused flashlight with magnifying lenses, the doctor peers into Brian's ear, checking for a clear ear canal and an intact eardrum.

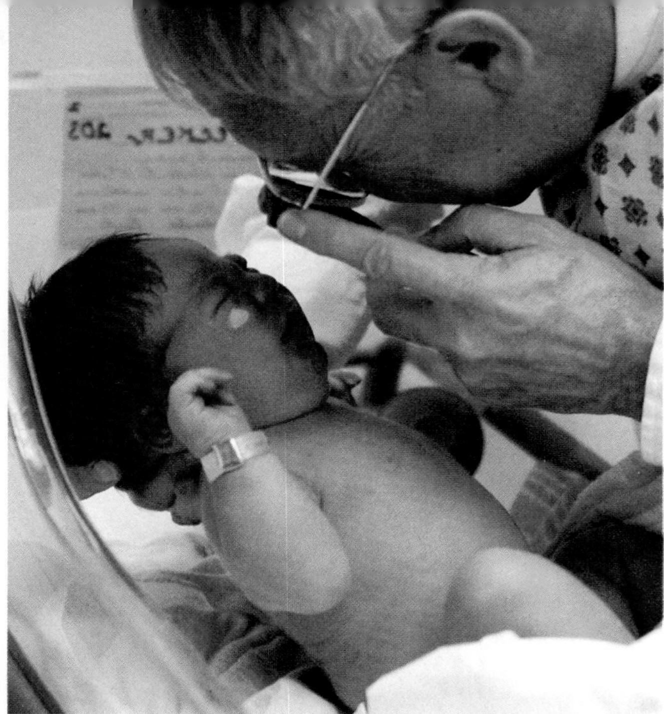

Brian squeezes his eyelids shut, thwarting the doctor's first attempt to examine the interior of his eyes with an ophthalmoscope. The test was made successfully on a later visit.

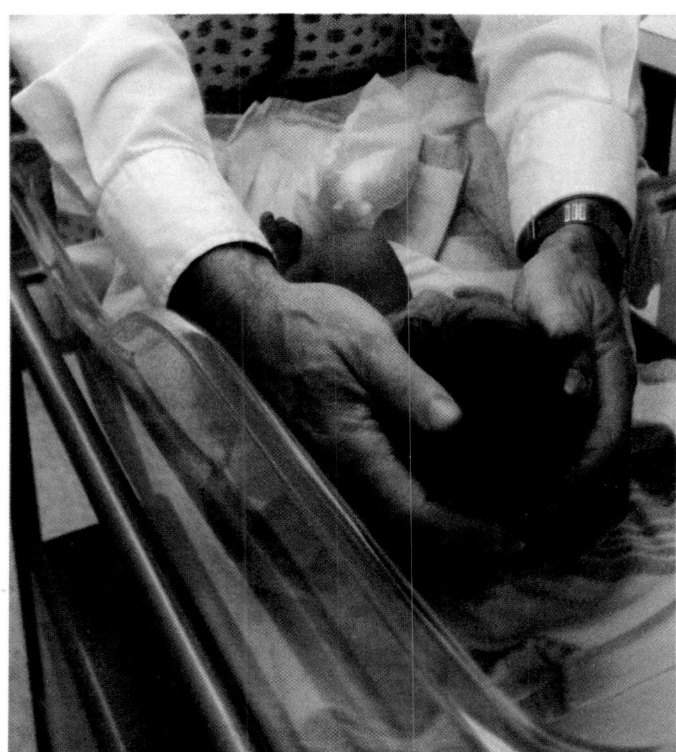

The doctor feels for Brian's "soft spots"—two gaps between a newborn's skull bones, covered only by membrane, skin and hair. The gaps remain for up to two years to allow for brain growth.

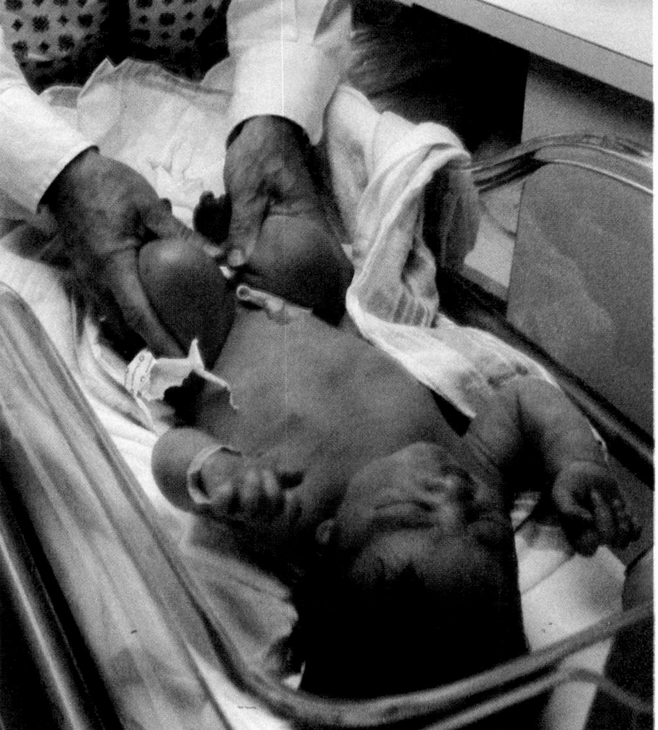

To check the vulnerable hip joints, the doctor gently flexes and turns Brian's knees while watching the angles of the joints. A telltale click would indicate a dislocation.

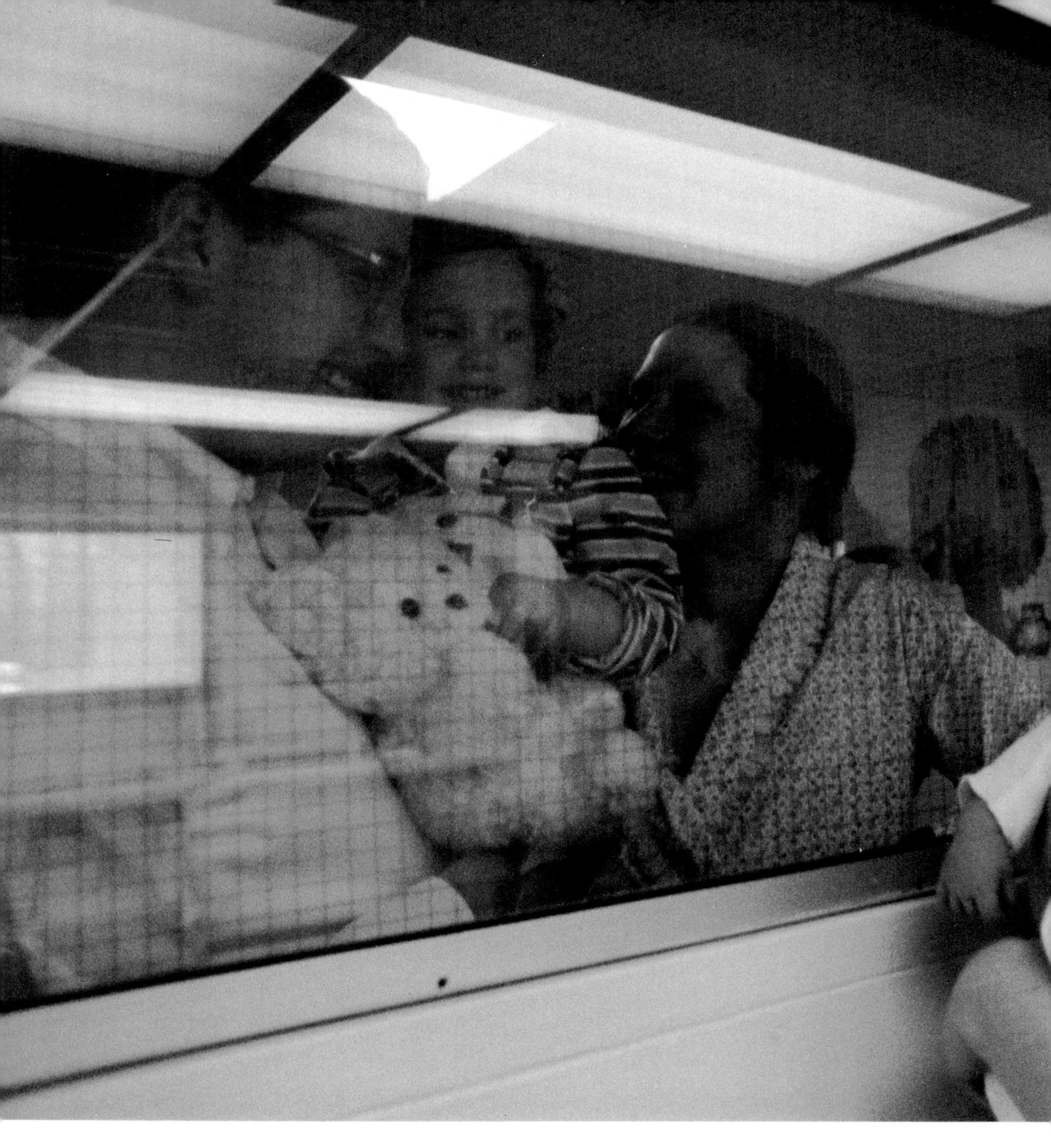

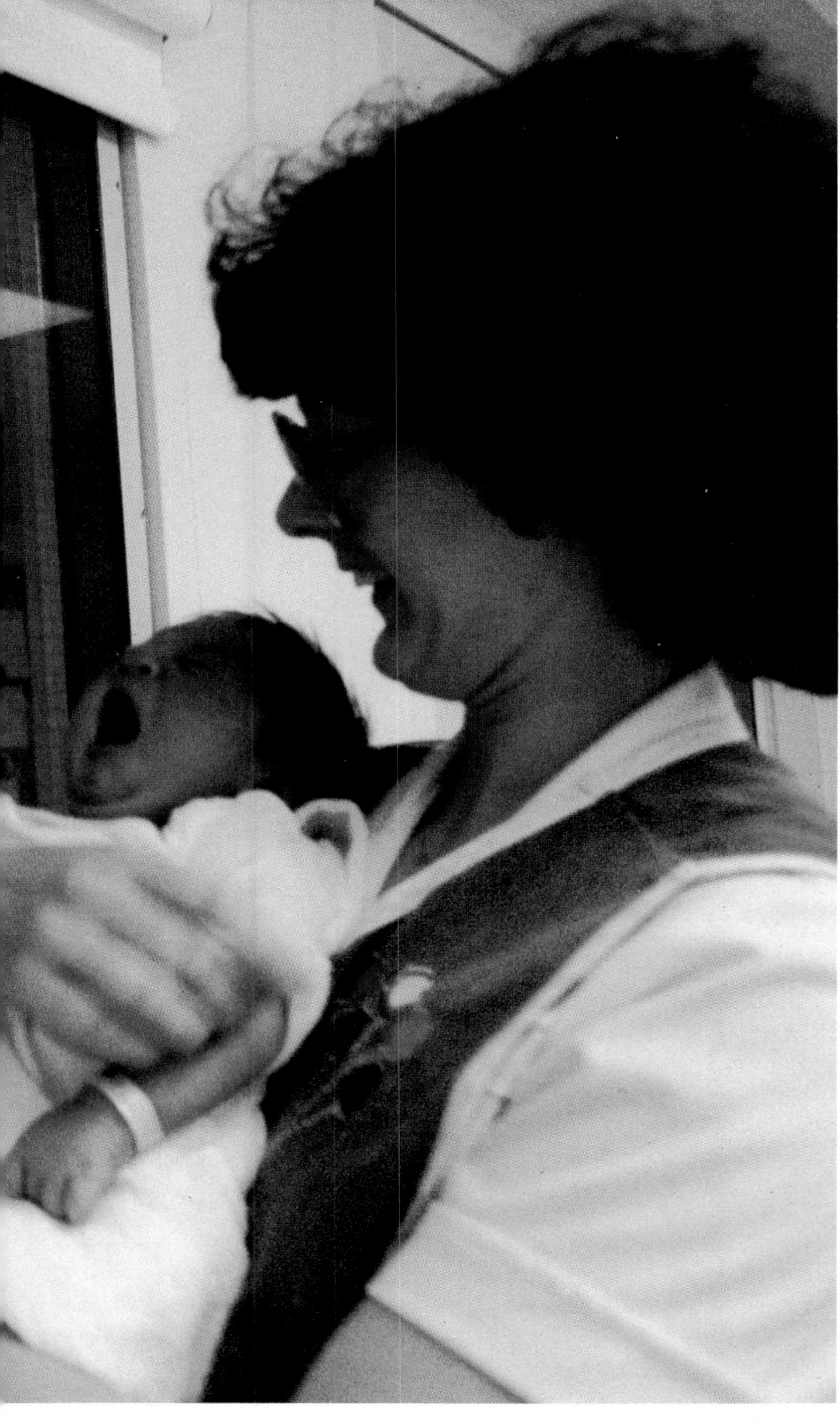

After months of anticipation, Jenny Becker gets her first glimpse of her brother, who greets her with a giant yawn. Elevated overnight to the status of big sister, she brought Brian a huge stuffed animal that she herself had chosen as a gift; her parents, in turn, gave Jenny a toy camera as Brian's gift to her. Still separated here by the glass nursery window, the Becker family was finally united at home the next day.

CHAPTER 4

Nurture for the first year of life

Beating the baby blues
Breast-feeding versus bottle-feeding
The switch to solid foods
Fitting the baby into the family
A newborn's store of knowledge
The pediatrician's well-baby care

With a newborn's arrival the excited anticipation of pregnancy and the drama of birth fade away, replaced by another kind of excitement and drama. During the next 12 months, the baby will change more radically than at any other time in his life. From a helpless alien with weak limbs and an overlarge head, emitting bewildered cries, he will be transformed into an active member of the family, who can walk a little, feed himself after a fashion, and even utter a few sociable words.

During the first weeks, these enormous changes seem impossibly remote. "I was terrified," recalled Florida journalist Madeleine Blais, of her first day at home with her son. "I remember wishing more than anything that this baby were a little older, a little less needy: three, four years old, wearing overalls, eating some cookies and asking in clear comprehensible English if he might also have some juice please."

Obviously, the responsibility of shepherding a new human being through the first jam-packed months of development is formidable. Babies depend totally on their parents for every need: food, shelter, even simple mobility. But infants are far tougher than their dependence and apparent fragility imply; they arrive equipped with potent survival mechanisms that make them physically and psychologically resilient.

Typically, it is the new parents, particularly the mother, who are unsettled or even shocked by the reality of living with an infant. Still weak from delivery, a mother suddenly finds herself alone with a demanding stranger in the house. During the first few weeks at home with a new baby, many women are subject to unaccountable mood swings, frequent tears and a feeling of exhausted despair. "There's just no escape," said one mother, of her first few weeks at home with a new daughter. "Things that ordinarily wouldn't bother you—like a dog barking—suddenly assume enormous proportions. I sometimes found myself wishing that God would just reach down from the sky and pluck me away."

The technical term for these symptoms is post-partum depression; the colloquial, more expressive name is "the after-baby blues." In part, they are due to physical changes that occur in the mother after delivery. Blood volume drops by 30 per cent, hormone levels change dramatically, lacerations or incisions are healing. Internal organs forced out of place by the growing fetus shift back into position. And the uterus shrinks from a two-pound mass of muscle to a normal two or three ounces, in a process that takes from five to six weeks and is often accompanied at first by cramps called afterpains.

These physical adjustments are complicated by emotions that can affect both parents: feelings of anticlimax following the birth, anxieties about caring for the baby and even fears about strains on the marriage. Also present is a more-or-less steady state of fatigue that is probably the most distressing aspect of the after-baby blues. "Pure exhaustion," says Elizabeth Whelan of the American Council on Science and Health, "is the primary factor in post-partum depression."

Exhaustion is an inevitable result of coping with the round-the-clock demands of a new baby; the best way to minimize its effects is to cut down on extra work. "Just let the house go," advises one mother. "You can clean it later." Visitors

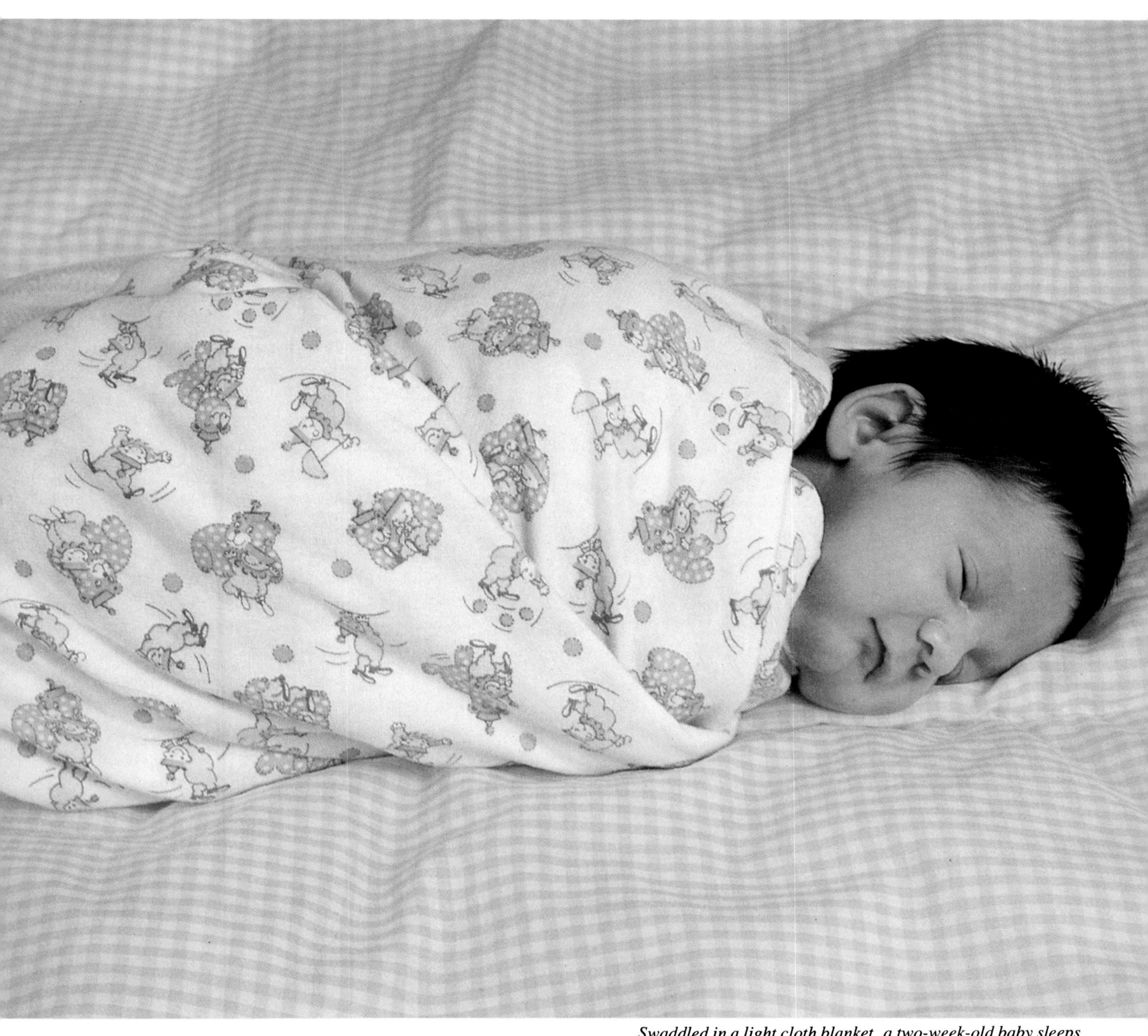

Swaddled in a light cloth blanket, a two-week-old baby sleeps peacefully. Swaddling restrains the limbs and inhibits reflex jerking movements that might otherwise disturb the infant's rest; it also gives a sense of warmth and physical contact that is especially soothing during the first month of life.

who do not take on some of the housework or attend to other children can be fatiguing. A common strategy for many new mothers is to turn off the phone and let the world go by for the first few weeks. "Everyone wants to see the new baby," commented one mother. "But you have to accept the fact that you're just not up to snuff."

Beating the baby blues

To lessen the risks of physical complications due to fatigue, Dr. Alan Guttmacher of New York City's Mount Sinai Medical School laid out a timetable for getting back into a normal routine. Among his recommendations are:

- Bathe or shower at least once a day. Warm, shallow baths ease the discomfort of hemorrhoids and, by stimulating circulation in the area of an episiotomy, help it to heal.
- For the first three to four days, try to avoid stairs; if possible, climb no more than one flight a day. Rest in bed for most of the afternoon, and take a two-hour nap.
- At four days, reduce the afternoon rest period to two hours, begin climbing stairs again and exercise lightly with five- to ten-minute walks.
- After 10 days, resume light housework and going out to dinner or the movies.
- Wait two weeks before doing heavy housework, three weeks before driving a car or marketing.

Thanks to antibiotics and sterile delivery practices, post-partum infections of the reproductive tract are now rare, but they do occur. Symptoms include a temperature of 100.4° F. or more for two days after delivery, chills, headache and loss of appetite; any of these signs should be discussed with a doctor. Breast infections, indicated by tender, hard, reddish areas over part of a breast, sometimes arise after delivery, and also call for immediate professional attention.

To reduce the danger of infection, doctors advise against using tampons until at least two weeks after delivery, or douching before the post-partum examination, generally scheduled for six weeks after the birth. For the same reason, many doctors advise against resuming sexual intercourse before the post-partum checkup.

But psychological as well as physical factors may affect a couple's sexual relationship after the birth of a child. Women often find that anxiety about the baby and insecurity about their changed appearance drastically diminish sexual interest. Fathers, too, are often confused by their wives' new role or seemingly altered personality. Psychologists find that such common stresses can persist for several months. They counsel couples to talk openly about their feelings and allow time for gradual readjustment.

No matter how soon a couple resumes sexual intercourse, they must use birth control. Although it generally takes about six weeks for a woman's reproductive tract to return to normal, she may ovulate several weeks sooner. Breast-feeding mothers are somewhat less likely to conceive than those who bottle-feed, but the notion that a woman cannot conceive while she is nursing a child is a very dangerous one. Though it may be from two to 18 months (five is average) before a nursing mother menstruates, she may be ovulating regularly all along; the absence of menstrual flow may be due to changes in the body's chemistry.

The choice of a contraceptive may be limited during the first month or so. Condoms are acceptable. A diaphragm must be refitted, generally about six weeks after delivery, and most doctors will wait at least six weeks before inserting an intrauterine device. Every mother should consult a doctor before resuming the use of oral contraceptives, and nursing mothers should wait until their milk is well established, because the synthetic hormones in birth-control pills can interfere with milk production. Even then, the Pill remains controversial for a nursing mother: Some pediatricians would advise her not to take the pills at all, since the steroids they contain can pass into her milk and may affect her baby's long-term growth and development. But the American Academy of Pediatrics found no significant effects of the Pill on nursing infants and in 1981, in a policy guideline, declared that a nursing mother can use the Pill safely.

Breast-feeding versus bottle-feeding

The problem of breast-feeding and the Pill is related to the larger, far more important problem of how to feed an infant. In the United States today, the feeding problem arises as a choice—whether to breast-feed the baby or bring him up on a bottle. No more than a century ago, that choice simply did not exist: Virtually all babies were fed with human milk and from the breast. Milk from dairy animals is largely indigestible to newborns, and babies whose mothers died were unlikely to survive without a wet nurse. In 1915, however, the first commercial baby formulas, based on modified cow's milk, were put on the market. By the middle of the century, bottle-feeding became the norm for American mothers; in 1955, only 18 per cent of all babies were being breast-fed at the time they left the hospital.

Then the tide turned. Pediatricians found that breast-fed babies tend to be somewhat healthier than their bottle-fed counterparts, with fewer allergies, respiratory infections or serious intestinal disorders. In one long-term study, adults who were breast-fed as infants proved to be less prone to obesity and the high cholesterol levels associated with heart disease. Accordingly, doctors began to urge mothers to breast-feed their babies. In 1980, more than half of all newborns were breast-fed, and today a woman whose mother was encouraged to bottle-feed her children (and was considered old-fashioned or eccentric if she did not) may find herself under considerable pressure to breast-feed her own child.

There is no question that human milk is the ideal food for a human infant; it is uniquely formulated to provide all of the nutrients a baby needs, in the correct proportions and in a readily digestible form. The protein in cow's milk, for example, consists primarily of a substance called casein, which is converted by human digestive juices into tough, cheeselike, almost indigestible curds. By contrast, human milk contains only a fourth the protein of cow's milk, but has a low percentage of casein. Breast-fed babies rarely become constipated, possibly because virtually all of the protein they receive is absorbed, leaving little to solidify in their intestinal tracts.

Human milk contains more of the vitamins A, C, D and E than cow's milk, and higher concentrations of lactose, an energy-yielding sugar. On the other hand, the concentrations of certain minerals in cow's milk far exceed a baby's needs. Because cow's milk contains more than three times as much calcium, six times as much phosphorus and more than three times as much sodium as breast milk, it places an abnormal load on an infant's immature kidneys.

Finally, human milk contains substances that protect babies from disease during the months when their own biological defenses have not fully developed. So-called IgA antibodies, for example, help prevent intestinal and respiratory infections (a major cause of serious illness and death in newborns) and also may play a role in preventing allergies. Babies are unable to manufacture enough of these antibodies—and the only source for them is mother's milk.

Despite the benefits of human milk, doctors stress that no mother need feel troubled about her child's nutritional welfare if career pressures, illness or her own inclinations lead her to bottle-feed her baby. To be sure, she will have to exercise extra care in certain areas. Formula manufacturers now fortify their products with vitamins and attempt to adjust water, fat, sugar and mineral contents to approximate human milk. If a child begins to show signs of allergic reactions, the formula should be changed, usually from a milk-based to a soy-based preparation. Unfortunately, there is no substitute for the protective immunological benefits of mother's milk.

Demand and supply at the breast

A woman's milk-producing system swings into action when her baby is born, even if she does not intend to use it. Delivery triggers the release of a hormone called prolactin, which stimulates milk glands distributed throughout the breasts to begin manufacturing. As milk is produced, it collects in tiny reservoirs. While the first batch of milk is being made, the breasts secrete colostrum, a yellowish, transparent liquid that accumulates during pregnancy. The ideal first food for an infant, colostrum is somewhat easier to digest than milk and full of nutrients and antibodies.

The first true milk generally appears about two to four days after delivery. It comes in faster if the baby nurses at the breast, because sucking stimulates nerves that trigger the release of another hormone, oxytocin, which contracts the breasts' milk reservoirs, forcing the fluid into the nipple area. This so-called let-down reflex is constantly repeated, so that the more the baby sucks, the more milk the mother produces.

During the early days of nursing, several minutes of vigorous sucking may be needed to stimulate the let-down reflex. Once the milk supply is well established, the reflex goes into action almost instantly. In some women the reflex works so efficiently that milk may spray from an uncovered breast.

But the delivery of milk to the baby is surprisingly slow; indeed, first-time mothers are often shocked to discover just how time-consuming breast-feeding can be. During the first few weeks, a baby may want to nurse as frequently as every two hours. Such seemingly inexhaustible hunger does not mean that the mother is not producing enough milk. Normally, the supply is equal to the demand, but a newborn's stomach holds only about two tablespoons of liquid, and it empties rapidly because breast milk is digested rapidly.

Even if a baby's needs seem excessive, it is good to feed him pretty much on demand for the first few weeks. His demands will soon fall into a pattern. By their second month, most babies cut back to six to eight meals a day; after their third, most settle into a routine of three to five times a day.

These early, virtually incessant demands pose a double problem for the mother: They take a physical toll on her body, and they take this toll at a time when she needs extra energy to produce milk and to replenish the nutrients it contains. The problems of keeping her strength up and her milk plentiful have evoked a bewildering variety of solutions. In China doctors have urged nursing mothers to include plenty of pork fat, shrimp heads, rice wine and blow-fly larvae in their diets, and folklore abounds with similarly exotic foods presumed to ensure a flourishing milk supply. In the United States doctors generally recommend a standard balanced diet and plenty of liquids. One change for most women is an increase in calcium to a level of at least 1,200 milligrams a day—the amount in a quart of cow's milk or about five ounces of cheese. Calcium is a major component of human milk; if a woman's diet is low in the mineral, her body will withdraw it from her bones to make up the deficit.

As a rule, any food that a mother can eat safely will not harm her baby. However, mothers often discover that some foods give their milk an objectionable flavor or quality. One baby, for example, became sick whenever the mother ate garlic—a reaction apparently inherited from the father, who suffered from stomach cramps whenever he ate garlic. Other women find that foods that make them gassy (cabbage, broccoli and Brussels sprouts are common culprits) have the same effect on their babies.

Common drugs, among them some seemingly benign nonprescription medicines, can have far more serious effects. No nursing mother should take any drug without first discussing it with her doctor. Drugs that are always off limits for nursing mothers include diuretics, anticoagulants, antithyroid drugs, and laxatives containing cascara or senna. Aspirin, antihistamines and milk of magnesia are generally considered safe in moderate use. But addictive narcotics such as morphine, taken by the mother, can produce an addicted baby. Small amounts of alcohol or caffeine seem to have little adverse effect on a baby. However, a mother who drinks enough to become intoxicated will make her baby tipsy as well.

A common physical problem in breast-feeding is engorgement. As the milk comes in for the first time, many mothers find their breasts suddenly becoming overfull and very painful. Eventually, pressure from the engorged tissues clamps down on the milk ducts and prevents any milk from escaping at all. Because a baby cannot grasp and suck at the swollen nipple area, the only cure for engorged breasts is to remove some excess milk manually. Soften the breasts with a hot bath or hot compresses; support the base of a breast in one hand, and with the other, stroke downward all around it to start the milk moving into the ducts. Next, cup the base of the breast in one hand, with your thumb about halfway up the top of the breast. Run your thumb firmly downward; when it reaches the dark areola around the nipple, press in upon the breast. Do not squeeze the nipple; that will close the ducts.

For times when the mother cannot be available to feed her baby herself, breast milk can be collected and stored in sterile bottles. It can be safely stored for up to 48 hours in the refrigerator, or frozen for months at a time. Several hours before using frozen milk, thaw it in the refrigerator, warm it under running tap water and shake it to remix the cream. Thawing or heating the milk in hot water will curdle it.

Breast-fed babies should not be introduced to a bottle and

Mastering the art of nursing

Babies are born ready for nursing, but a first-time mother may need some training to prevent a potentially serene experience from turning into an exasperating session that leaves the baby hungry and the mother harassed. The so-called letting down reflex that releases breast milk to the nipple area demands relaxation and comfort. Proper support, for example, is more important than many mothers realize; the weight of an incorrectly supported eight-pound baby can strain the mother's arm and abdomen muscles within minutes.

The pictures shown here and on the following pages illustrate a variety of techniques for holding a baby and helping the baby to nurse. The techniques are designed for the mother's comfort and the baby's satisfaction, a combination that gives nursing time a rarely equaled sense of closeness and fulfillment. A bottle-fed child can get much the same warmth and security from being cuddled during a feeding. And both bottle- and breast-fed infants will probably end a meal in the same way—with a hearty burp to expel air bubbles sucked in along with the milk.

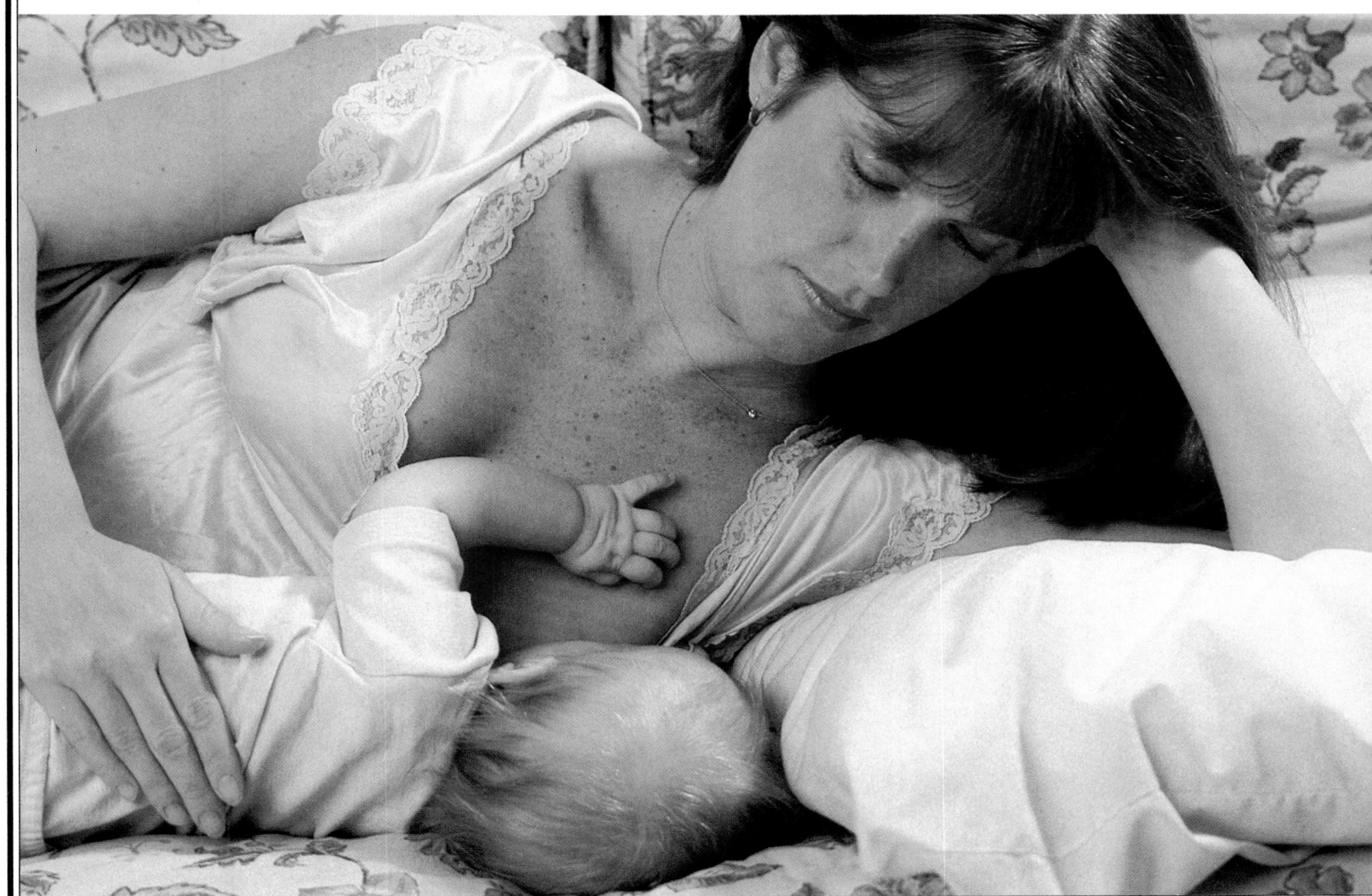

Propped up by pillows at her back and under her arm, a nursing mother lies on her side, rolling slightly forward to bring her breast level with her baby's mouth and accessible to the baby's hand. Often recommended for late-night feedings, this reclining position may also be the best in daytime nursings for a mother who is sore from an episiotomy or a Caesarean section.

The best positions for baby, breast and bottle

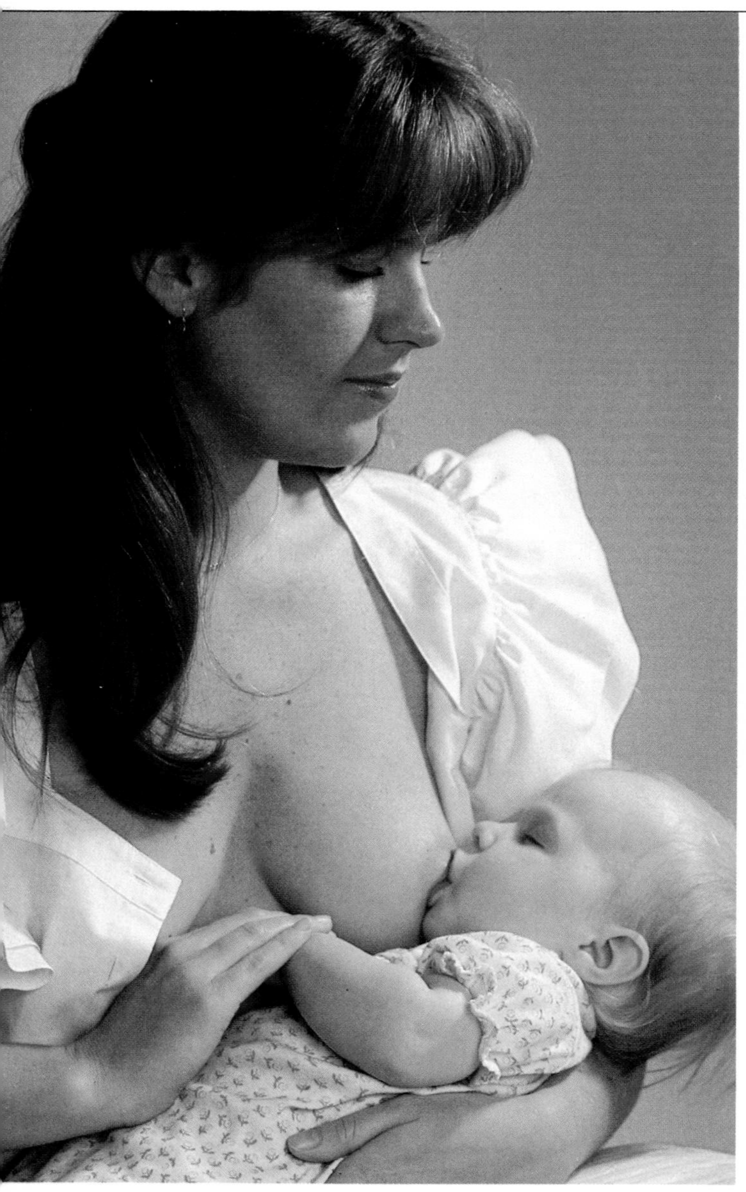

In this classic sitting position, a pillow on the lap helps to support the baby at breast level. The infant's mouth should cover the nipple and all or part of the areola; rhythmic pressure upon this area, rather than true sucking, presses the milk out.

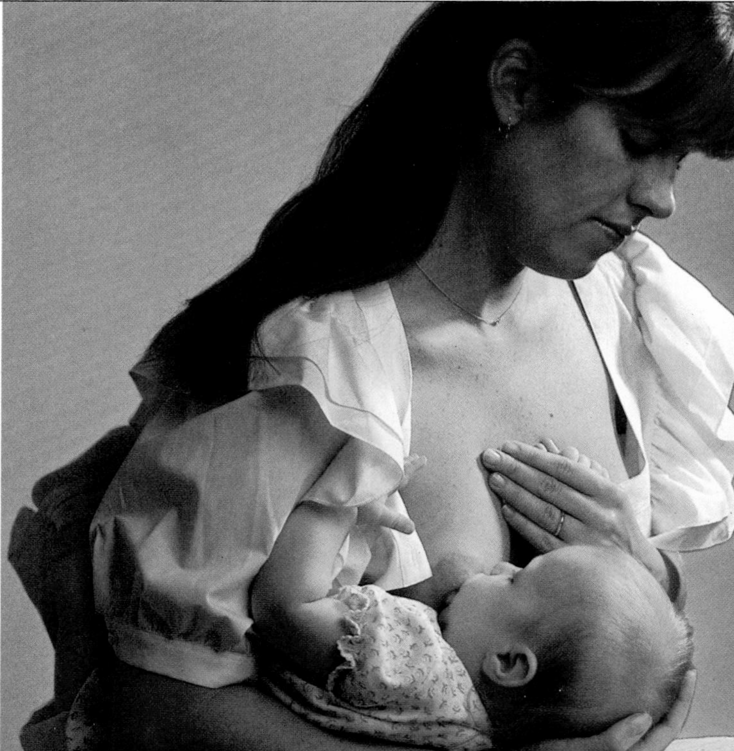

In an alternate sitting position often called the football hold, the baby is cradled at the side of the nursing breast. Because the baby does not press against the abdomen, this position is often adopted by mothers whose abdomens are tender after a cesarean section; it can also be used to nurse twins simultaneously.

To make it easier for the infant's small mouth to take hold of the nipple at the beginning of a feeding, the mother compresses the nipple between her thumb and forefinger. This baby girl has already turned her head toward the breast and opened her mouth in the instinctive "rooting reflex."

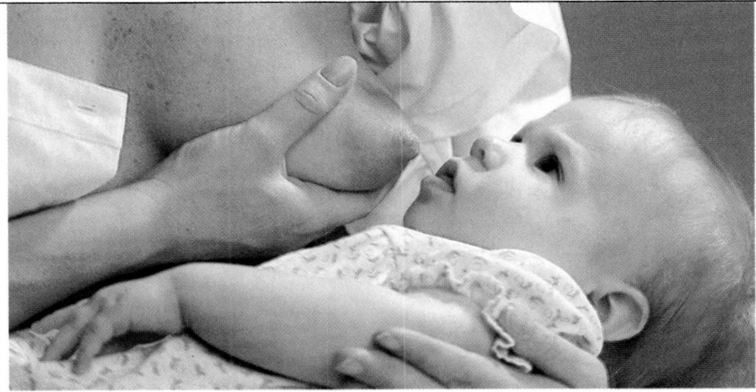

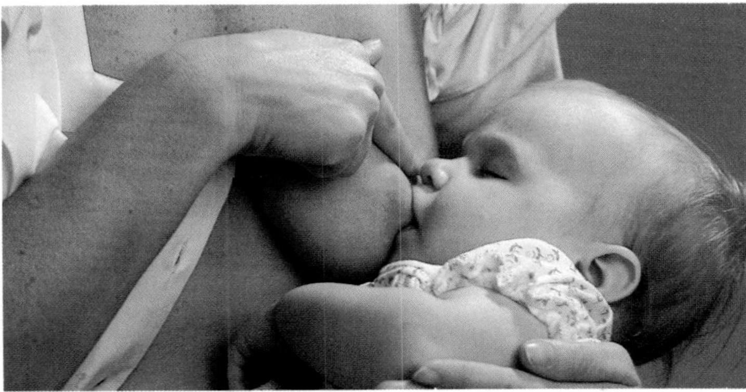

To make sure the nursing infant has room to breathe through her nose, the mother clears an airway by pressing the area immediately above the areola slightly back and down. This precaution is particularly important in the first few minutes of a feeding session, when the breasts are full.

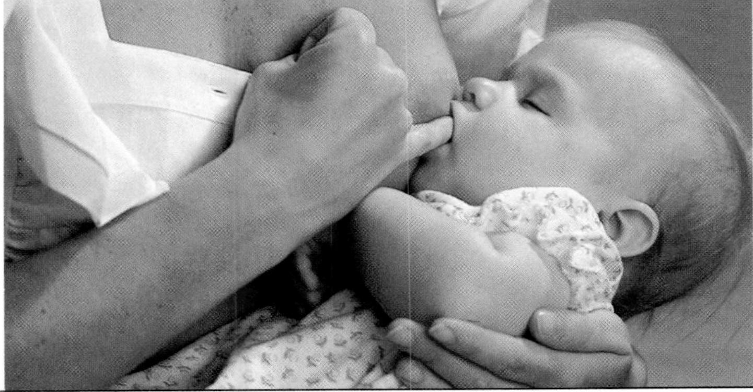

To remove this tenacious baby from the breast at the end of feeding, the mother inserts a fingertip between her nipple and the baby's lips to break the seal created by the child's mouth. Simply pulling the breast away usually causes an infant's jaws to clamp down harder, and may result in cracked or sore nipples.

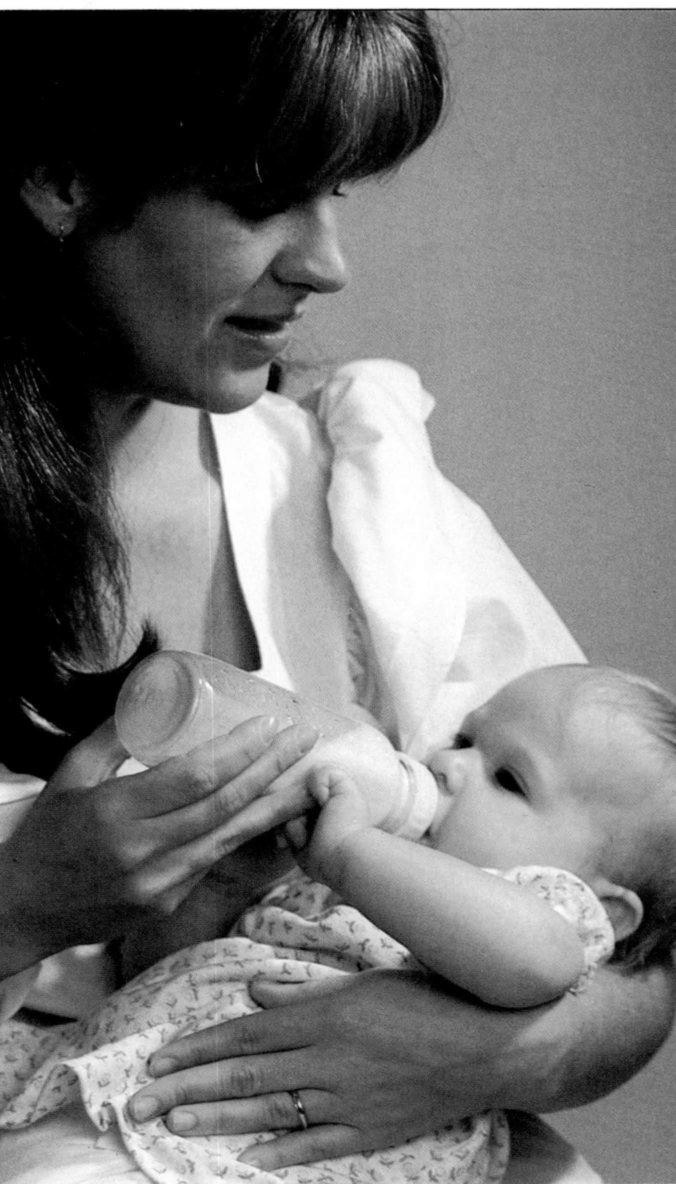

For a feeding from a bottle, which yields a faster flow of milk than a breast, the mother slightly raises her daughter's head to reduce the risk of choking. In addition, the mother holds the bottle at a slant to keep the nipple full of milk and free of air.

Coaxing out air bubbles

In an alternate method sometimes preferred for larger children, the mother sets the baby stomach-down across her lap and holds the child steady with one hand while patting with the other. A protective lap pad or diaper is indispensable: Milk as well as air is usually expelled from the baby's tilted stomach.

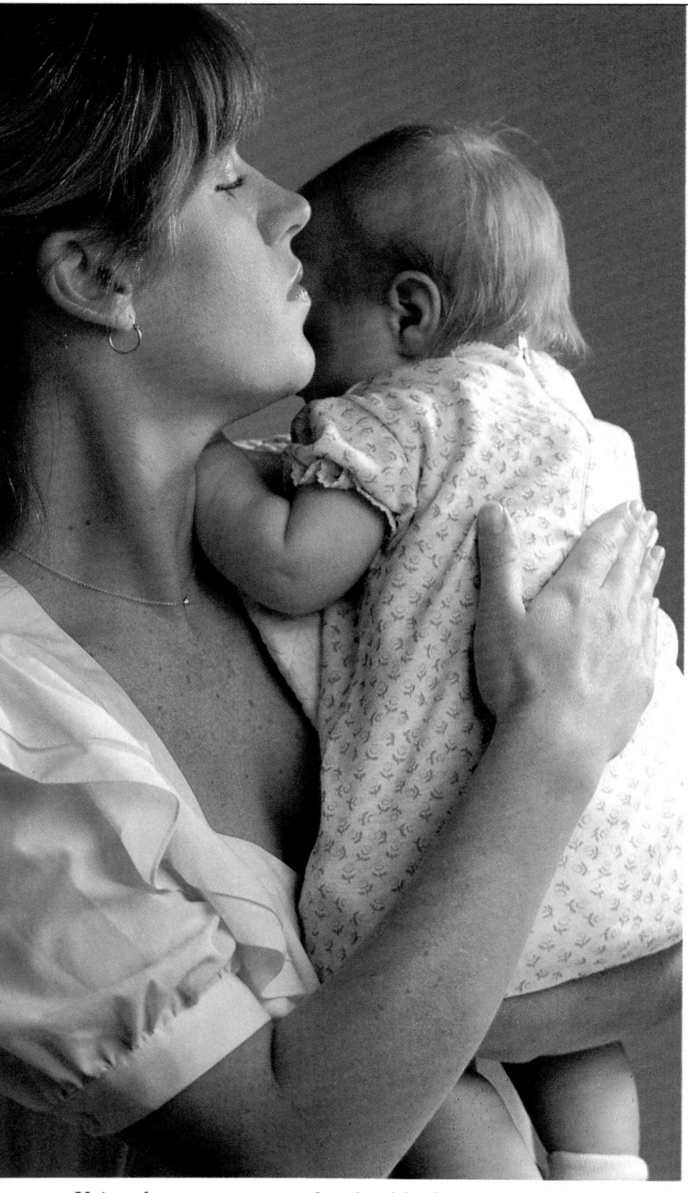

Using the common over-the-shoulder burping position, a mother gently pats her child's back to bring up any air bubbles that were swallowed during a feeding. Vigorous thumping is not necessary: It does not bring air up faster.

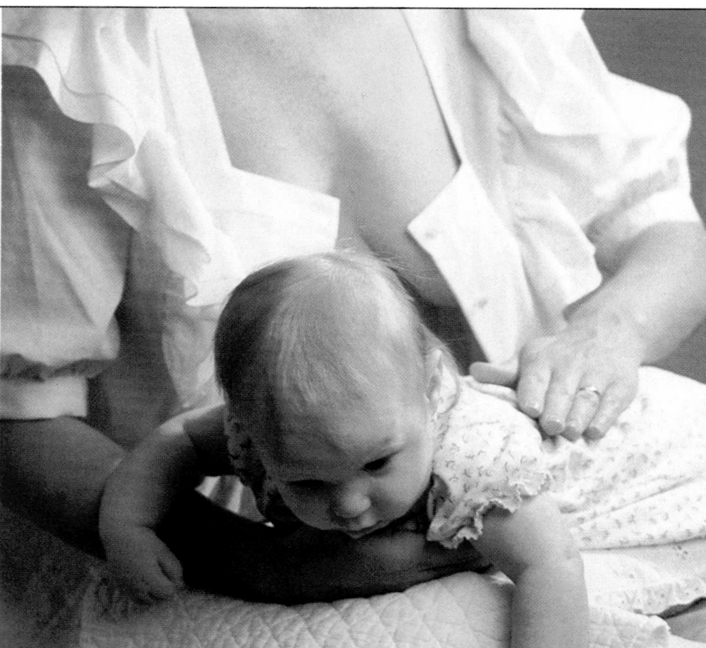

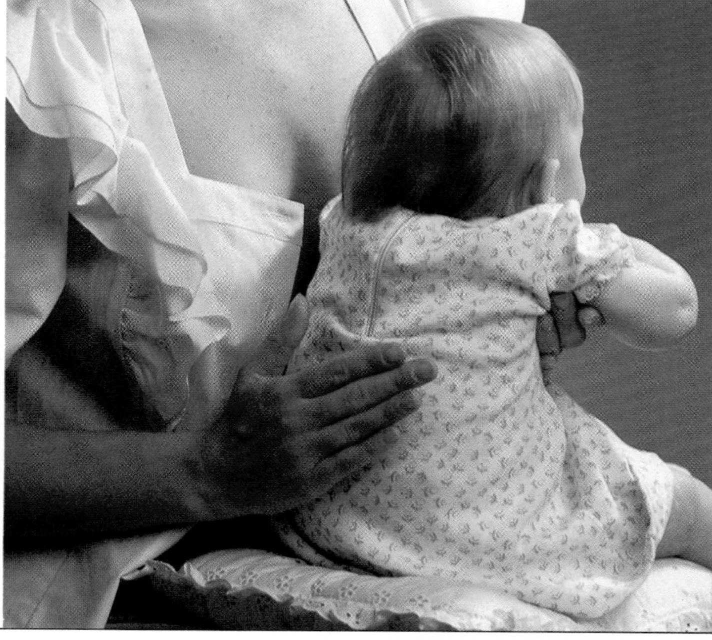

The baby is seated upright on her mother's lap in a position especially suitable for burping very young infants. The mother's hand, here shown supporting the baby's chest, can also be cupped around an infant's chin and jaw to brace a wobbly head.

an artificial nipple before the age of about two weeks. Letting them drink from bottles earlier deprives the mother's breasts of the stimulation they need to produce milk, and because milk flows faster from an artificial nipple, a very young baby may prefer the bottle and refuse the breast. Once the baby has become an experienced feeder at the breast, a mother can give him (or have someone else give him) an occasional bottle-feeding of breast milk without disturbing his normal breast-feeding routine; if she does not have enough expressed breast milk on hand for a complete bottle feeding, she can fill the relief bottle with a commercial formula.

Formulas that simulate mother's milk

Before the 1960s, some 80 per cent of all bottle-fed babies drank evaporated milk, diluted and sweetened at home. Today, most parents have switched from such brews to formulas designed to simulate human milk. These commercial brands come in four forms, varying in cost and convenience. Powdered formula, the least expensive and easiest to store, must be measured precisely and mixed with water; dissolving the powder generally requires a good deal of stirring and shaking. Liquid concentrates cost more than powder, but are easier to measure and mix. Premixed, ready-to-feed liquid formula is more expensive still, but can be poured directly from a can into the bottle. Premixed formulas sealed in sterile disposable bottles are the most convenient of all—the parent simply attaches a nipple at feeding time—but can be prohibitively expensive when used full-time.

Most bottle-fed infants eat less frequently than breast-fed; eight three-ounce bottles are usually enough for a 24-hour period. On the other hand, preparing the bottles is a time-consuming chore. Traditionally, everything from the formula itself to the spoon used to stir it is sterilized to kill bacteria. Two sterilization methods are commonly used: aseptic, in which materials are sterilized before the formula is mixed; and terminal, in which sterilization takes place afterward. The first is somewhat faster, the second somewhat safer.

To prepare formula by the aseptic method, boil all your equipment—bottles, bottle tops, screw-on nipple rings and such gear as a measuring cup, a bowl or pitcher, a can opener for canned formula, a funnel and long-handled tongs—in a covered pan for 10 minutes. Boil the nipples separately for three minutes (longer boiling weakens the rubber) in a smaller covered pan. Drain the pans, boil mixing water for five minutes and mix the formula. After being poured into the bottles, the formula can be refrigerated for up to 24 hours, to be used as it is needed.

For terminal sterilization, you will need a special bottle sterilizer or a pan deep enough to hold all the bottles upright; if you use the pan, you will also need a small cake rack to raise the bottles above the bottom of the pan, so the heat will not crack them. Wash the bottles and fill them with formula; attach clean nipples and bottle caps loosely so that steam can escape from the bottles; then pour in two or three inches of water, cover the pan and boil the bottles for 25 minutes. Allow the pan to cool for two hours before uncovering it.

Most parents heat bottled milk before feeding it to their babies, but recent studies have shown that babies happily drink formula at refrigerator or room temperature. They do object, however, to temperatures that vary from feeding to feeding; parents should decide on one method and stick to it.

During a feeding, stay with the baby and hold the bottle *(page 85)*. Never leave an infant alone to suck on a bottle propped beside his head. Babies younger than five months have little control over their head and neck muscles. If milk flows from the nipple faster than a baby can swallow, he often cannot cough it up or turn his head to the side, and may begin to inhale, or aspirate, the liquid. Aspiration is a leading cause of accidental death in newborns.

Do not confuse aspiration with the act of swallowing air, a harmless event whose effects are relieved by periodic burping *(page 86)*. Babies also spit up some of their food, almost as a matter of course. The valve at the top of the stomach has not developed sufficiently to seal the organ, and milk in this area may rise through the throat to the mouth, then dribble down the baby's chin. This can be messy, particularly if the baby spits up several times during a single feeding, but it is not in itself a sign of illness. Even true vomiting, when the baby expels most or all of the stomach's contents, is not a cause for immediate alarm if it occurs only occasionally and is not accompanied by such other signs of illness as fever.

After feeding and burping a baby, discard any leftover milk. Small amounts of saliva seep into the bottle as the baby sucks, carrying bacteria that can multiply to dangerous levels in a few hours.

The switch to solid foods

Parents were once encouraged to introduce solid foods as early as possible, often with the argument that the food would fill a baby up and help him sleep through the night. However, nutritional experts have found that a baby who eats solid foods regularly by the age of two months (an estimated 96 per cent of all American infants do so) takes in 35 per cent more calories than the recommended daily allowance. Equally important, according to the experts, is the fact that breast milk or iron-fortified formula is the only food a baby needs for the first four to six months of life, and the only food most babies should have until they are at least four or five months old.

An infant's facial anatomy is tailored for sucking rather than chewing. The tongue is disproportionately large, forming a broad, muscular pad against the mother's nipple, and the sucking muscles are three times as strong, proportionately, as an adult's. At six or seven months, the baby's facial configuration has changed. The muscles used for chewing are better developed; the tongue is proportionately smaller, and mobile enough to push food to the teeth for chewing. This is when a baby is physiologically ready for solid foods, and the time when most of them should first have it. To be sure, there are exceptions to the rule. Many doctors recommend that any baby who takes more than a quart of formula a day or feeds often from the breast and still cries for food should have small portions of mushy semisolid food.

Special iron-fortified baby cereal mixed with formula or expressed breast milk is the traditional first solid. Before the age of six months, a baby should have only two teaspoons of cereal a day; when he is clearly ready for more, he can have more cereal and a few spoonfuls of puréed, strained fruits. Introduce new foods one at a time, about a week apart. If the baby vomits a new food up, or shows such signs of intolerance as a rash, do not be alarmed; try it again in a few weeks.

At around seven to eight months, a baby's system can usually handle a wide variety of foods, including commercially prepared puréed vegetables and meat and small portions of the family's regular meals ground up in a food processor or blender. Season homemade foods with a light hand; spices can irritate an immature stomach, and babies quickly develop cravings for sugar and salt—tastes that can later contribute to tooth decay, obesity and high blood pressure.

Fitting the baby into the family

A new baby always calls for major adjustments in a family's routine. For months, the entire household will seem to revolve around the newcomer's needs, made abundantly apparent through loud, insistent cries. During the first seven weeks of life, an average baby cries more than two hours a day. These cries are always distressing to parents and to anyone else who hears them. Nature has apparently designed an infant's squalls to be peculiarly unnerving; to no one's surprise, researchers have found that the sounds produce muscular tension, an elevated heart rate and soaring blood pressure in an adult.

A baby's specific needs are not always easy to identify. Some cries can be classified according to the pattern of the sounds. A basic cry of hunger, the most common of all, may have the pattern of an indrawn breath, a pause and a rhythmically rising and falling wail. A cry of pain is generally a series of sharp inward gasps, each followed by a rising shriek and a pause. Other patterns indicate fatigue, loneliness or the discomfort of a wet diaper.

In theory, parents learn to decipher their babies' cries. In practice, reading the message of a baby's cry is more often a matter of eliminating causes than of interpreting signals. In general, the sooner you respond to a baby's cry, the sooner he will calm down. Despite popular belief, prompt attention to a crying baby is unlikely to produce a spoiled child. Studies have shown that if a parent responds readily to a baby's cries during the early months of life, the child is less likely to cry frequently or for long periods when he is a year or so old.

Some crying babies can be soothed by being wrapped snugly in a blanket *(page 79)*. Other babies calm down if they are patted on the back, rocked or walked, and some like the sound of music; child-care experts suggest that rhythmic sounds or movements remind a baby of life in the womb.

But there are times when nothing works at all, and a baby who cries frequently for no apparent reason can have a devastating effect on a parent. One father, who faced the problem at its worst, recalled: "When Lisa was about two and a half months old, she started to cry every night when I got home. She cried from six to midnight, every night. We tried everything, feeding her, rocking her, giving her toys. The only thing that seemed to help was walking her, the faster the better. By midnight I would practically be running up and down the hall with her. And it went on like that for six weeks."

Such nightmarish hours of ceaseless crying are part of a larger pattern called colic. Typically, a colicky baby cannot settle down after an afternoon or evening feeding, and either cries immediately afterward or erupts into frantic screams within an hour after bedtime. Almost any remedy—feeding, cuddling, burping—may check the crying momentarily, but it resumes almost at once.

No one knows the cause of colic. Many doctors believe that the ailment arises from the immaturity of a baby's digestive or nervous system, yet a premature baby is no more likely to get it than any other. A colicky baby should be seen by a doctor, to rule out other illnesses, but if the baby does turn out to have colic, the only cure is time. The condition typically lasts four to eight weeks; then the screaming stops, often as suddenly as it began.

Though a baby's cries always disrupt his parents' sleep, his own sleep is unlikely to be disturbed by much of anything. Up to the age of four months or so, babies will sleep a total of about 16 hours a day. During the first weeks of life, newborns drift almost randomly in and out of sleep, waking when they are hungry, dropping off when they are full, and spending a good deal of time suspended between the two states. At about six weeks of age, the difference between sleep and wakefulness is more distinct; during at least one period during the day, a baby is likely to be wide awake for an hour or two. This is the time to start adjusting his sleep patterns to fit those of the rest of the household.

Many babies have their most wakeful periods in the afternoon. They sleep after breakfast, wake for lunch, nap for a couple of hours, then wake up and remain alert into the early evening. After an evening meal, they sleep soundly until a late-night feeding. Parents whose babies naturally adopt this pattern may find that if they give this final feeding just before they go to bed themselves, the baby needs to eat only once in the early-morning hours. Gradually, they stretch the period between the last feeding of the night and the first one of the morning so that these feedings eventually coincide with their own bedtime and wake-up time.

Not all babies take readily to this routine. Some feel most alert and playful between six and 11 p.m. If that pattern is inconvenient for the rest of the family, you can alter it by deliberately keeping the baby up during the afternoon, so that he will begin to sleep more soundly in the evening.

Equally valuable is a routine that teaches the baby the difference between night and day. A bedtime ritual—changing the baby into night clothes, feeding him his last meal of the day in a darkened room, then putting him to bed and wrapping him warmly—eventually becomes associated with nighttime sleeping, as opposed to nap time. And keep a middle-of-the-night feeding as low-key and brief as possible. Gather everything you will need ahead of time, so that you will not need to move around the room when you go in to feed the baby. When he cries for his nighttime feeding, go in immediately, before he can wake up completely.

By the time they are four months old, most babies are sleeping in a pattern that includes an eight-hour nighttime stretch. But the point at which a baby reaches this happy stage varies, and probably depends more on physical development than on age. "The nurses at the hospital told me that as soon as Noah weighed 13 pounds, he'd start sleeping through the night," said one mother. "And that's exactly what happened."

Many parents feel that a new baby should be bathed daily —but newborns frequently have an aversion to baths. The contact of clothing on their skin helps them feel secure; its absence can frighten them. Being placed naked in a tubful of water can literally terrify them. In their fear, they may begin

Bathing a baby safely and well

A baby's first bath can be distressing for parent and child alike, but the procedure shown here is safe, simple and, after a few sessions, generally enjoyable for both parties. From the start, try to work in an easy, confident way, and keep up a soothing flow of chatter to relieve the infant's uneasiness or fear. Remember, too, that a very small baby does not need a full-scale bath. Until the stump of the umbilical cord drops off, limit washing to a thorough wiping, concentrated in two regions: the head, particularly around the face and neck to remove traces of milk and dribble; and the diaper area, to clean off irritating residues of urine and stools.

For true bathing, the safest and most convenient vessel is a small basin at waist height. An inflatable baby bath *(below)* provides extra cushioning, but even the kitchen sink will do; cover the faucet spout with a washcloth and turn it aside to protect the baby from bumps, then line the sink with a diaper to make its surface less slippery. Keep the room warm (75° to 80° F.) and draft-free, and prepare the vessel with a few inches of water that is comfortably warm when tested with your wrist or elbow—not your hand, which is accustomed to hot water. Everything you need—mild soap, washcloth, towel, hairbrush and clean clothes—should be at hand; never leave the baby while you fetch a forgotten article.

Before undressing the baby, wash his head. Moisten the washcloth with clear, warm water and wipe over the eyes from the nose outward, using a separate part of the cloth for each eye; then gently wipe the baby's face. Clean the outside of each ear with a washcloth-covered finger, but do not swab out the ear canal. Rub gently across the fontanel, the membrane-covered "soft spot" in the baby's skull. Once or twice a week, wash the baby's hair. Hold the child tucked under one arm like a football, with his head over the bath basin; wet his hair with the washcloth and work up a lather with soap or a mild shampoo. Rinse the hair thoroughly with repeated applications of a wet washcloth.

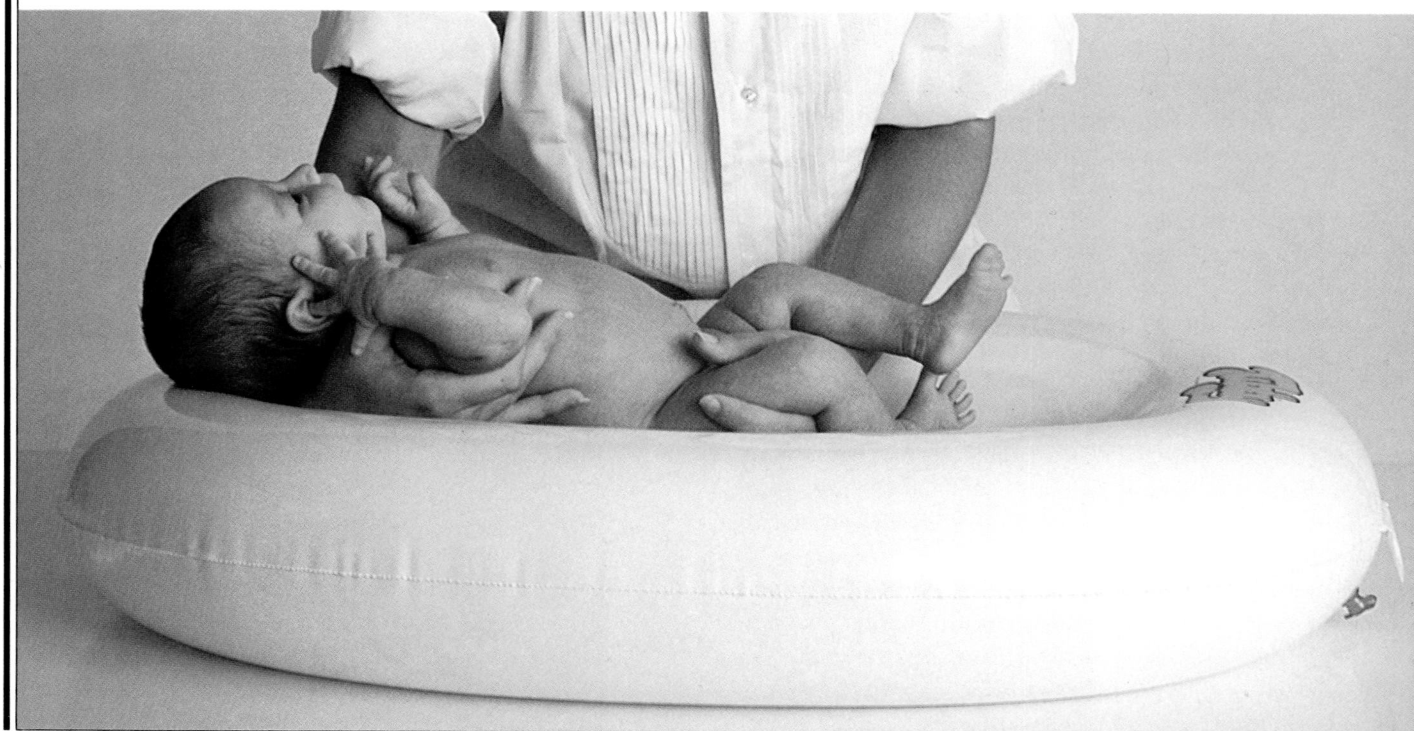

IMMERSING THE BABY

Cradle the baby on your forearms, maintaining a secure grip at the shoulder and thigh; the hand you will use for washing should be under the legs, while the other hand provides support at the neck. Gently lower the baby into the water. After a minute or so, slowly slip your hand from under the baby's legs.

WASHING THE FRONT OF THE BABY

Lather the washcloth, then soap the baby gently on the front of the torso and around the arms and legs. To avoid spreading diaper residues, start with the cleanest areas and work toward the most soiled, making sure to clean within the folds of skin. Rinse the washcloth and wipe the soap off, going over the skin at least twice.

WASHING THE BACK

Raise the baby to a sitting position, grip his shoulder securely with the hand you have been using for washing, and use the other hand to soap and rinse his back. Return the baby to the original position.

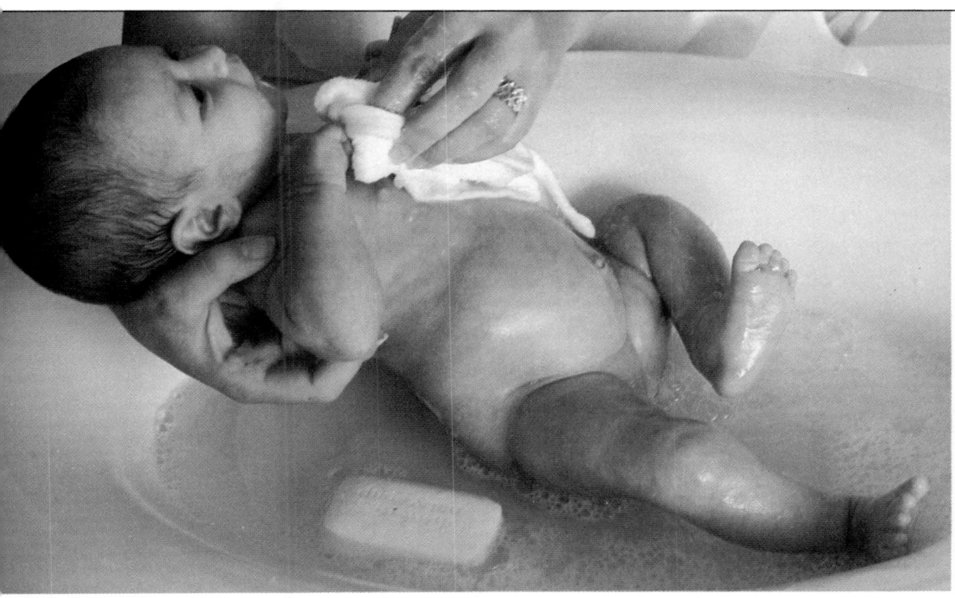

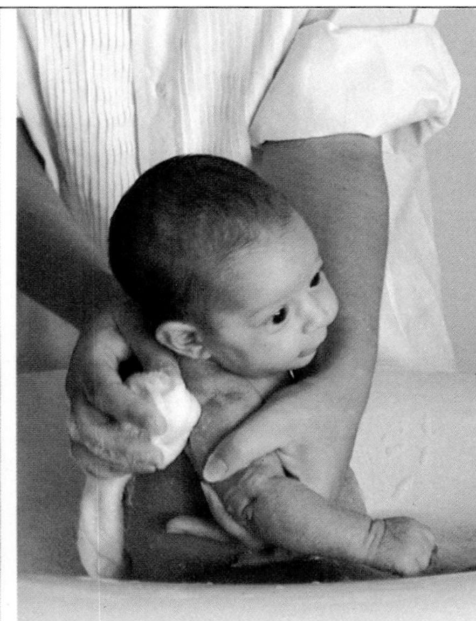

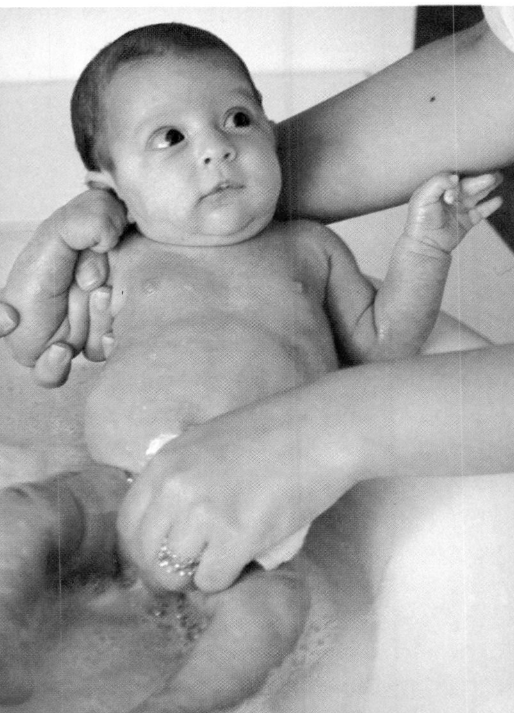

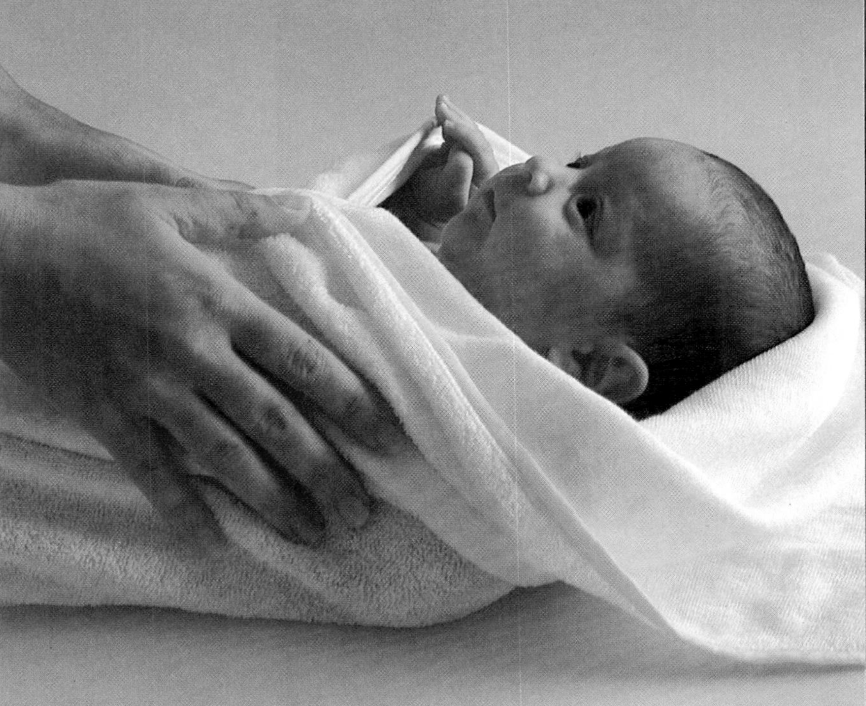

CLEANING THE GENITALS

Wash both surfaces and crevices in the area. For a girl, wipe from front to back to keep feces away from the vagina and urinary tract. Wash under an uncircumcised foreskin only if it can be pulled back easily.

DRYING OFF

Remove the baby from the bath, maintaining a firm grip on his wet, slippery skin, and wrap him immediately in a large towel to protect him from chilling. Dry the baby by patting the towel gently; rubbing can irritate the skin. Check to be sure that all skin folds are free of moisture, then put on clean clothing.

to thrash about, making the difficult job of holding their slippery bodies all but impossible.

Because baths can be traumatic experiences for both a newborn and a parent, it is often best to defer them until the baby has had a few weeks to settle down. Some doctors, including Benjamin Spock, suggest that if an infant seems particularly apprehensive, it will not hurt to postpone bathing him until he can sit up with support. In any case many pediatricians recommend that parents give the first bath only after the baby's navel has healed, sometime between one and two weeks after birth.

In the meantime, infants should be given frequent sponge baths, and their bottoms should be cleaned carefully several times a day—wiped off with a damp cloth if they are wet; washed with a soapy cloth, then rinsed with a wet one after a bowel movement.

For the first day or so after birth, a baby passes a blackish-green, tarry substance called meconium. Then, as his digestive system switches over to milk or formula, the stools become runny, and may look peculiar to an uninformed parent. In fact, greenish-brown or bright-green transitional feces, sometimes containing mucus or curds, are all normal.

Breast-fed babies' stools remain loose and are usually pale or orange-yellow. They may be produced frequently, perhaps after every feeding and several times in between. But the pattern can change suddenly to once a day or even once in several days. A bottle-fed baby generally has fewer bowel movements, and his stools are comparatively solid.

Because breast-fed babies are unlikely to get diarrhea or become constipated, the appearance of their stools and the timing of bowel movements are rarely causes for concern. But a bottle-fed baby who goes for two to three days without a movement, or whose stools suddenly become loose and runny, may have diet problems; ask a doctor about changing the formula. Diarrhea, which may signal a dangerous intestinal infection, always calls for immediate professional help.

Babies urinate frequently—it is impossible to keep them perfectly dry all the time—and most do not seem to notice or care if they are a bit damp. Nevertheless, a diaper sodden with urine or feces should be changed at once. It is irritating and uncomfortable; also, it is an invitation to diaper rash, caused mainly by bacteria that multiply rapidly in a warm, wet diaper. Skin chafed by the diaper is especially open to bacterial invasion, and the condition can progress from mild chapping to severe inflammation and infected sores.

To prevent diaper rash, change the baby's diapers frequently and leave him undiapered as much as possible, to expose his bottom to air and free it from contact with bacteria. Each time you wash or change the baby, dry him carefully and thoroughly. Use plastic pants sparingly; they trap moisture on the baby's skin. A coating of petroleum jelly or a silicone or zinc oxide ointment will help protect the baby's bottom from moisture.

If a baby does develop a rash, as most do from time to time, intensify the preventive measures: more frequent changes, more time undiapered and no plastic pants at all. Do not use baking soda, a traditional home remedy: It can be absorbed through chafed skin and may make the baby ill. If sores develop, a pediatrician can prescribe a medicated ointment; protective ointments or jellies can retard healing and should not be used for the time being.

The time-honored ritual of sprinkling a baby's freshly washed bottom with talcum powder is now considered of dubious value. At best, powder absorbs moisture and reduces friction only temporarily, and it can be a health hazard. Most baby powders consist primarily of the mineral talc or of a talc substitute called zinc stearate. Both are dangerous when inhaled, and a generous dusting of powder can fill the air with tiny toxic particles. What is more, many powder containers closely resemble nursing bottles, and inquisitive infants often suck at the container tops, making baby powders a surprisingly common type of swallowed poisoning.

A newborn's store of knowledge

Tending to a newborn's physical needs takes up so much time and energy that parents may well wonder if eating, soiling, sleeping and crying represent all their baby can do. Until the mid-20th Century, scientists assured them that this was indeed the case. The newborn's world, announced psychologist William James in 1890, was one of "buzzing, blooming confusion.'' Generations of his successors agreed that newborn babies were passive, parasitic creatures who could hardly distinguish among sights or sounds, and responded only to a handful of bodily urges.

In recent decades, however, researchers have begun to see complex psychological and physiological patterns in an infant's development. One typical modern researcher, psychologist Robert L. Fantz of Western Reserve University, disagrees completely with James: ''The findings to date have tended to destroy the myth that the world of the newborn is a big, blooming confusion. The infant sees a patterned and organized world, which he explores discriminatingly with the limited means at his command.''

A newborn's sensory apparatus is programed to respond to people, and specifically to the people who generally give him most care. Infant hearing, for example, is keyed to the human voice: Babies move their limbs in time to the rhythms of human speech, and they are more interested in high-pitched, female voices than in low-pitched, male ones. They have limited vision, fixed in focus at eight to 10 inches—but they can see faces poised above their own when they are being held. And they are clearly attracted to faces. Their eyes linger longer on curves than on angles, and a pie plate painted with a crude hairline, eyes, a mouth and a chinline will hold their attention longer than one marked randomly.

Within two weeks, infants can identify their mothers, a skill that was once thought to take months to develop. In one British experiment, two-week-old babies were presented with four different test situations: their mothers, speaking directly to them; strangers speaking to them; the mothers speaking in imitation of the strangers' voices, and the strangers speaking with the mothers' voices. The babies responded strongly when their mothers spoke to them, less when the strangers did. The combinations of imitated voices with inappropriate faces provoked fearful tears.

Babies quickly learn to recognize their fathers, but with a difference. ''Amazingly enough,'' says pediatrician T. Berry Brazelton, ''an infant displays an entirely different attitude—more wide-eyed, playful and bright-faced—toward its father than toward its mother.''

Besides amassing evidence that babies are born with functioning senses, scientists have helped to explain why infants need emotional nurturing as well as food and warmth—a fact that mothers have always known instinctively, and one that was suggested about 700 years ago in a bizarre investigation into infant development inadvertently carried out by the 13th Century Holy Roman Emperor Frederick II. According to a chronicler of the experiment, the Emperor ''bade foster mothers to suckle the children, to bathe and wash them but in no way to prattle with them or speak to them, for he wanted to learn whether they would speak the Hebrew language, which was the oldest, or Greek or Latin, or Arabic, or perhaps the language of their parents of whom they had been born. But he labored in vain, because all the children died. For they could not live without the petting and joyful faces and loving words of their foster mothers.''

The subjects of the Emperor's experiment were victims of what doctors now call the ''failure-to-thrive syndrome.'' It often strikes institutionalized infants who get adequate physical attention but are bereft of playing and cuddling. Physical well-being is tied to a baby's emotional health because his brain and nervous system develop hand in hand with the rest of his body. Just as the baby needs adequate food for the growth of his bones and muscles, his senses need adequate stimulation for the development of his brain.

How and what a baby learns

A baby's physical development follows two simultaneous sequences, one from head to toe, the other from the torso to the fingertips. In the first, the eyes come under control, followed by the face and neck, the trunk, and finally the legs. Progressing outward, babies gain control over their arms and legs, then their hands and feet, and finally their fingers and thumbs. Similarly, their senses become progressively refined as their brain matures, and their interests broaden in another invariable sequence—from the people who tend them, to their own bodies and finally to objects.

The rate at which babies develop depends on a host of factors, from their physical condition to their personalities and temperaments. The generally accepted timetable for ac-

How to put a diaper on

A diaper's function is served equally well by the traditional cloth diaper or the more recently developed disposable type. Deciding between the two is a matter partly of convenience, partly of cost.

Reusable cloth diapers, such as the prefolded type shown in the top row of pictures, are the less expensive and the more versatile. They can be adjusted to fit a newborn or a toddler, and to give extra thickness in the area each sex wets most heavily—the back for a girl, the front for a boy. Their chief shortcoming is one of convenience: Hours must be spent in laundering, including pre-soaking and double rinsing to remove all traces of urine and soap. A diaper service will supply freshly laundered cloth diapers, but at a considerable increase in cost.

Disposables *(bottom pictures)* are more expensive than any cloth alternative. However, they offer an obvious advantage in convenience. In addition, they are certain to be clean and residue-free, and they are secured with tape tabs rather than sharp-pointed pins. Many parents who choose cloth diapers buy a stock of disposables for trips away from home.

Whatever your choice, avoid backaches by making diaper changes on a waist-high surface. Cover it with a comfortable, easy-to-clean mat (the example shown here is a fabric-covered sheet of foam rubber); have supplies close at hand, but out of the baby's reach; and be sure that the baby is thoroughly clean before you put on the fresh diaper.

USING A CLOTH DIAPER

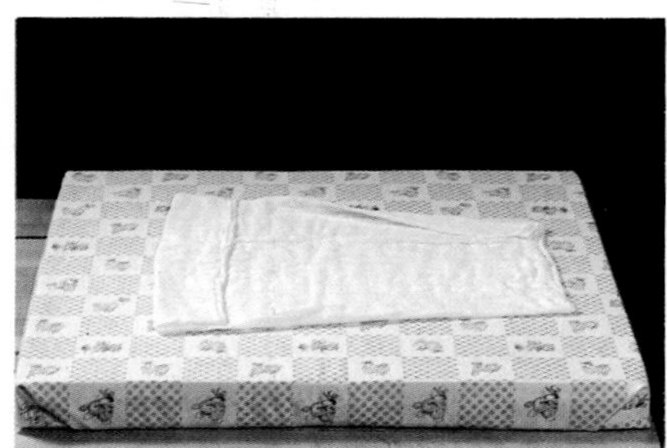

Spread the diaper. In this example, it has been folded over at the back end and in at the sides to fit the baby.

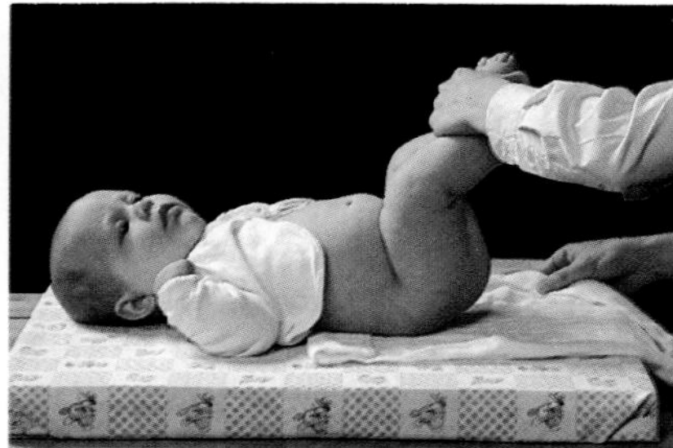

To adjust the baby's position, raise both legs in one hand, inserting a finger between the ankles as a cushion.

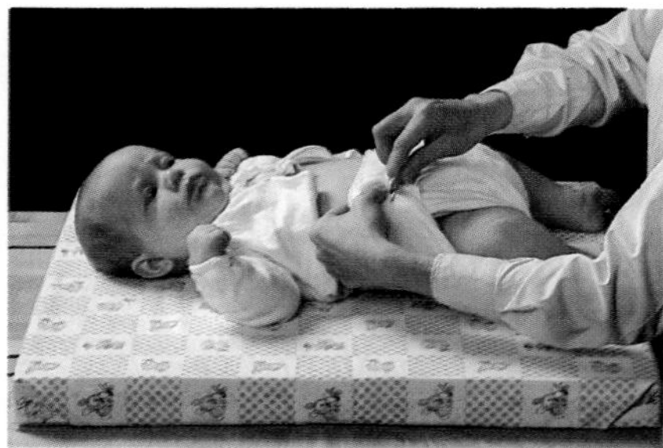

Bring the diaper up between the legs and pin the back edges over the front ones. Shield the baby's skin with your fingers.

USING A DISPOSABLE DIAPER

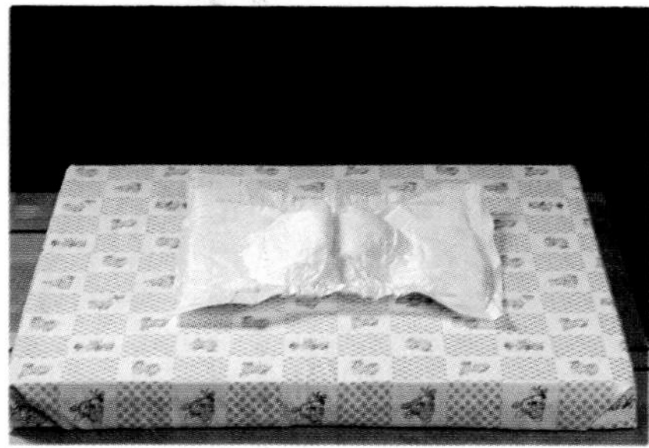

Spread out the ends of the diaper, leaving the center pleats still gathered to fit snugly between the baby's legs.

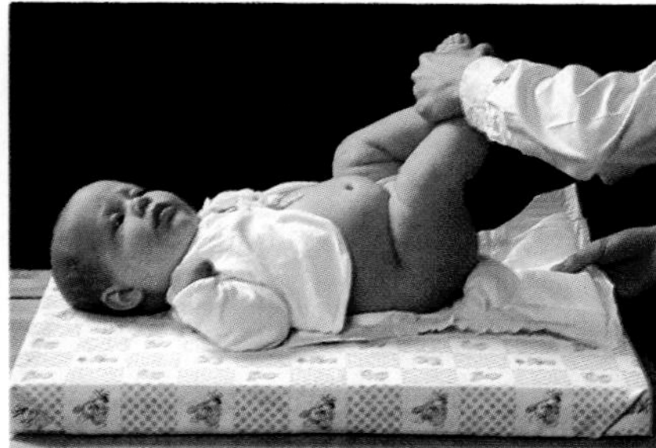

Place the baby on the end of the diaper fitted with tape tabs. Use a finger as a cushion between the baby's ankles.

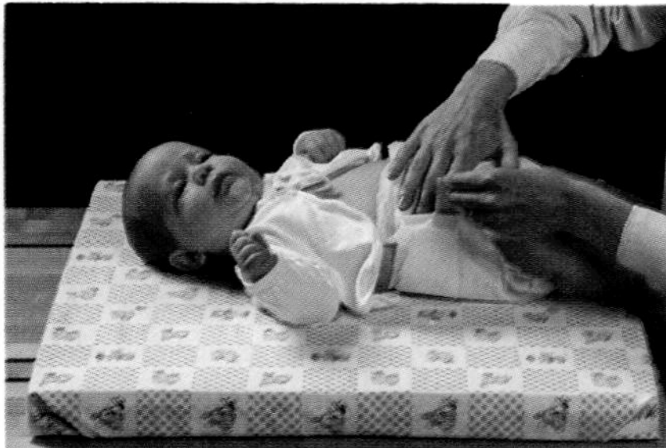

Tape the back edges of the diaper over the front. Finally, fold the plastic top in at the waist to seal in moisture.

quiring motor, language and social skills *(pages 98-107)* is based on statistical evidence; an infant may stray from it in either direction and still be developing normally. Whatever the rate of progress, no one should underestimate an infant's capacity for getting himself into trouble. Initially, a baby's movements are governed by reflex, and because these ungoverned motions can be strong and sudden, newborns should never be left unattended on a bed or a changing table, where a few sharp jerks can flip them onto the floor. Though they have no conscious control over their hands, their sucking instincts and grasp are strong; they may seize any small object that comes to hand—a diaper pin, perhaps, or a button—bring it to their mouths and suck it in.

During the third month of life, a baby's brain and nervous system undergo dramatic changes. His brain-wave patterns begin to resemble an adult's, a sign that the upper brain, which controls thought and conscious movement, is gaining ascendancy over the lower brain, which governs involuntary actions. Most of the early reflexes begin to fade at this point. As his senses become more sophisticated, a baby seeks more sophisticated ways of using them. His physical movements, though still crude, become more purposeful. Instead of gazing raptly at his mother's face, he may pat it with his hands, and he will bat at a mobile to make it move.

Toward the midpoint of their first year, most babies master the art of reaching for an object and closing their hand on it—a feat of perception and coordination impossible for a newborn, and one that indicates they are on the brink of another surge of physical and mental development. In the following months the shape of the baby's body changes noticeably, becoming in effect less babyish and more childlike. Longer and stronger limbs enable him to pull himself across a floor, then to crawl, and finally to haul himself upright, to take a few shaky steps.

Throughout the second half of the year, most babies become increasingly active, with a relentless energy that no adult can match. Olympic gold medalist Jim Thorpe, widely considered the greatest athlete of his day, is said to have tried to imitate all of a baby's movements in a typical 24-hour period. After four hours of following the infant's wiggles, kicks and rolls, the superbly conditioned Thorpe gave up in exhaustion. The baby kept at it for another eight hours.

Another significant sign of growth generally makes its appearance around the midpoint of the year—a tooth. A baby's first teeth, the sharp incisors at the front of the mouth, break through the gums easily, seldom causing more than minor discomfort. The larger, broader molars, which may erupt with real pain, generally do not appear until the end of the year or later. New teeth are sometimes blamed for fever, convulsions, earache, vomiting and diarrhea. In fact, none of these ailments is a symptom of teething. An increased interest in chewing, however, is a normal sign. Almost any attractive object may go into a teething infant's mouth for an experimental nibble—and with the baby's increased mobility and dexterity, virtually anything within sight may also be within reach.

Happily, at this stage, most infants have another outlet for many of their new interests: food. They are only marginally interested in food as a way of satisfying hunger, but they are fascinated by it as a plaything. Feeding himself offers a baby a chance to practice his manual skills, to indulge his passion to chew, and to satisfy his burgeoning curiosity.

The ingenious uses to which the baby puts his food—from dismantling a cookie, crumb by crumb, to squeezing a banana to a pulp and rubbing the pulp on his head—means that a lot of it will go to waste. But it is worse than futile, say experts, to urge him to eat all of a meal—or, for that matter, to eat neatly. "Many mothers," said Dr. Brazelton, "feel so compulsive about getting food into their babies, that they miss the obvious value of the baby's exploratory behavior with it." A baby who is restrained from playing with his food misses out on some experiments in motor development—and seems to realize that fact. Some become so enraged at having their fun spoiled that they may, in the end, sullenly refuse to eat anything at all.

Child-care expert Penelope Leach suggests that the best way to handle early feedings is to cover the baby with a bib, surround him with newspapers and let him go it alone, getting the food from his plate to his mouth in any way he chooses. The baby's interest in chewing will lead him to

These charts show typical patterns of growth in height and weight during a baby's first year. Measurements for 80 per cent of all babies fall within the colored bands; a measurement slightly above or below a band is not necessarily a cause for concern, but should be referred to a doctor for evaluation. For typical measurements during the next four years of life, see page 121.

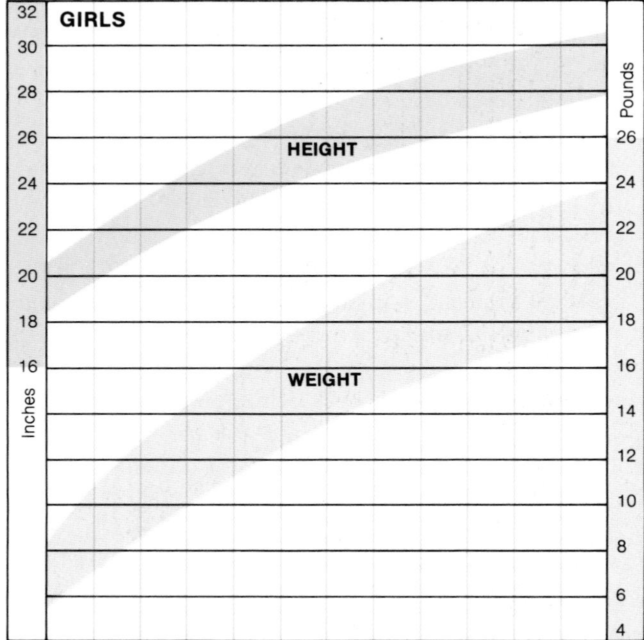

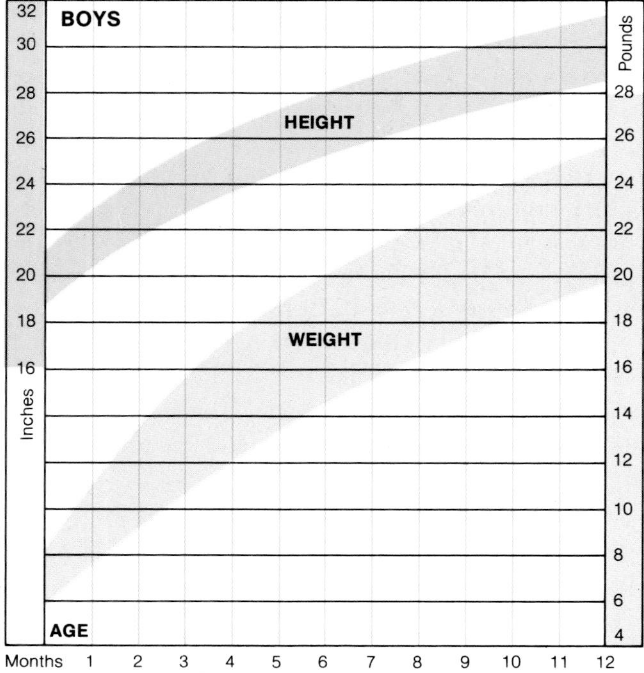

swallow enough food to nourish him. And as the novelty of mashing, spitting and smearing wears off, he will become more willing and more able to learn the eating habits that are acceptable to his elders.

The pediatrician's well-baby care

The rapid changes of the first year of life make it difficult for parents to be sure that their baby is developing normally. A pediatrician, however, is trained to make that judgment. Most medical specialists are consulted only when a patient is ill. A baby doctor has an additional role: One of his primary functions is to provide what is called well-baby care—the observation and assessment of a baby's development.

A typical well-baby visit consists essentially of a thorough physical checkup. A doctor, nurse or assistant generally interviews the parent about the baby's progress, to glean information that will alert the doctor to possible illness or growth problems. The baby is weighed and measured, and his weight and height are recorded on a growth chart; the pediatrician will compare the continuing record with statistical averages as the child grows. He will also measure the circumference of the baby's skull. A head growing at a normal rate indicates normal brain development. On the other hand, a head measurement that is not keeping pace may suggest that the brain is not growing properly, while one that is disproportionately large may signal a dangerous collection of fluid around the brain.

Well-baby visits also include sight and hearing tests. The doctor will check the baby's eyes to see that the pupils are equal in size and constrict when a light is flashed upon them; a failure to pass such tests of muscle and nerve development calls for the services of a specialized eye doctor. Hearing tests are harder to do because most types of hearing impairment do not present obvious physical signs. To check for possible deafness, the doctor will closely observe the baby's actions and ask the mother about the baby's behavior at home. Between the ages of three and six months, most babies begin to respond to noises in a recognizable fashion—waking up or quieting at the sound of their mother's voice, and turning their eyes and head toward the source of a sound.

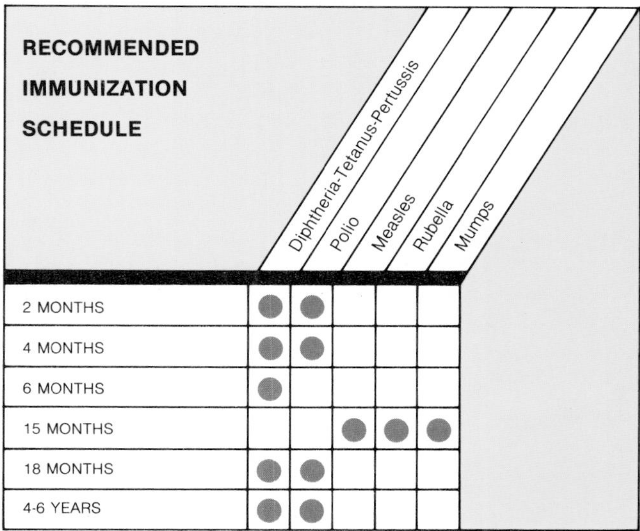

RECOMMENDED IMMUNIZATION SCHEDULE

	Diphtheria-Tetanus-Pertussis	Polio	Measles	Rubella	Mumps
2 MONTHS	●	●			
4 MONTHS	●	●			
6 MONTHS	●				
15 MONTHS			●	●	●
18 MONTHS	●	●			
4-6 YEARS	●	●			

An immunization schedule recommended by the U.S. Public Health Service protects children against a variety of diseases, all serious and potentially fatal. Parents may be required to furnish proof of these immunizations before enrolling a child in school, but a specific shot may be deferred if the child has an illness with fever at the time given in the schedule.

Nevertheless, it may take months to determine whether a child has a substantial hearing defect. All infants make the same sounds when they are very young, and parents who might otherwise suspect a hearing problem may be reassured by the sound of their child's voice, on the assumption that a baby who experiments with sounds must be hearing them as well. But a child who does not go on past the babbling stage or who gradually seems to lose interest in making any noise at all is likely to be having hearing trouble. If the pediatrician finds such signs of deafness, he will send the child to another specialist, an audiologist, for a full evaluation.

A final, but crucial, aspect of well-baby care is immunization. The practice of vaccinating children against such diseases as smallpox and polio has virtually eliminated the kinds of epidemics that once devastated entire populations. Many parents—and even some health-care professionals—have been lulled into the belief that the diseases themselves have been eradicated, but that is not the case. The lethal microbes that cause them still exist, posing a threat to young children and making the vaccination as important as ever.

The chart on page 97 lists the standard schedule of vaccinations for children from infancy to six years. Babies less than a year old are routinely given only two types of vaccine—polio and what is known as DTP, a combination of vaccines for diphtheria, tetanus and pertussis (whooping cough). The polio, diphtheria and tetanus vaccines produce relatively few adverse reactions, but the pertussis component of the DTP shot often causes such side effects as mild fever and irritability. What is worse, there have been scattered cases of far more severe side effects from the pertussis vaccine—high fever, convulsions and, in some cases, permanent brain damage.

As a result, DTP shots have become increasingly controversial in recent years. But the U.S. Centers for Disease Control, the American Academy of Pediatrics, and most doctors are convinced that the risk of the disease far outweighs the risk of the vaccination. Pertussis is a truly severe disease, particularly dangerous to infants under six months of age; it can cause major brain and lung damage, and may be fatal.

In the United States, the pertussis vaccine has all but wiped out the disease. During the 1930s, before the vaccine came into use, as many as 265,000 people fell ill with whooping cough every year, and some 7,000 died; today, the annual toll is 1,000 to 3,000 cases, and five to 20 deaths. In Great Britain, by contrast, a vast, inadvertent medical experiment showed that the disease can still be as dangerous as ever. In 1974, after three decades of nationwide pertussis vaccination, unfavorable publicity led the British people to refuse the vaccine. By 1978 the rate of immunization had dropped from about 80 per cent to about 30 per cent—and between 1977 and 1980 an epidemic of whooping cough swept the British Isles, with more than 100,000 cases reported.

Through the immunizations he gives and the assessments he makes, a pediatrician adds professional reassurance to ordinary parental care. Generally, he provides the only medical attention babies need during the first 12 months of their lives, for babies grow like the proverbial weed, quickly and under almost any set of circumstances. Parents often find that before they have a chance to savor fully such milestones of infancy as toothless grins, halting steps and shaky sips from a cup, their squalling infant has become a one-year-old—no longer a baby, but a child. ❋

A year's "swift season of growth"

It may be that nothing in all of human life is more deceiving than the apparent passivity of a newborn infant, such as the one shown at right. This tiny, helpless, crib-bound creature is in fact a complex individual, endowed with a giant capacity for learning. Over the next 12 months, in a learning spree without parallel in the animal kingdom, he will change from a babe in arms to a walking, talking, probing, playing child.

Dr. Arnold Gesell of Yale University, a pioneer in the study of child development, called the first year of life a "swift season of growth," and wrote that its transformations "far exceed those of any other period" of life after birth. Working with observations of thousands of children in studies spanning more than 50 years, Dr. Gesell and other researchers recorded specific stages of development in this crucial year. The picture essay on the following pages, based largely on data assembled by Dr. Victor C. Vaughan of Temple University School of Medicine, summarizes much of this research.

The essay describes and illustrates a typical child's patterns of behavior in three major areas at eight critical points in the year. First, it follows the steps by which the child learns to use and coordinate muscles to achieve mobility and to control the objects in his world. Next, it describes his social behavior, including his responses to change and his increasing give-and-take interactions with other people. Finally, it traces the evolution of the peculiarly human gift of language, from the newborn's all-purpose cry to the child's mastery of the first true words in his vocabulary.

All these chronological steps are approximate, subject to wide variations in perfectly normal behavior. Children who are precocious in some areas may be slow to develop in others, and on any given day a child may perform poorly because of hunger, fatigue or distractions; indeed, it is unlikely that a child will match all the patterns through the year. Still, the essay as a whole provides parents with a reliable set of criteria for observation.

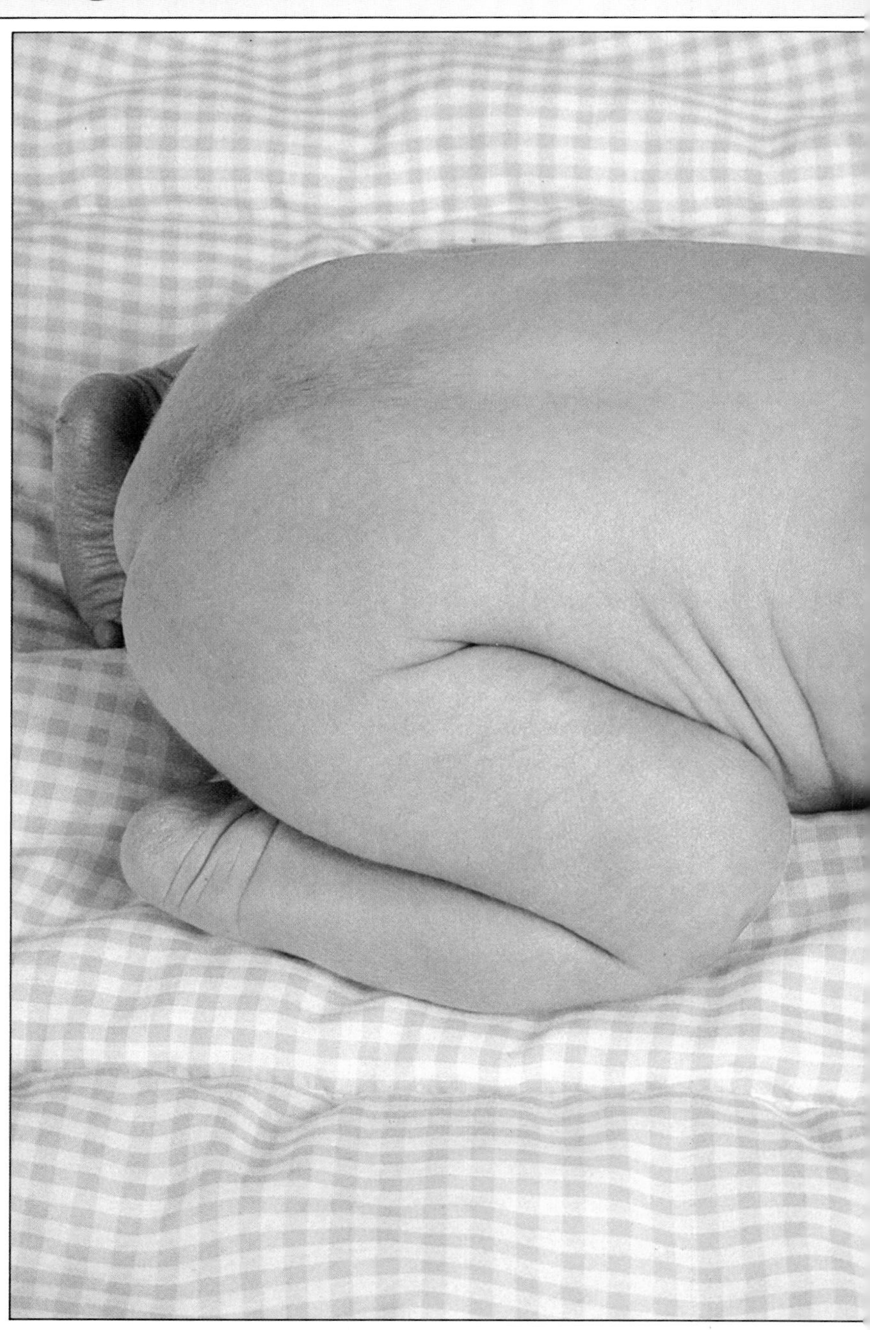

THE NEWBORN INFANT

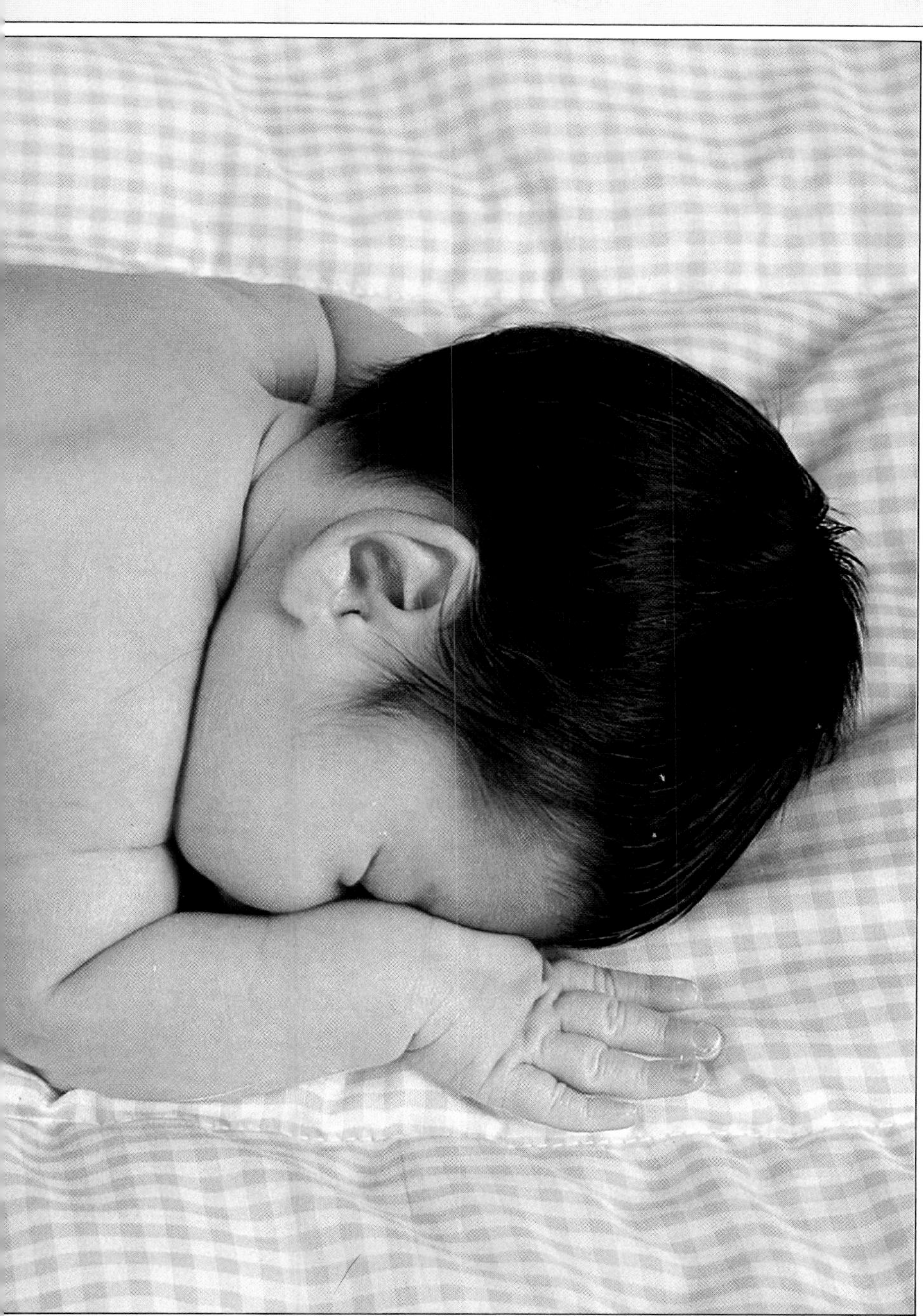

Muscle control

Lying on his stomach, the newborn sleeps with legs drawn up and arms bent toward the body in a symmetrical posture *(left)*. He can turn his face to one side to avoid suffocating, but if he is lifted to a testing position called ventral suspension, in which he is supported horizontally by a hand under his abdomen, his head will sag downward. On his back, he lies stiff, with arms and legs similarly bent.

Many of his movements are simple reflexes, which will gradually evolve into more deliberate, voluntary motions. The dramatic Moro, or startle, reflex, for example, may be stimulated by a sudden noise or movement: The infant tenses and flings out his arms and legs, then rapidly brings his arms together and clenches his fists. This clasping motion may be a survival mechanism from a remote primate ancestry, in which newborns grabbed for a tree limb or a mother's hairy body to avoid a fall. Other reflexes are described and illustrated on pages 61-63.

Social behavior

Shown a series of drawings of simple shapes in a variety of patterns, the newborn will stare briefly but intently at the one most resembling the human face. Tests indicate that the newborn can distinguish between voices and prefers high-pitched, female ones; as early as the first week of life, he will turn his head more readily to the sound of his mother's voice uttering his name than to an unfamiliar voice or his mother's voice uttering other words.

Language

The newborn communicates almost exclusively by cries that vary little in intensity and manner. His language capacity is marked more by receptivity than by utterances: In learning to recognize his mother's voice and his own name, for example, he is acquiring the foundations of linguistic awareness.

AT FOUR WEEKS

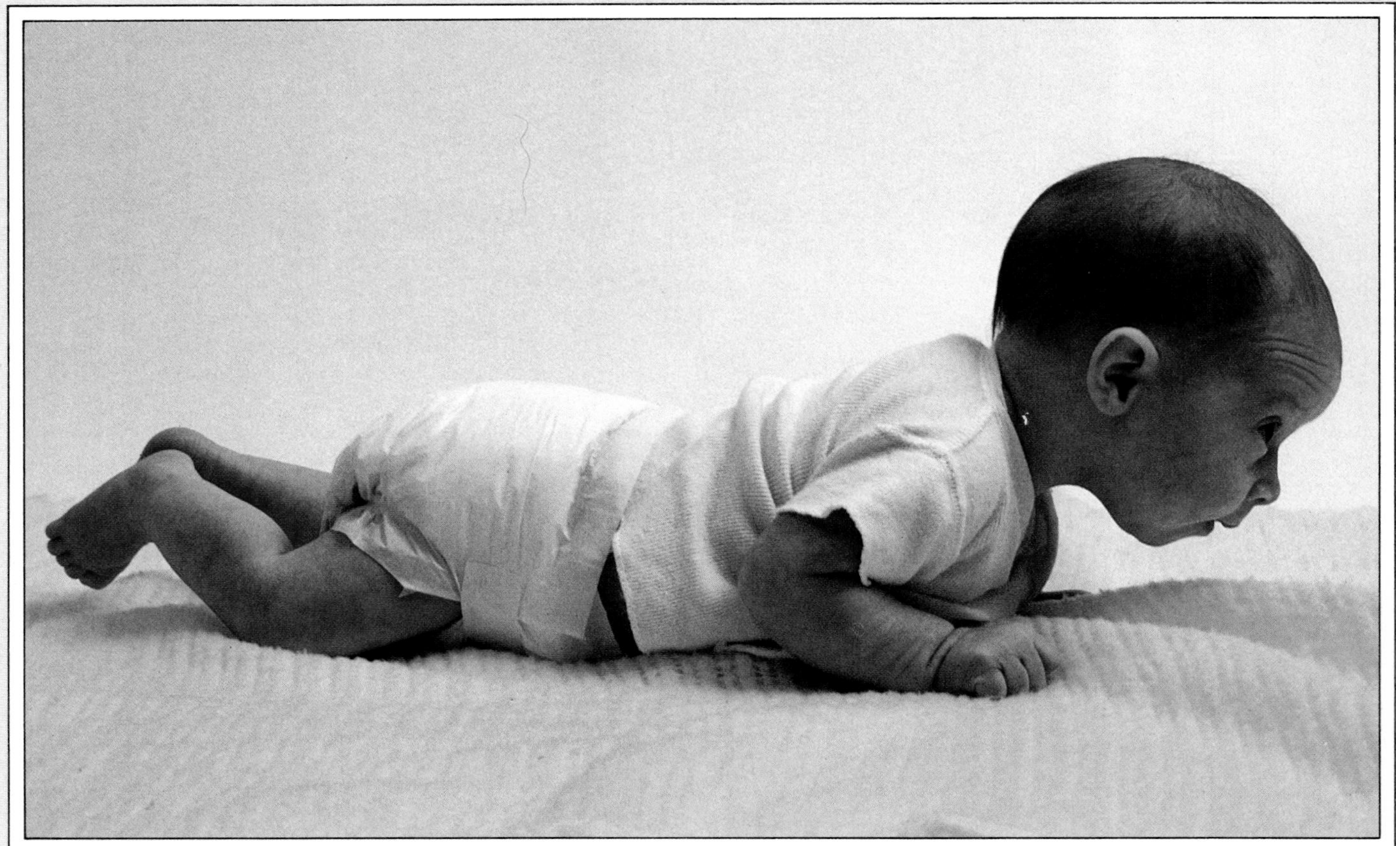

Muscle control

When lying down, the infant assumes relatively relaxed postures. If he is placed on his stomach, he can extend his legs slightly, raise his chin above the mattress and turn his head *(above)*. On his back, he tends to assume a reflexive position, with a pattern of flexed and extended limbs aptly called the fencing posture *(pages 61 and 63)*.

In ventral suspension, the infant can momentarily lift his head level with the line of his body, but when he is pulled into a sitting position his head lags behind and wobbles uncontrollably. At this age he exhibits long staring spells, as his eyeball muscles come under increasing control. He will gaze at windows, ceilings or people, and will follow the path of an object as it is moved across his field of vision. If a bell is tinkled nearby, he will suspend all muscle activity to listen—a kind of auditory fixation or "staring" at sound.

Social behavior

Held face-to-face in his mother's arms, the four-week-old will move his body in time to her speech rhythms as she talks to him; these movement patterns are so distinct that an experienced observer can match a taped voice to a motion picture of a baby's movements. The beginnings of a social smile may also be seen—a marked facial brightening used by the infant to greet someone, as opposed to earlier faint grimaces with no social meaning.

Language

The cries that were insistent and similar in the first weeks are beginning to be differentiated, so that parents may be able to distinguish between cries of hunger, pain and the like. In addition, cries are supplemented by occasional mews and brief throaty sounds, not communicative in themselves, but precursors of pleasurable social babbling.

AT EIGHT WEEKS

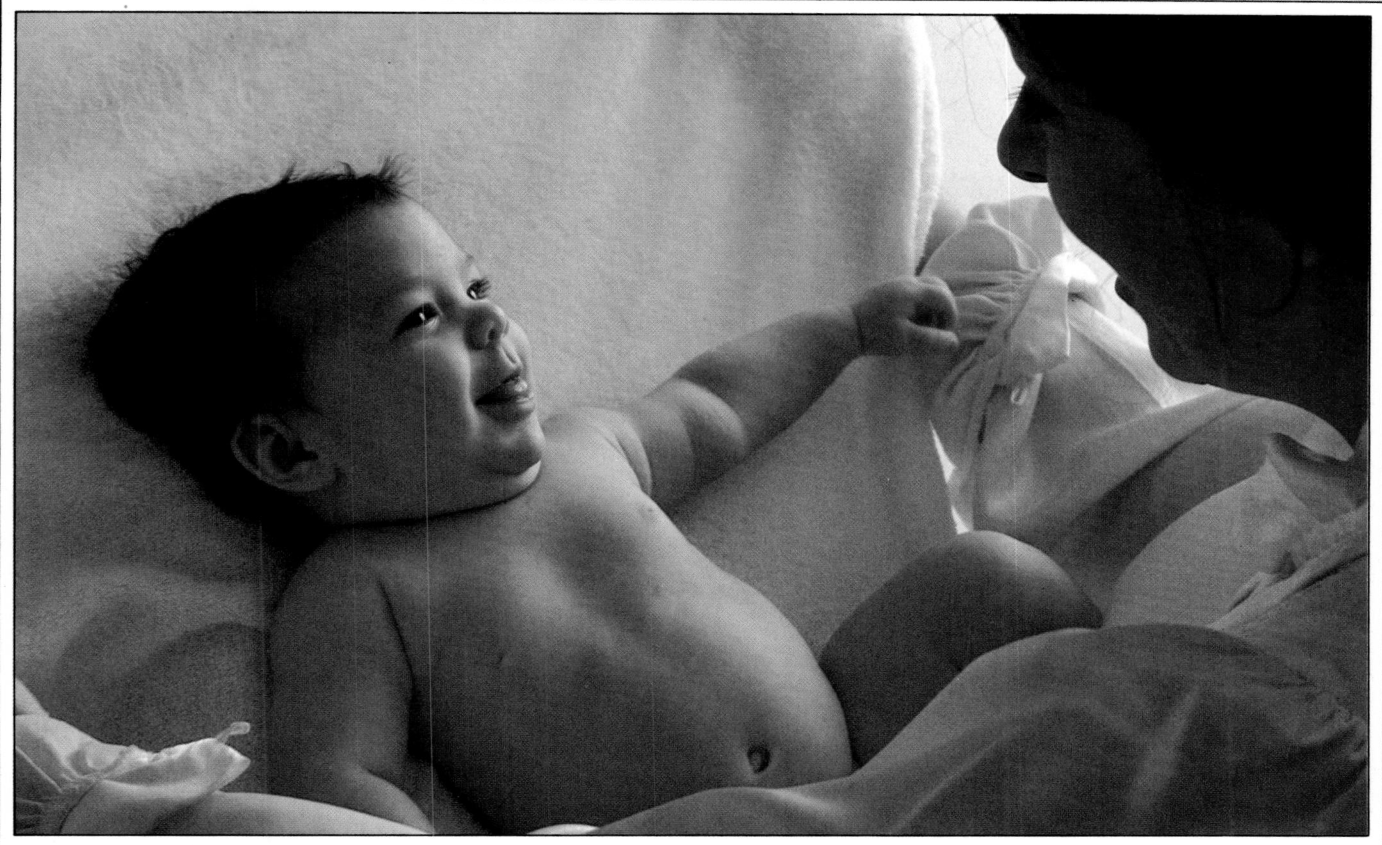

Muscle control

Propped on pillows or lying on his back, the infant can now track an object over a much wider range: If the object is shown to him at an angle of 90° to his eyes and then carried over him from side to side through an arc of 180°, he will follow it with his eyes and head all the way.

There are no big changes in the stomach-down position, though he can control his head better and raise it farther from the mattress. When held in the ventral suspension position, he can now hold his head up steadily at the level of the rest of his body, but it still lags behind his body when he is drawn up to a sitting posture. The early grasp reflex is beginning to disappear; with improving hand-and-eye coordination, an active grasp is gradually taking its place.

Social behavior

The eight-week-old infant will smile regularly on social contact with his mother *(above)* or another visitor. Research findings indicate that such smiles are elicited by the infant's discovery that he has control —at first inadvertently, then predictably —over some aspects of his environment. Typical acts of control include summoning his mother to his crib with noise or activity, and setting a nearby toy or other inanimate object into motion.

Language

The infant's varied cries are now clearly distinguishable from one another, and signal a wider range of meanings; a parent can interpret not only basic cries of hunger, discomfort or pain, but also cries of simple fussiness or fatigue. Other sounds, often described as cooing, may be made in response to voices. The infant who produced small throaty noises at four weeks can now make such sounds as ''ooh'' and ''aah''—building blocks of linguistic development.

AT TWELVE WEEKS

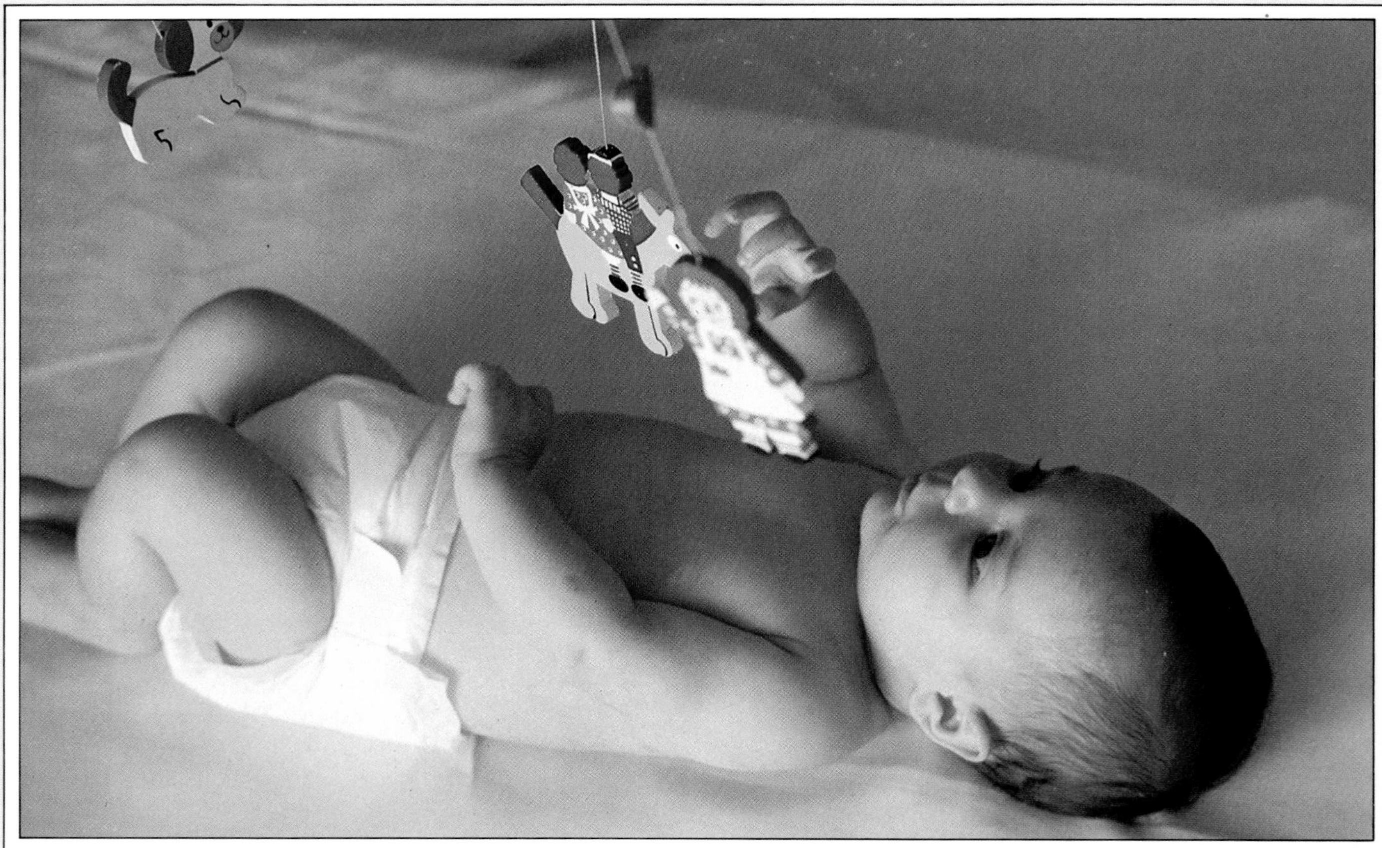

Muscle control

When lying on his back, the baby frequently shifts from the fencing posture to respond to persons or objects around him. The automatic grasp reflex has now given way to a conscious though still-imperfect grasp. If an object is placed within his reach or offered to him, he will try to seize it *(above)* but is unlikely to connect with it; if he does succeed, he will soon drop the object. He will also wave excitedly toward a toy that is held beyond his reach, in a nonsocial gesture that has no relation to an older baby's deliberate "bye-bye" wave. The automatic startle reflex is now fading; when startled, the baby may simply cry or try to withdraw.

When lying on his stomach, the baby can raise his head and chest from the mattress with the support of his extended arms. In the ventral suspension position, he now lifts his head above the line of his body. Supported in a sitting position, he now has partial control over his head, though it tends to tilt forward a little and bob erratically.

Social behavior

In his mother's arms or in his crib, the baby pays relatively extended attention to someone who talks or plays with him—a clear advance upon his capacity in earlier weeks, when he was easily distracted. He is now clearly aware of pleasant sounds and may enjoy listening to music. If he is fussing, a rhythmic or continuous sound—whether a piece of music or the whine of a vacuum cleaner—may quiet him.

Language

In a time of especially rapid development, the infant makes delighted squealing or chortling sounds when entertained by another person. He now begins to assemble vowel sounds into compound noises such as "aah, ngah," uttered with obvious pleasure in response to social contact.

AT SIXTEEN WEEKS

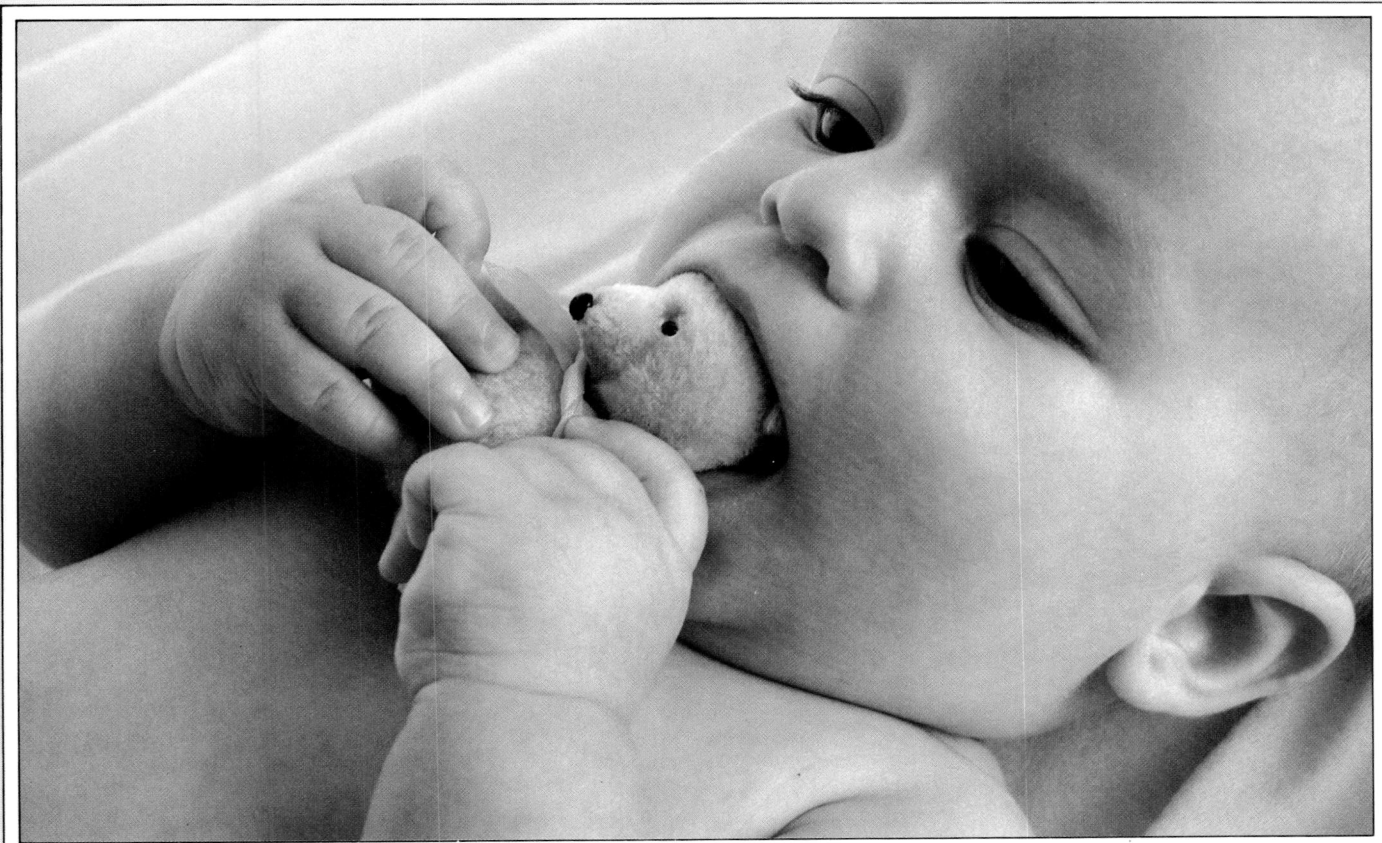

Muscle control

In an important turning point of development, the baby organizes groups of movements. When offered a sizable object, for example, he will seize it firmly and probably bring it up to his mouth for exploratory tasting and sucking *(above)*. He will not, however, investigate a small object such as a raisin if it is placed before him.

Lying on his back, the baby usually assumes a symmetrical posture rather than the fencing posture. When he lies on his stomach, his legs are now fully extended. He lifts his upper body high off the mattress, with his head sometimes held nearly vertical. When he is pulled by his hands to a sitting position his head no longer lags, and he can hold it steady. The baby enjoys sitting upright, partially propped up with pillows. And when pulled up and held erect, he pushes down with his feet—not in the newborn's reflexive stepping in place, but in his first attempts to balance his body.

Social behavior

The smile continues to evolve as the baby's chief tool of social exchange, but other expressions also come into play. If he is pleased, he will laugh aloud, and if a person amusing him leaves, he may change expression, fuss or cry. He becomes excited at the sight of his food, waving his arms and legs. He fully recognizes familiar faces, especially his mother's; at the sight of a stranger, his expression may become sober.

Language

The baby now listens to a nearby human voice, and uses his own laughter as a more elaborate kind of vocalization than the earlier coos and vowel sounds. His repertoire of sounds expands and refines as he purposely experiments with bubbles, chuckles and gurgles, exercising the oral and breathing apparatus that underlies articulate speech.

AT TWENTY-EIGHT WEEKS

Muscle control

If placed in a sitting position, the baby can now remain there for brief periods on his own, though his back is slightly rounded and he requires light support at the hips *(right)*. Held erect, he may carry most of his weight on his feet, bouncing up and down.

When lying down, he has remarkable mobility. He can roll over completely, from his stomach to his back and onto his stomach again. He will pivot on his stomach to reach for an object; such squirming motions foreshadow later attempts to crawl.

Using his improved control of posture and motion, the baby spends much of his time in manually exploring his world. With a grasp in which the thumb is pressed against the side of the forefinger, he can hold a large object such as a rattle, and can transfer it from one hand to the other. He still cannot pick up a raisin-sized pellet, but he will rake at it vigorously with his fingers.

Social behavior

The baby laughs at the sight of himself in a mirror, and will pat his image. For company, he almost invariably prefers his mother, and when held in her arms, may fuss at the approach of strangers. The picture at right captures two typical features: pleasurable patting and the fixation on the mother. At this stage the baby may develop so-called separation anxiety, and cry when his mother leaves the room. He is also conscious of changes in tone when someone is speaking to him; if a smiling companion suddenly frowns, the baby will immediately stop laughing or smiling.

Language

Repeated sequences of vowel sounds such as "ooh-ooh" or "aah-aah" are typical vocalizations, and the baby will babble to anyone who talks to him. His interest now in the tones and inflections of adult speech is a preparation for his later understanding of words.

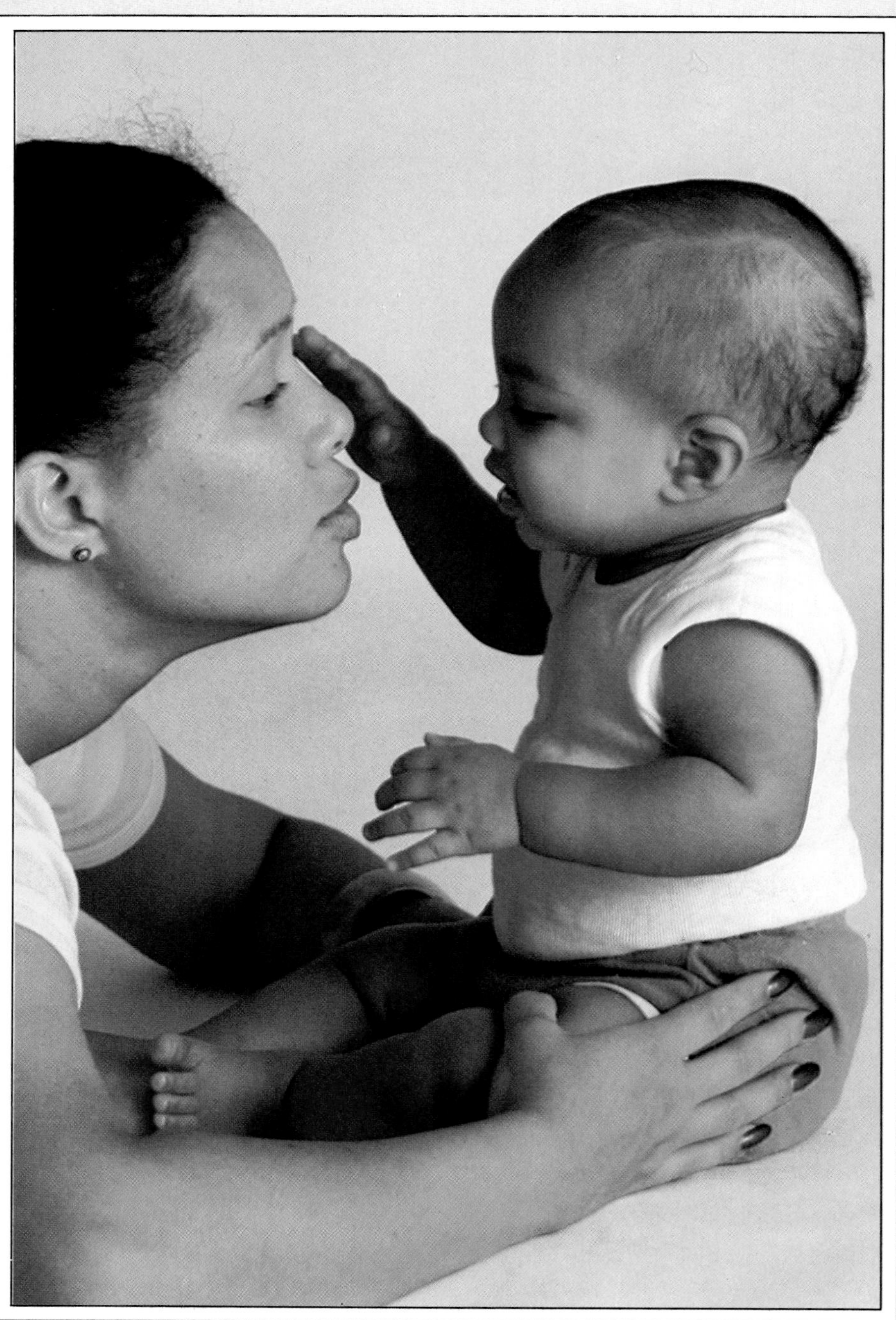

AT FORTY WEEKS

Muscle control

The baby can work up to a sitting position and sit up without help indefinitely *(right)*. He performs this feat at every opportunity; in fact, he rarely lies down except to sleep. When sitting, he holds his back straight; he can also lean over and recover his balance. The baby pulls himself to his feet by using the sides of his crib; if his hands are held, he may take a few wobbly steps. The usual mode of travel, however, is creeping or crawling.

He uses his hands in new ways. For example, he now grasps raisin-sized objects, using his thumb and forefinger in a pincer movement, while steadying the heel and palm of his hand against the surface on which the object rests. He will explore a hollow object such as a small bell by poking the interior with his forefinger.

Social behavior

The baby is less dependent on his mother's immediate presence, partly because he can follow her around more easily, and partly because he is learning that a person or object out of his sight has not really vanished. If a toy is shown to him, then covered with a cloth, he will confidently uncover it; the same lesson is embodied in the game of peek-a-boo. Another game the baby enjoys is pat-a-cake, for he has learned to imitate such gestures as clapping hands. He likes to have people around him; he may wave them bye-bye, but generally prefers that they stay. He will release a toy if a person gives it a gentle tug.

Language

A growing dexterity of tongue and lips and a newly developed ability to stick out his tongue are developments that will help the baby become articulate in time. At this point, however, his own use of language has progressed only to repetitive consonant sounds, such as "da-da" and "ma-ma," with no real understanding of their meanings.

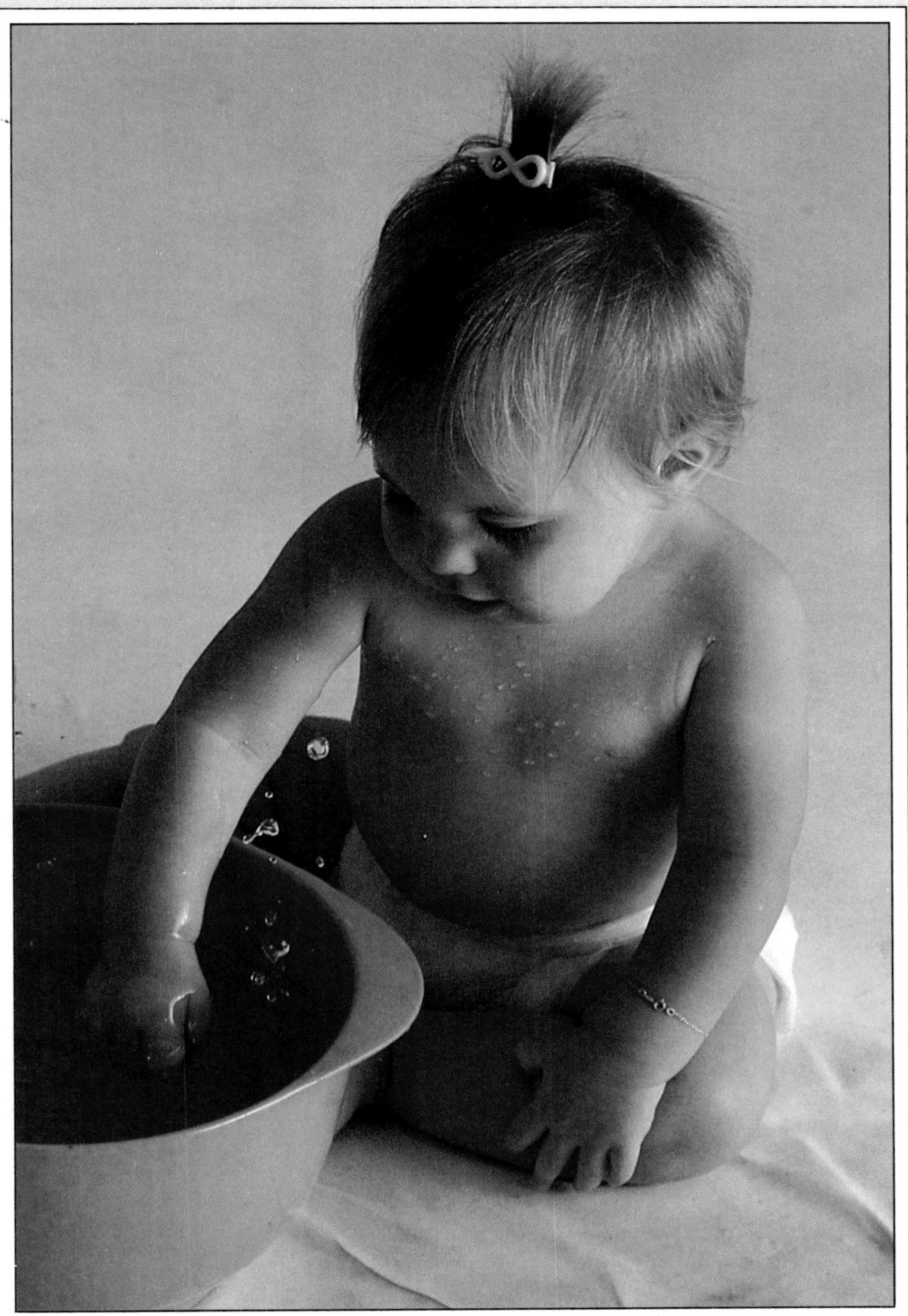

THE ONE-YEAR-OLD CHILD

Muscle control

Although a one-year-old still creeps, and does so with surprising speed, he has an ungovernable urge to get up on his feet. With an assist for balance, the child can rise from the floor and stand erect *(far right)*. From that position he may move around the room sideways, bracing himself on chairs or low tables, in a form of locomotion called cruising. Alternatively, if one hand is held, the child can get around slowly by himself.

Manual dexterity has improved significantly. He now uses an unassisted pincer movement of thumb and forefinger to pick up a raisin-sized object, without needing to steady his hand. He can place an object into a container, turn a bottle upside down to empty it, and hold one object briefly over another in a forerunner of tower building. Given several cubes, he will place them on a table one after another—the rudiments of counting.

Social behavior

The child now willingly hands over a toy held in his hand if he is asked, or even at a simple gesture *(right)*. Increasingly involved in the family's social life, he takes part in such simple games as ball rolling. He is often the center of attention, and may repeat a performance that draws a laugh the first time around. He feeds himself with his fingers, and when he is being dressed will help by holding out an arm for a sleeve or a foot for a shoe.

Language

The child now fully distinguishes and understands such once-meaningless sounds as "ma-ma" and "da-da," and may know a few other words, too. He understands what is meant by "give it to me" when an object is asked for, and is beginning to obey such simple commands. He echoes familiar words when they are repeated for him, and he listens intently to new words he is about to acquire.

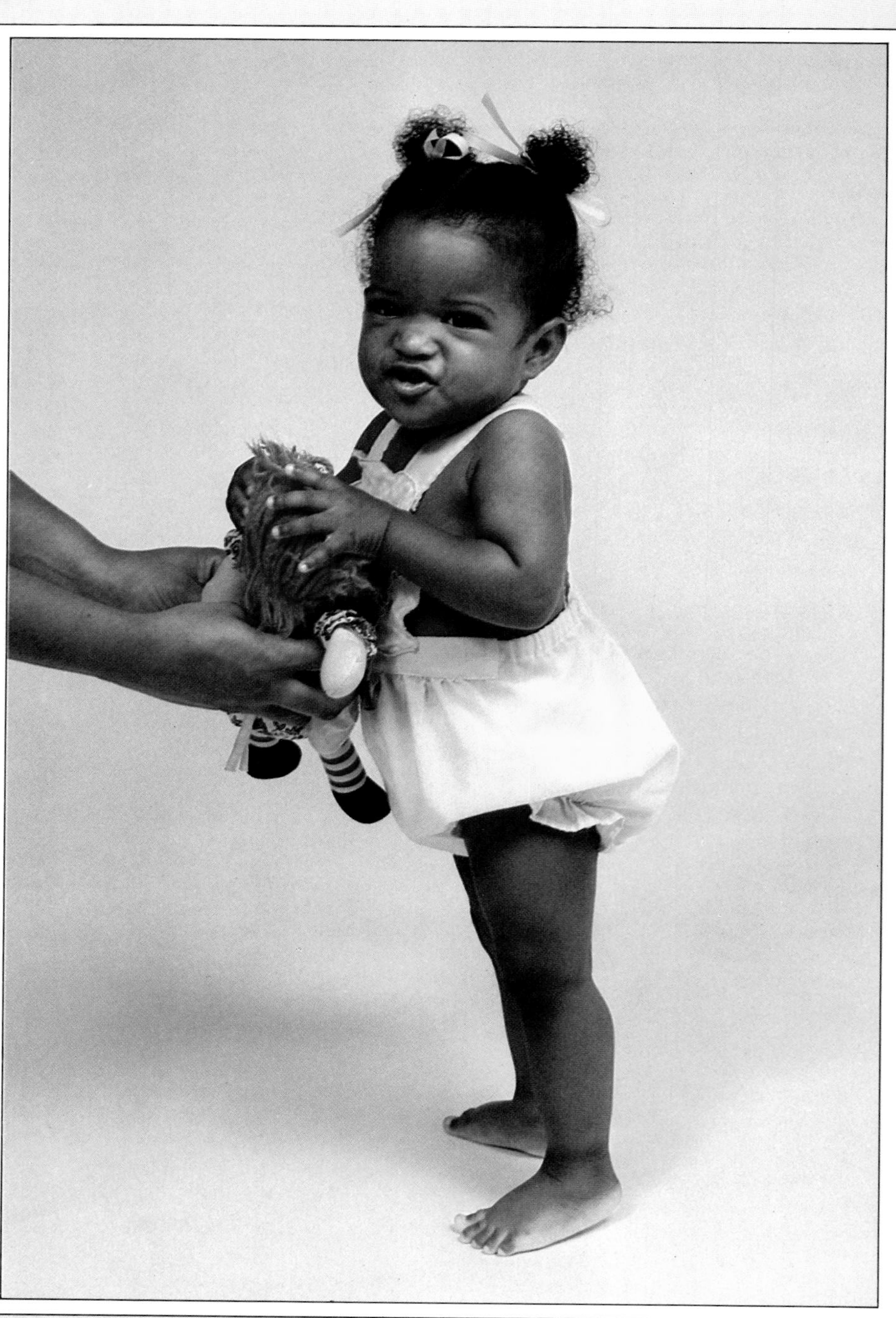

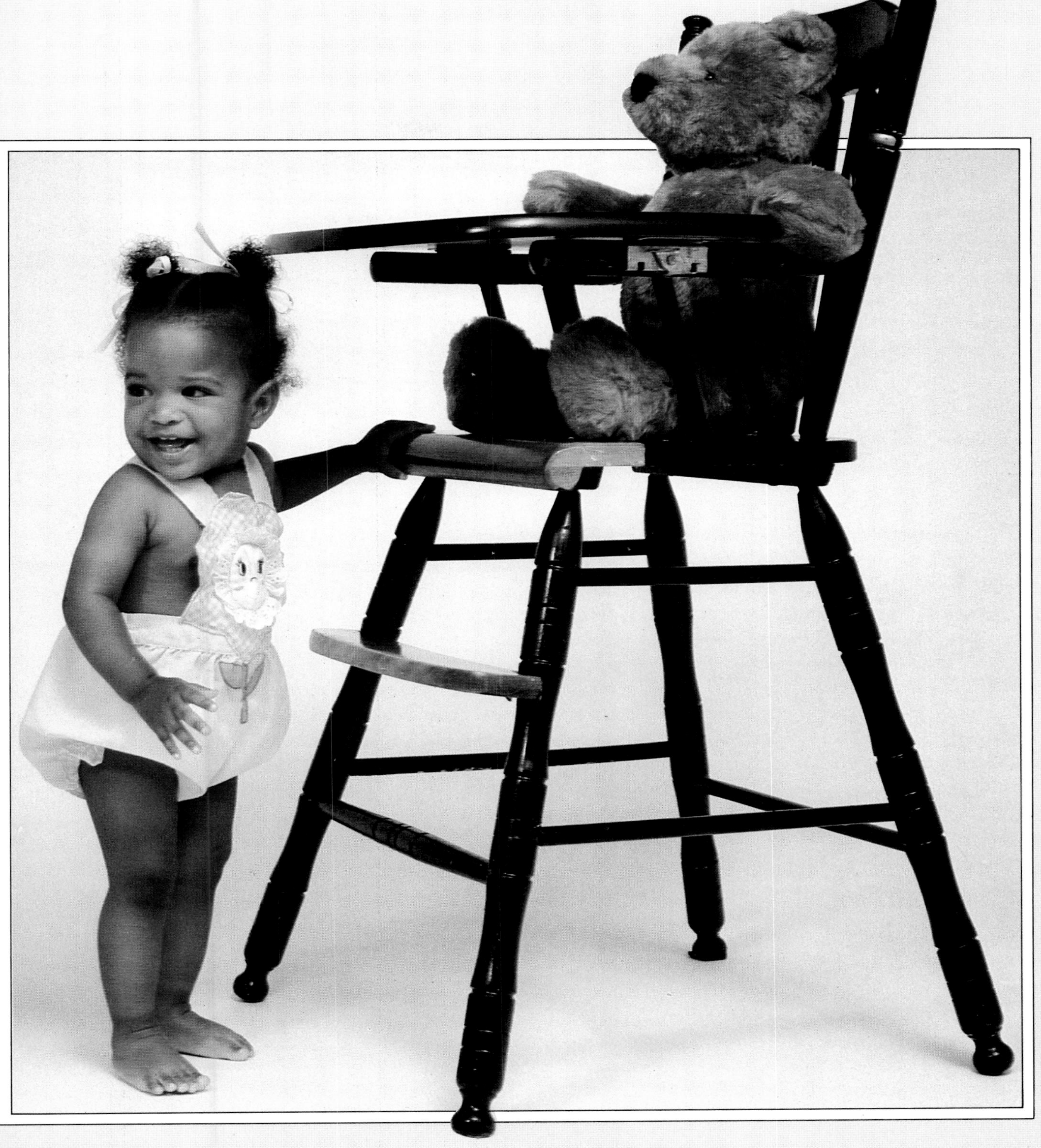

CHAPTER 5

The years from one to five

Safeguards against accidents
Teaching a finicky eater what to eat
Winning the bedtime battle
Toilet training: a job of patient persuasion
Discipline: learning to live by the rules
Mastering humanity's greatest skill—the use of language

At 15 months Susan is happy, healthy—and difficult. When her mother tries to restrain her long enough to change and dress her, she squirms and cries, "No! No!" At breakfast, she may accept several spoonfuls of cereal, then send the bowl clattering to the floor. If her father urges her to drink her milk, she may take a few dutiful sips—and turn the cup upside down on her head. Set free, she toddles off uncertainly, tripping and falling as she goes. She constantly asserts her independence, but when her mother leaves the room for a moment, Susan dissolves into misery and begins to wail.

Susan's parents sometimes wonder if they will survive this ornery stage between infancy and childhood. But changes come rapidly. By her second birthday, Susan will dash about sure-footedly and enjoy run-and-catch games. Mealtime will be less of a battleground; she will have learned to appreciate food more for eating than for playing. By three or four, she will be ready to venture outside her home and mingle with other children and adults, perhaps at a nursery school. As a preschooler, in contrast to her balky, self-centered one-year-old self, Susan will be affectionate, cooperative, and eager to please—at least, most of the time.

Between the ages of one and five, the period that forms the subject of this chapter, a healthy child develops from a person-in-the-making to a fully human being. Much of the progress is almost automatic. In a normal environment, all healthy children learn to walk and talk when their bodies and minds reach specific levels of maturity. At around the age of two and a half, they sense that it is time to forsake diapers for the potty. To a large extent, their bodies tell them how much sleep they need and how much food to eat.

But the process of development is not entirely automatic. With limited judgment and experience, children cannot protect themselves from accidents and illness, and parents must do this for them. During the first half of the period, parents train a toddler in such skills and habits as taking meals, sleeping and using the toilet in ways and rhythms that conform to those of the rest of the family. In the second half, other problems come to the fore: Parents teach the child how to behave toward others and how to tell right from wrong, and enforce these teachings with discipline. Toward the end of these preschool years, they are likely to concern themselves with the youngster's ability to use language effectively. To parents, caring for a young child often seems like several full-time jobs.

Safeguards against accidents

First and foremost, however, parents are a child's protectors. They must defend him from physical hazards as he explores a rapidly widening world. They also must safeguard him against hazards to health, making sure he has regular checkups, is immunized against preventable diseases, and is screened for defects that could impair his development.

Of the two kinds of hazards, the physical are by far the more pervasive and dangerous. Accidents are the greatest threat to children over one year of age; in the United States, more children die from them than from the five leading dis-

Jingling a tambourine, a toddler moves joyously to the sound of music. By the age of two years most children enjoy such dance movements as turning in circles, swaying, swinging the arms and bouncing the body from the knees.

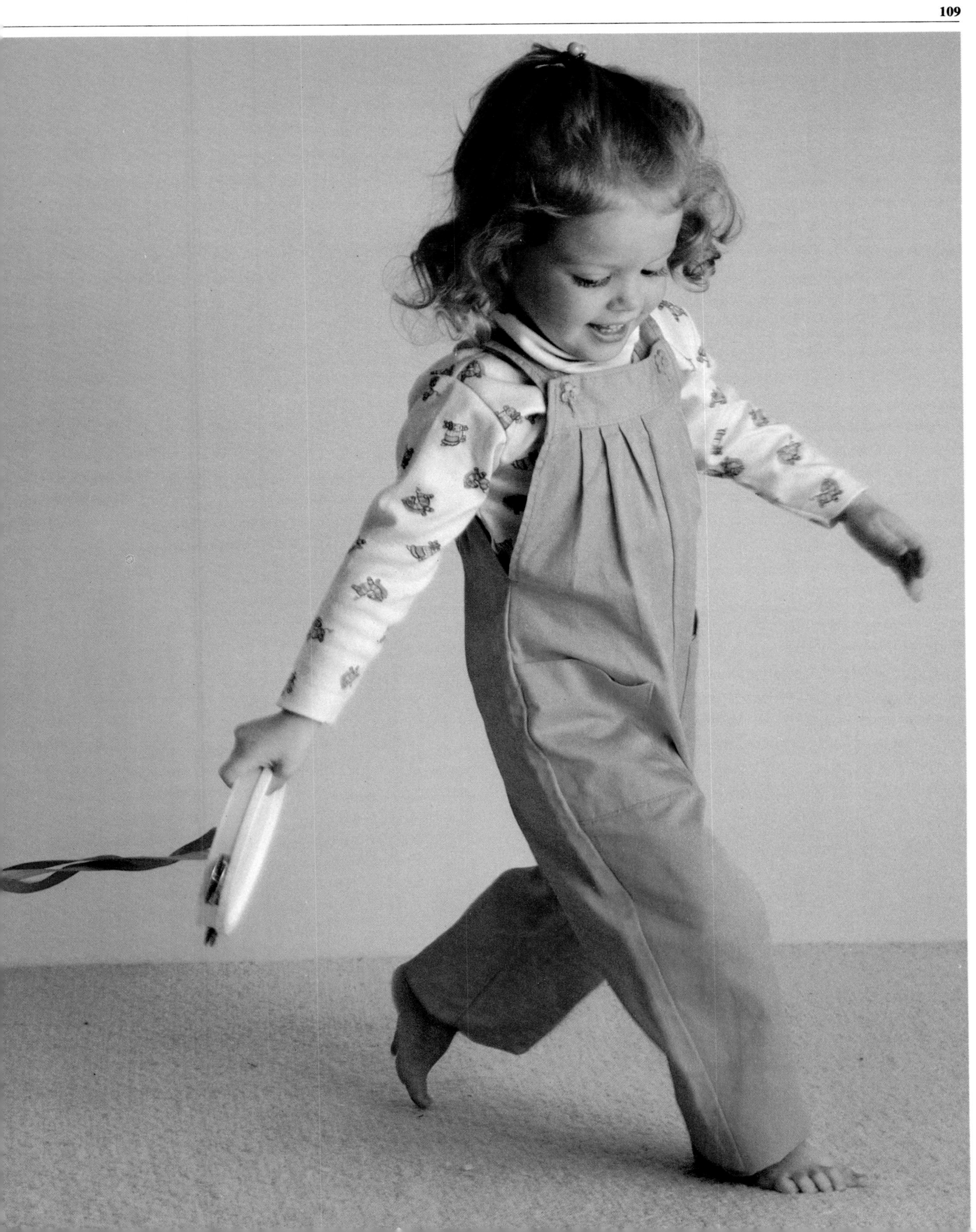

eases combined. Never take safety for granted, even if you think your children are grown-up enough to understand the rules. Throughout the preschool years, a child's motor skills greatly exceed his judgment, and the time to start baby-proofing the house is as soon as the infant begins to get around under his own power—usually at about nine months of age. From then on, his range of movement increases rapidly. Between the ages of 12 and 16 months, the child takes his first unaided steps and becomes an adept climber, able to clamber from chair to counter to cupboard. Medicine cabinets and upper kitchen shelves are no longer beyond reach.

Toddling children are avid explorers, examining as many as a hundred objects or spaces in an hour. They are literally into everything—yet their muscle control is poor. Toddlers who have just begun to walk cannot always put on the brakes to avoid falling, or steer well enough to avoid an obstacle. Their memory is short. They may trip repeatedly over the same step because they simply forget it is there. They plunge ahead with no recollection of past warnings and no forethought about the consequences. The word "No!" has little meaning at first, and an independent child may decide to ignore it if the forbidden action is attractive enough. One mother's most vivid memory of her toddler was discovering him astride his tricycle, about to pedal down the stairs. In such situations, obviously, the only solution is to snatch the child from danger, then try to direct him to safer activity.

At this stage of omnivorous curiosity, children will put almost anything into their mouths. Unlike adults, they are not repelled by foul smells and tastes. In studies conducted during the 1960s, Dr. Burton White, a child-development expert at Harvard University, gave a group of young children a variety of foodstuffs. All tasted much the same; they differed chiefly in their scents, which ranged from chocolate or floral to extremely unpleasant smells, such as that of rotten eggs. Dr. White found that the amounts the children swallowed were in no way related to the odors of the substances.

For a parent, the object of accident prevention is to give a young child as much access to the home as possible while protecting him. Ideally, the parent would know what a toddler is doing at all times. At the least, parents should check every room for poisons, electrical outlets, flammable materials, sharp objects, and anything that could conceivably smother a small child *(right)*. The hazards are not always obvious; some contents of food cupboards, for example, such as vanilla or almond extracts, are powerful poisons if swallowed straight from the bottle. Think also about hazards associated with visits away from home or visitors to your home—the pills on Grandmother's nightstand, or the cosmetics and matches in an unattended purse.

Next to the home, the most dangerous place for a child is the family car. Every year, more than a thousand children under the age of five die in automobile accidents, and another 70,000 are injured. According to experts at the American Academy of Pediatrics, about 90 per cent of these deaths could be prevented, and about 80 per cent of the injuries prevented or reduced, by the correct use of seat belts. Never hold a child on your lap in the front seat: In a collision at 30 miles per hour, the child would be ripped from your arms and crushed against the dashboard with as much force as if he had been dropped from a third-floor window. No matter how short the trip, every infant and toddler should be strapped into a carrier appropriate to his size and weight *(page 112)*. Children who are more than four years old or weigh more than 40 pounds should wear regular seat belts.

Like all aspects of child care, a concern with safety must be kept in balance. On the one hand, do not let yourself become so obsessed with protecting your child that you stifle his creativity and freedom to explore. Minor cuts and scrapes are a normal part of childhood; the child who never has a mishap is an overprotected child. On the other hand, be prepared for the worst. Despite all precautions, active young children are always at risk of serious injury—broken bones, deep cuts, poisoning, burns, electric shock, choking, animal bites. Every parent should know the specific first-aid measures for dealing with such emergencies.

The roles of the doctor and dentist

Safeguarding a child's health is relatively easy for modern parents, mainly because medical advances have greatly reduced the risk of childhood illnesses. Even healthy children,

How to childproof a home

Though minor accidents are a part of growing up, many can be prevented. Far more important, of course, is the prevention of serious injuries such as burns or poisonings. Because most childhood accidents occur at home, parents should take steps to render this environment safe for a child's combination of mobility, curiosity and inexperience.

Ways to prevent the most common home accidents are given below. Some precautions apply to the house as a whole; others are listed for the rooms or areas that are most hazardous for a child. All together, the items constitute a "childproofing" checklist.

General

- Block unused electrical outlets with childproof caps, heavy electrical tape or furniture.
- Never leave an extension cord plugged in unless it is connected to an appliance.
- Unplug appliances when they are not in use, and coil their cords out of a child's reach. Keep appliances away from water and potential sources of water, such as faucets.
- Keep matches and lighters out of reach and set a screen in front of a fireplace.
- Install smoke detectors and fire extinguishers on every floor of the house.
- Use nontoxic interior paints.
- Keep doorways and halls well lighted and free of obstacles.
- Avoid slippery floors by keeping wax to a minimum and by wiping up spills as soon as they occur.
- Anchor carpets and rugs in place.
- Check floors daily for small, swallowable objects and for tripping hazards.
- Make sure that balconies and porches have sturdy guard railings.
- Open windows from the top rather than the bottom; do not permit a child to sit on window sills or to lean against screens. Never set a crib under a window.
- Never leave an infant alone in a baby carrier on a table, counter or chair.
- Dispose of plastic bags as soon as you have emptied them; if a child puts a plastic bag over his head in play, he can suffocate.
- Place purses and brief cases out of a child's reach; they often contain objects or medicines that are dangerous if swallowed.
- If the telephone rings while you are working with a potentially dangerous substance, such as a cleaning agent, take it with you to the telephone.

Child's room

- Make sure the slats of the child's crib are less than three inches apart, and always keep the sides of the crib raised and locked. As the baby grows, lower the level of the mattress.
- Never leave a pillow or loose bedclothes in an infant's crib; they can interfere with the baby's breathing.
- Never leave a bottle propped in the mouth of an unattended infant.
- Never leave an unattended baby on a changing table. Everywhere in the changing area, keep diaper pins and other potential hazards out of the baby's reach.
- Use a toy box with a lid equipped with hinges that keep it from snapping shut.

Kitchen

- Do not leave a small child unattended in a kitchen.
- Keep knives and other dangerous utensils out of a child's reach.
- Use extra care around the stove. Turn pot handles toward the rear of the stove, so that a child cannot grab them. Fry foods and boil liquids on back burners only; use the front burners for low-heat cooking.
- Keep high chairs away from the busy areas of the kitchen, such as stoves and counters.
- Store household cleaners, soaps, vitamin supplements, food extracts and other dangerous substances out of a child's reach. Take the same precaution with such foods as dried beans and peanuts, which can choke a child.
- During meals, keep hot foods at the center of the table where a child cannot reach them; never pass hot food over a child's head.

Bathroom

- Do not leave a small child unattended in a bathroom.
- Store medicine, household cleaners and toiletry items, including hair-care products and cosmetics, out of a child's reach.
- Install abrasive treads in a tub or shower.
- Always test the temperature of bath water before bathing a child in the tub; it should be about 90° to 100° F.—body temperature.

Storeroom or workroom

- Instruct a child to stay away from these areas; if possible, keep them locked.
- Keep paints, solvents, insecticides, laundry soaps, bleaches and other dangerous substances in their original, labeled containers and out of a child's reach.
- Store potentially dangerous tools where a child cannot reach them. Disconnect power tools that are not in use.
- Remove the door of an unused refrigerator or freezer, or seal the door shut with fiber-reinforced tape and turn it toward the wall.

Garage

- Keep the garage locked when not in use.
- Keep all potentially dangerous tools and substances out of a child's reach.
- If you install an electric garage door, use one with sensors that open the door automatically if it strikes an object while closing.

Stairs

- Install safety gates at the top and bottom of a staircase to prevent falls.
- Instruct an older child not to run, play or sit on the stairs.
- Keep stairs free of clutter.
- Make sure the stairs are well lighted and have a sturdy handrail.

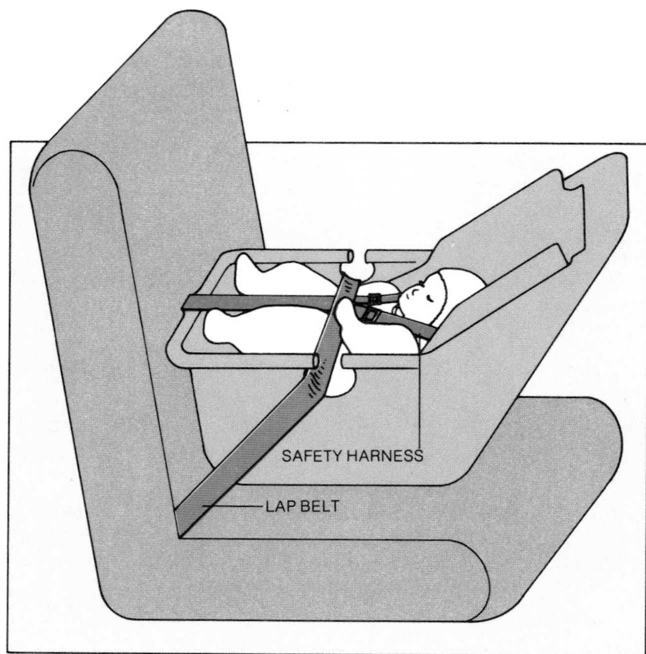

During the first year of life, a baby in a car should be protected by a rear-facing, semireclining safety seat; the example shown here, anchored to the car seat by the vehicle's lap belt, secures the child with a safety harness in a tub-shaped cradle. The best place for any child is the middle of the rear seat, but the high back of this carrier makes it safe for front-seat riding.

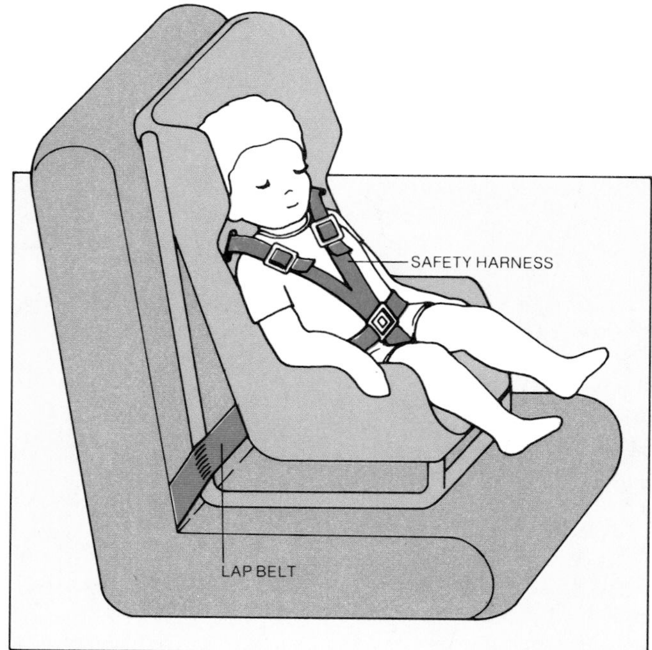

Designed for toddlers from about one to four years old, this forward-facing safety seat, like the one at top, uses both a lap belt and a harness; several manufacturers offer convertible models that can be reversed for the infant position. For children more than four years old and heavier than 40 pounds, the automobile's regular seat belt provides adequate protection.

however, need professional health care and regular examinations by the doctor. After periodic checkups during the first half year of life, these so-called well-baby visits to the pediatrician need not be made on a tight or burdensome schedule. The American Academy of Pediatrics recommends a visit every three months between the ages of six and 18 months, a yearly visit between the ages of two and six, and a visit every two years thereafter.

To some extent, the pediatrician will use these checkups to confirm findings already made by the parents. For example, a doctor will check that a child's height and weight are within the normal ranges for his age—but by using the charts on pages 96 and 121, the parents themselves can make these checks between visits to the doctor. By contrast, only regular visits can ensure that a child is properly immunized against a host of diseases that were once childhood scourges—polio, diphtheria, tetanus, whooping cough, measles, mumps, and rubella (commonly known as German measles).

These diseases are now so rare that some parents believe they no longer pose a threat and that vaccinations are no longer important. This is not true. The organisms that cause the infections are still plentiful, and are fully capable of causing a fatal or crippling illness. To be protected against them, children must be immunized according to a specific schedule between two months and school age *(page 97)*. It is the parents' responsibility to keep a permanent record of their children's immunizations. Pediatricians do not keep such records indefinitely; at most, they are required to maintain a file for seven years after a patient leaves their care.

Finally, regular well-baby visits give the doctor an opportunity to screen a child for defects of hearing and sight. Certain common problems must be identified and treated early. After about the age of six, for example, treatment for "lazy eye" and cross-eye can at best be little more than cosmetic. The brain by then has learned to suppress the images it receives from the defective eye and will continue to do so; as an adult, the victim will never be able to use both eyes together for clear, three-dimensional vision.

Equally important in the preschool years is the care of a child's teeth. Even in the primary or so-called baby teeth, hidden decay must be diagnosed and controlled; if decay has led to cavities, they should be filled. These first teeth hold space in the jaws for the permanent ones, which first erupt around the age of six. If primary teeth are lost prematurely, the permanent teeth may erupt too early, without well-developed roots to hold them in place. Moreover, the gaps left by the lost primary teeth can permit the remaining teeth to shift position, so that the permanent teeth grow in crooked.

A parent can make four main contributions to a program of dental care: Limit a child's intake of sugar; clean the child's teeth daily, or make sure that the child does so; strengthen the teeth's resistance with fluoride; and take the child to the dentist for regular checkups.

When the bacteria most responsible for tooth decay come into contact with sugar, they produce a gummy substance, dextran, that glues them to the teeth and to each other. If the bacteria are undisturbed, they form large colonies, and the glue traps both food debris and dead cells shed by the lining of the mouth. All of these substances form a meshlike mass, called plaque, which acts as a blotter every time a child eats, soaking up food and liquids that the bacteria then process at leisure for 20 minutes or more. As the bacteria digest sugar, they produce acids that adhere to the surface of the teeth, slowly dissolving the enamel.

Because bacteria can form new colonies in the mouth within 24 hours, plaque should be removed from tooth surfaces at least once a day, and preferably after every meal. Wipe a baby's first tooth with a clean washcloth or gauze pad. As other teeth erupt, brush them gently with a soft brush (no toothpaste is needed) and floss between them to remove the plaque. At two and a half, a child generally has all his baby teeth; from then on, under close supervision, he can use toothpaste and his own soft toothbrush. You will still have to do the flossing, however; a child will not master that skill until he is about five.

Another way of preventing tooth decay is to strengthen the teeth's resistance to bacterial acids. Fluoride, a compound of the natural element fluorine, has exactly that effect. When swallowed, fluoride is incorporated into a child's developing teeth, and it armor-plates the enamel. When fluoride is deposited upon the teeth, it is absorbed by the plaque, where it attacks bacterial colonies and interferes with their ability to produce acid. For maximum effect, a two-pronged attack is best. Children should take fluoride internally through drinking water or, if their drinking supply is not fluoridated, in drops or tablets. They should also use it externally in the form of toothpaste and mouth rinses.

A child's 20 primary, or "baby," teeth break through the gums at the approximate ages indicated below. Though these teeth are temporary (all are shed between the ages of six and 12), an infected tooth can spread decay and cause permanent damage. Until a child learns to use a toothbrush, parents should clean the primary teeth with a soft brush or a cloth pad.

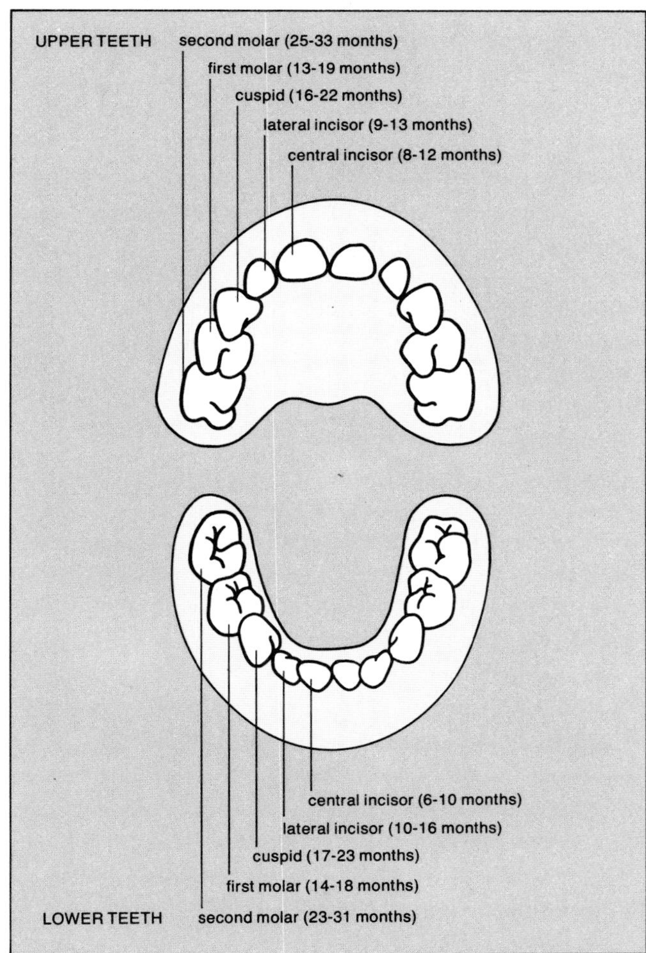

Finally, however thorough you are at home, there is the need for regular professional checkups. Because teeth are vulnerable to decay from the moment they erupt, a child should make his first dental visit at about the age of two, when all primary teeth have appeared; according to the National Institutes of Health, subsequent visits should be made at six-month intervals up to school age. At every visit the dentist might fill cavities caused by hidden decay, install spacers for teeth that are delayed in eruption, or correct a child's bite with orthodontic braces. But the visits are important even when the dentist finds no need for any dental therapy. Treatments and the disorders that call for them are irritating at best, and often painful. Introducing a child to the dentist under pleasant circumstances helps to develop a positive attitude toward dental care that will last a lifetime.

Teaching a finicky eater what to eat

Ultimately, of course, the goal of all child care is to teach children to take charge of their own bodies. In a child between the ages of one and three, particularly, parents must instill the basic habits that favor good health and social development. Three areas of special concern—and of almost inevitable conflict between parent and child—are eating, sleeping, and toilet training.

Teaching a young child how and what to eat is at once an opportunity and a source of anxiety for parents. The eating habits a child acquires in the preschool years will shape many of his future likes and dislikes. But toddlers are balky and finicky eaters, who often seem to appreciate food mainly as a tool for asserting a newly felt sense of independence. It is not surprising that these are years when eating problems abound.

You can take much of the pressure off yourself and your child by accepting the fact that eating behavior that may seem bizarre to you is natural for your child. Decide in advance not to be overconcerned if your child insists on using his fingers when you know that he is capable of wielding a spoon, or eats nothing but cream-cheese-and-jelly sandwiches for days at a time, or refuses to eat anything at all for a spell. Focus instead on helping your child to enjoy eating and avoid the two major nutritional problems: obesity and tooth decay.

Persuading a child to eat is not one of these major problems. If your child's height and weight are within the normal ranges for his age, if he is active and alert, and if his skin, hair, and teeth look healthy, then he is getting enough to eat. Young children simply are not big eaters. What is more, they may well eat less at 18 months than they did at six or eight months. Their reduced intake is perfectly normal: Weight gain is only a third as much in the second year of life as in the first, and a child gets part of his energy by burning off some of the fat that he stored in his body during infancy. Thus the toddler's daily food requirements are modest. They can be met with one small serving of meat or one egg; a pint or more of milk; three to four tablespoonfuls of vegetables or fruits, plus fruit juice; and half a cup of cereal or two slices of bread.

A child need not eat such a well-rounded diet every day. It is, in fact, unlikely that he will accept daily servings from each of the major food groups. Nevertheless, you can be sure that your child will not starve or become malnourished so long as a variety of nutritious food is available to him. In a famous study a Chicago physician, Clara Davis, permitted infants of weaning age to choose without prompting from a variety of solid foods. At each meal, a nurse placed six to eight dishes containing vegetables, fruits, meats, eggs, cereals and milk in front of the babies, but made no attempt to feed them or to attract attention to any one food. When a child reached for a particular food or began eating it with his fingers, the nurse would offer him some with a spoon, but she could not comment on what the babies ate or did not eat. Over a year's time, Dr. Davis found that the babies chose food in sufficient quantity and variety to sustain themselves splendidly. Their appetites and preferences fluctuated considerably, but over the long run they ate diets that were well balanced by any nutritionist's standards.

At home children are not very different from these laboratory subjects. Bread or crackers, cheese and a piece of apple may not seem much of a meal to an adult, but the combination is nutritionally balanced. Keep in mind that no one food is absolutely essential. If children eat fruit, they do not really need vegetables. They may not like to eat eggs, but the egg in a pancake or a pudding is just as nutritious. Even the child who does not drink much milk can get enough calcium from cheese, yogurt, and the milk used in such foods as cereal, sauces, creamed soups, custards, cocoa—and ice cream.

A dentist who turns fear into fun

"A child is curious, and I try to play on that curiosity," says Virginia dentist Edward Hindman. In the course of a checkup, shown here and on the following pages, Dr. Hindman introduces his young patients to the mysterious tools of his profession, each with its disarmingly playful nickname. With the toddler's attention engaged and his fears overcome, the checkup goes smoothly, and the patient leaves with a souvenir, such as a tiny racing car, from the doctor's "treasure drawer."

Other dentists have their own chairside manner, but, like Dr. Hindman, most encourage parents to bring a child in soon after all of the primary, or baby, teeth have emerged. Many of these teeth come in crooked or wrongly spaced, and in more than half of the youngsters they show signs of decay. Both conditions are potentially dangerous: Primaries maintain the correct spacing for the permanent teeth, and an infected primary can harm the permanent tooth developing under it. Finally, the dentist teaches and encourages home tooth care—brushing and flossing after meals; the control of diet, particularly decay-promoting sweets; and the possible use of a fluoride supplement when the water supply does not contain sufficient fluoride to harden tooth enamel against decay.

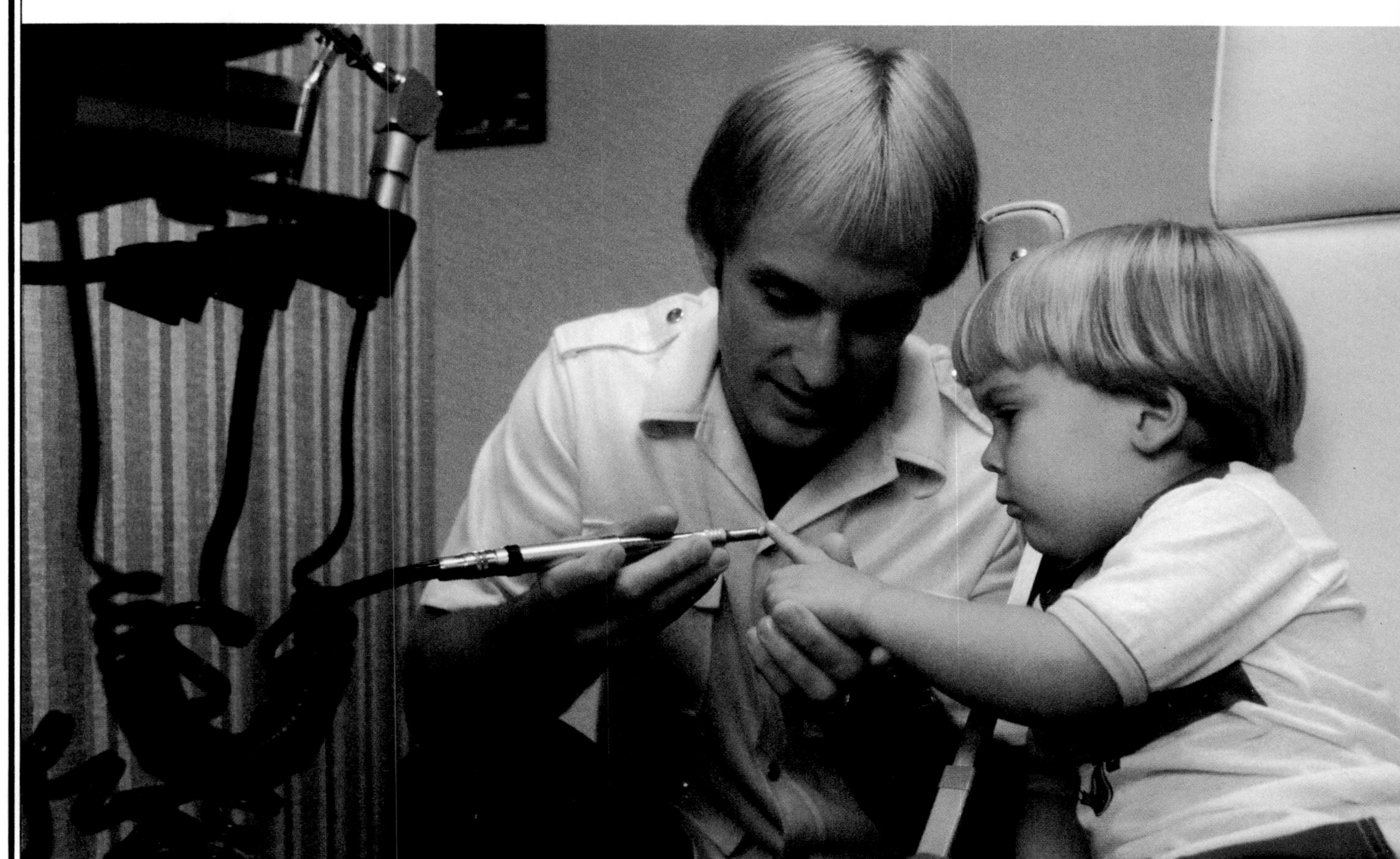

Before cleaning the teeth of young Jeffery Lozito for the first time, dentist Edward Hindman demonstrates the low-speed drill he will use for the job. Introducing the instrument as "Mr. Choo Choo," he lets Jeffery touch the flexible rubber tip, first with the motor off, then with it on. The dentist has introduced himself by the name Jeffery will use in future meetings—Doctor Ed.

Doctor Ed helps Jeffery shoot water into the rinsing basin with ''Mr. Squirt''—a power syringe—explaining to the youngster that the device will clear away food particles and saliva bubbles with a jet of water, or air, or a fine spray combining both.

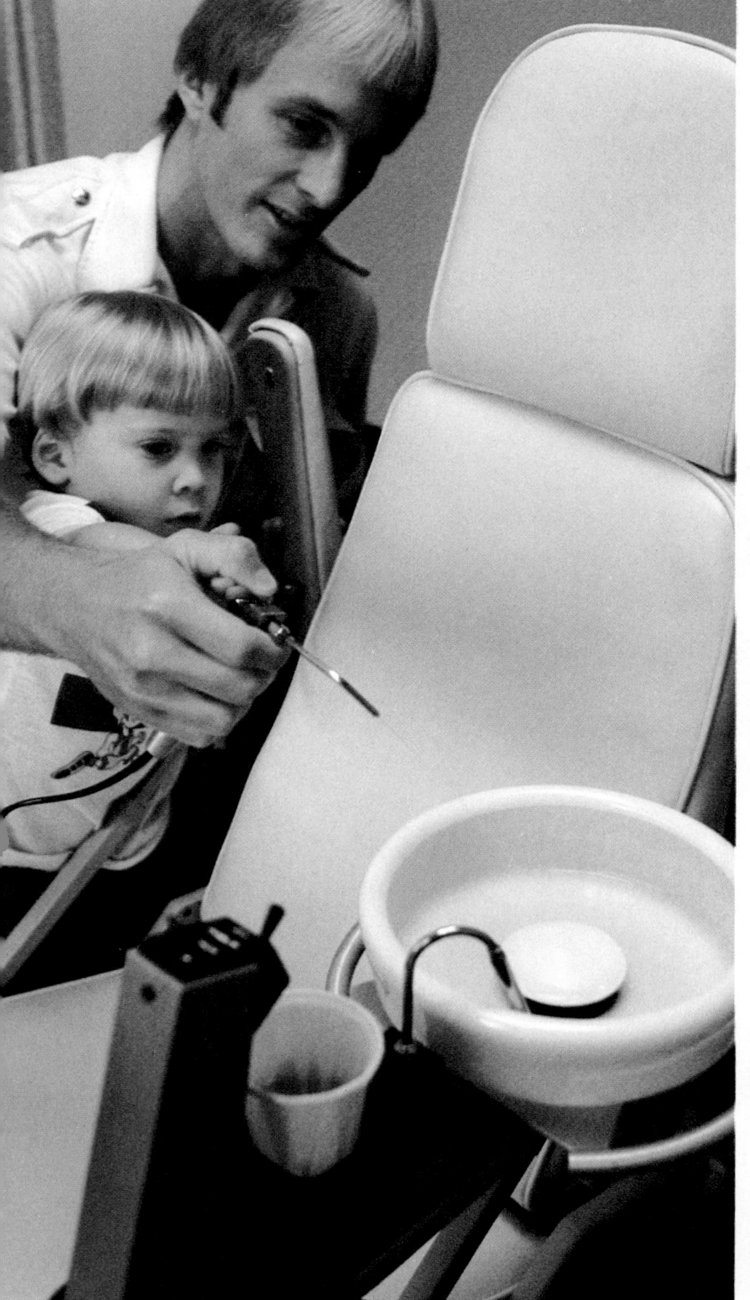

The dentist demonstrates a dental probe, ''Mr. Tooth Toucher,'' by tapping the probe on his thumbnail. He explains that he will tap each of Jeffery's teeth in this way to test for decay; to show how the instrument will feel, he will tap the boy's nail as well.

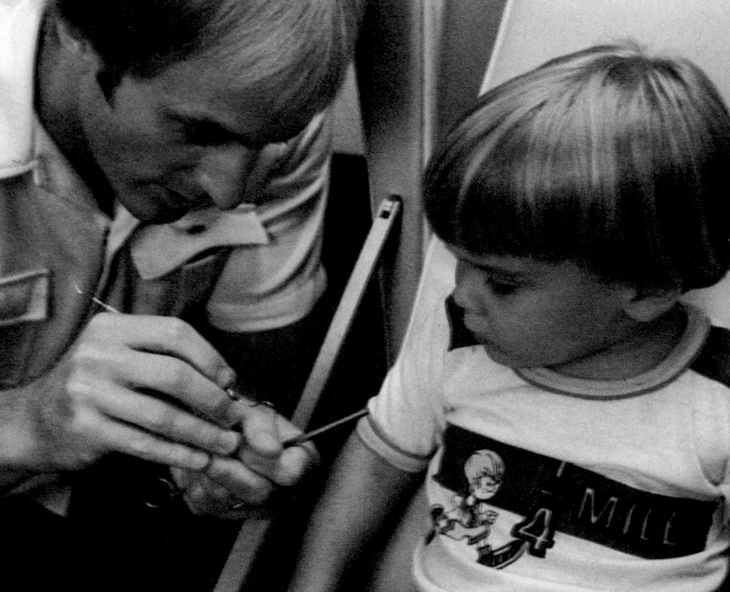

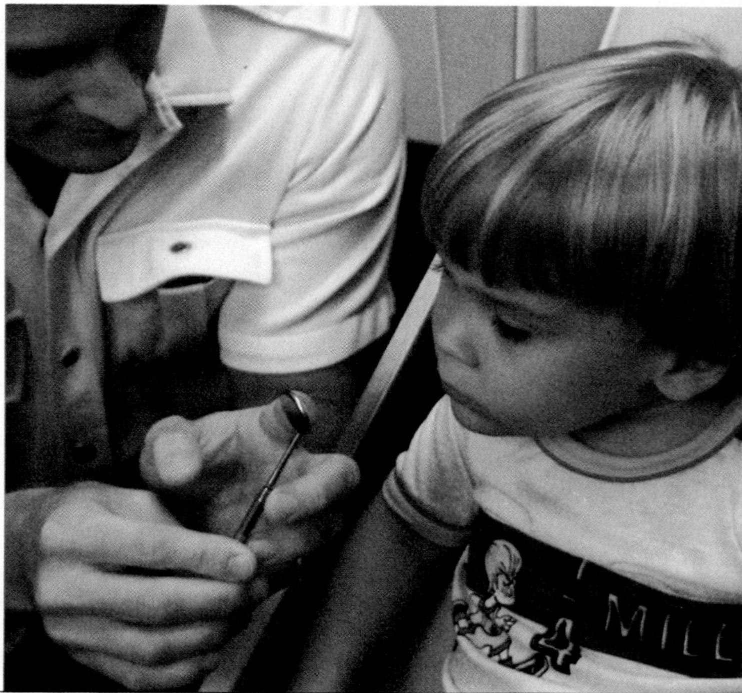

To capture the child's interest, Doctor Ed points out an Indian-head trademark on the back of ''Mr. Mirror,'' before going on to explain how the tool will help him to see all of Jeffery's teeth from many different angles.

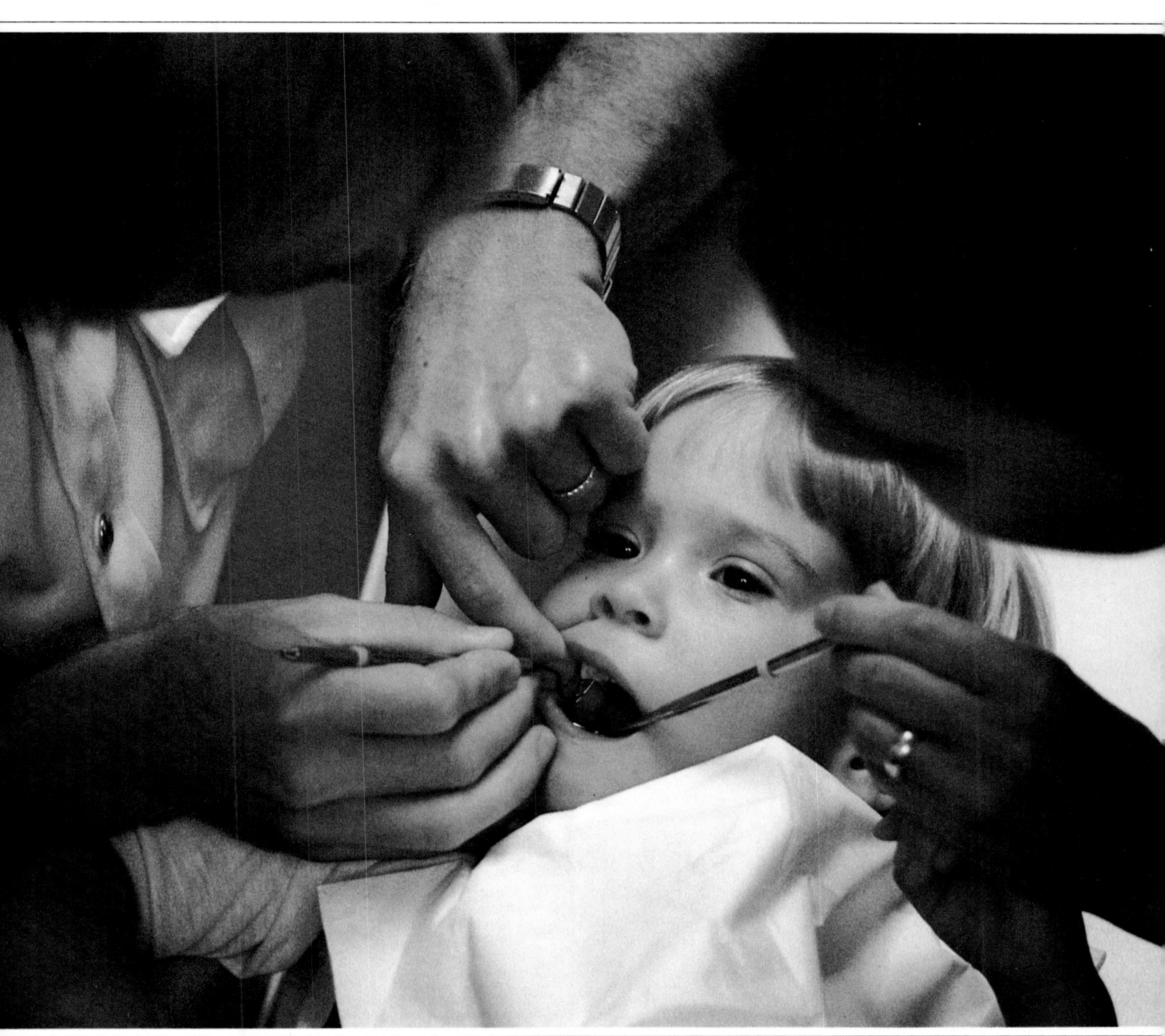

As Jeffery's mother watches in the mirror, the dentist points out a small cavity in an upper molar, which he will fill on a later visit. Throughout the checkup Mrs. Lozito has been nearby, remaining quiet but always standing where the child could see her.

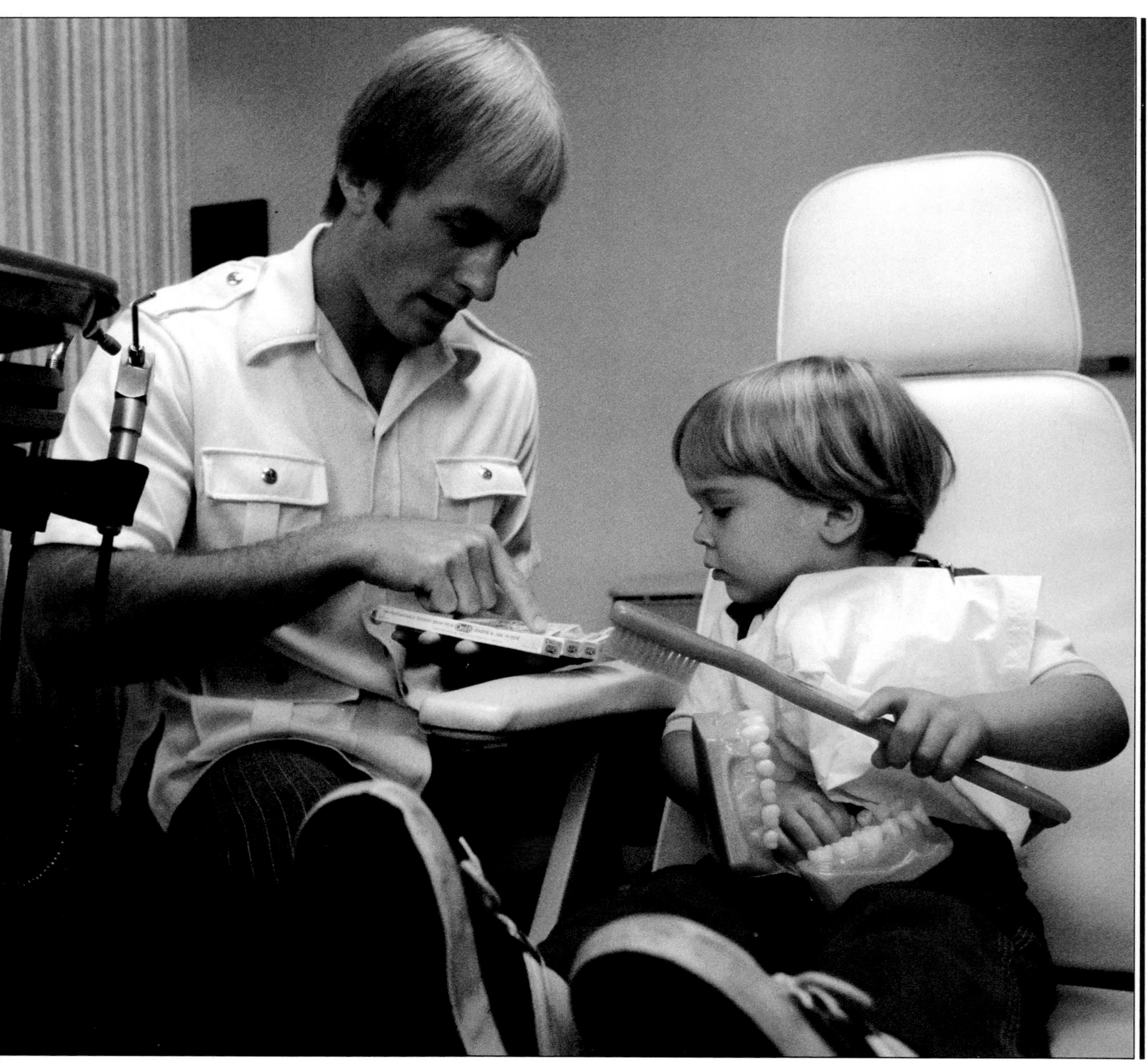

Having taught Jeffery proper toothbrushing technique with two giant models—a toothbrush and a set of dentures called "Big George"—Dr. Hindman offers the boy a real toothbrush to take home. Told to pick his favorite color from the assortment in the doctor's hands, Jeffery took two—a green and a blue.

One reason the infants in Dr. Davis' experiment fared so well is that she did not offer them candy or other junk food. But parents, too, can control a child's food selections, particularly during the preschool years. Such foods as cheese, fruit, raw vegetables, or leftover portions of meat and poultry provide more nutritious pick-me-ups than typical processed snack foods, which are full of the empty calories that lead to obesity, and the sugar that fosters tooth decay.

From the standpoint of dental health, the worst possible foods are soft, sticky sweets, such as caramels or chewy baked goods. Even dried fruits, often touted as health foods, are dangerous. According to Dr. Andrew Christopher of Georgetown University Dental School: "Parents should not feed their children snacks of raisins, prunes, or other dried fruits. These foods become wedged in the grooves of the teeth, where they dissolve slowly, giving the teeth a sugar bath all day long. In the fresh version of those foods—grapes, plums, fresh apricots and apples—the sugar is much less concentrated. The juice in fresh fruit increases the flow of saliva, so that much of the sugar present is washed away."

Withholding all sweets from a child would be both unfair and unrealistic. Instead, choose sweets that dissolve quickly—pieces of chocolate, for example—urge the child to eat all that you give him at one time, and encourage him to wash it down with water or milk. Better still, serve sweets as part of a regular meal, so that other foods dilute the sugar's effect.

Whatever the type of food being offered, the best way to encourage healthful eating habits is to keep calm and matter-of-fact. Allow your child as much independence as possible in deciding how much he wants to eat and how he wants to eat it. Give him small portions—one tablespoonful of each food for a toddler—and let him ask for more if he wants it. In this way, the child regulates his own food intake, and if he does eat all you give him, he will enjoy a sense of accomplishment. Coaxing him to clean his plate and rewarding him when he does is the wrong way to solve an eating problem: It paves the way for the more serious problem of overeating. Similarly, bribing him by withholding dessert until he finishes his spinach will only strengthen his conviction that dessert is far more desirable than spinach.

Introduce new foods when a child seems hungriest, and do it without fanfare or any sign that you consider certain foods more important than others. "One way to get a child to like vegetables is to pretend that they are adult foods that the child is being permitted to try," advised University of Iowa pediatrician Dr. Samuel Fomon. "All of a sudden he gains interest and enthusiasm for vegetables."

Strengthening a child's independence also means encouraging him to feed himself as soon as he can. Let a toddler use his fingers whenever he pleases and offer him foods in easy-to-pick-up pieces, but always have a spoon handy for him to experiment with. Acquaint him with its use by offering him a few spoonfuls of food, then hand him the spoon. Most one-year-olds want to try a spoon, and many children handle it well by age two. After that, children are eager to graduate to a fork, but no child should be allowed to use a sharp dinner fork or a knife until he has the dexterity to keep from hurting himself—usually not much before the age of five.

The messy job of "learning to eat like big people" is actually hampered by an undue concern for neatness and adult manners. "The more you try to impose rules and regulations on eating and table manners, the clearer it becomes to the toddler that the mealtable is a marvelous place for a fight," says child psychologist Penelope Leach. "Soon your child knows that it is one place where he or she can always get your attention and concern." A far more valuable lesson for a child to learn is that eating, as part of the social exchanges of a family meal, can be a pleasant experience.

Winning the bedtime battle

Aside from regular mealtimes, perhaps the most important routine of a young child's day consists simply of going to bed. Here, firm rules are necessary, partly to make sure that the child gets enough sleep, partly to prevent bedtime from becoming a nightly battle. Children vary considerably in the amount of sleep they need; according to the U.S. Department of Health and Human Services, a healthy two-year-old may require as few as eight or as many as 17 hours. Most toddlers, though, sleep about 11 or 12 hours a night, and one or two additional hours during daytime naps.

At around 18 months of age, a child goes through an awkward stage when two daytime naps are too many and one is not quite enough. A period of quiet, structured play, such as listening to a story or assembling a puzzle, can give such a child the extra rest he needs. By the age of three or four, children stop taking naps during the day. But whatever a child's sleeping pattern, it is easy to tell whether he is getting the right amount of sleep. If he wakes very early in the morning, he probably should go to bed later at night. If he gets cranky, less coordinated and either underactive or overactive late in the day, he probably needs more sleep.

The hour of going to bed, however, should not be changed arbitrarily or often. Even when they are tired, about half of all toddlers balk at being put to bed, and the most effective way to minimize the struggle is to set a regular bedtime and stick to it. Though the child may grumble, he will secretly feel more secure with a firm schedule. Establish a bedtime ritual that helps the child settle down at the end of the day. Quiet, relaxing activities—a bedtime story, a chat about the day's events, perhaps a back rub—allow a child to slip into a passive state that makes sleep possible. This quiet time with a parent also reduces the sense of isolation from family activities that a child being trundled off to bed is bound to feel.

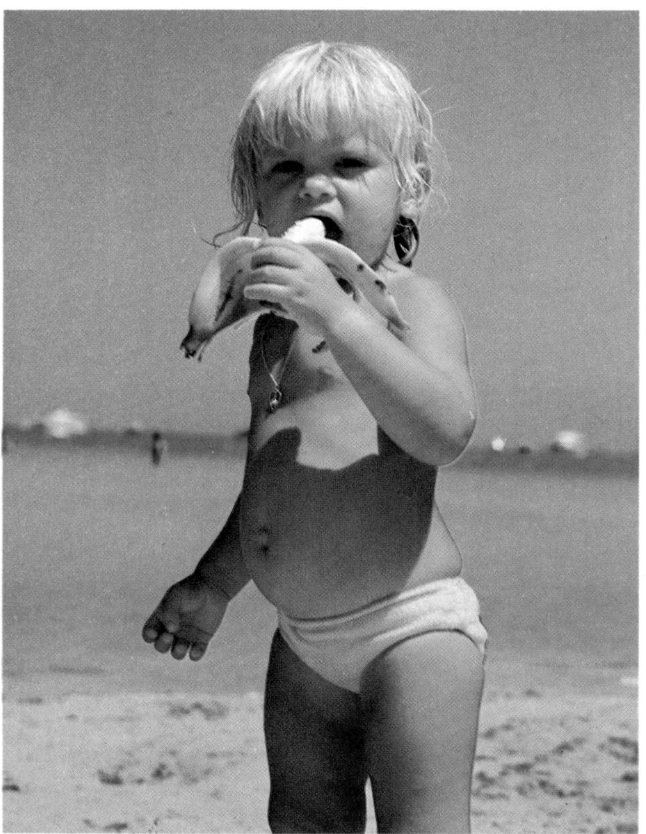

A preschooler pauses in mid-play to eat a banana—a nutritious snack that curbs her hunger between meals. Fruit and raw vegetables, nourishing and pleasant to eat but low in calories, make good snacking substitutes for such high-calorie, low-nutrition foods as candy, soft drinks and pastry.

Despite your best efforts, your child will surely test the rules by refusing to settle down. Respond by making it clear, firmly but calmly, that it is time for him to be in bed and that you expect him to stay there. If a child begins to cry in his crib when you put him to bed, go back to his room, say good night and leave immediately. If his crying continues, return every five minutes or so to let him know you have not abandoned him; but simply repeat your good night and leave at once; do not stay in his room or take him back to the rest of the family. "I have known it to take a week for this policy to work," says Penelope Leach. "I have never known it to take longer except when the parents weakened."

An older child who can climb out of a crib or is using a regular bed may get up repeatedly on the pretense of needing a drink or having to go to the bathroom. Tend to his needs, then lead him back to bed immediately. If he rejoins the family and attempts to charm you into letting him stay up a bit later, calmly march him back to bed until he gets the message that his stalling tactics will not work.

Nighttime fears and bad dreams are as common among young children as not wanting to go to bed in the first place. Fear of the dark, for example, is almost universal, and in a child's vivid imagination, toys, wallpaper designs and even furniture can become scary monsters when the lights go off. One obvious solution is to leave a dim light burning in the child's room. Another, which can be made part of the going-to-bed ritual, is to encourage pleasant thoughts at bedtime by playing a game in which you ask the child to close his eyes, take a deep breath, and think of his favorite place.

A child who wakes up in fear during the night often wants to join his parents in their bed. If you permit him to do so, you encourage him to form a habit that is hard to break. The best course is simply never to take a child into your bed. When he appears in your room, make sure he is not sick, take care of his needs, then return him to his own bed.

More serious is the problem of a child who wakes in the midst of a nightmare. Bad dreams are especially frightening to preschoolers, who have real difficulty in distinguishing fantasy from reality. If you hear your child scream or cry out in the night, get to him as soon as you can. The sight and touch of a parent will calm him, and he may drop back to sleep before he screams himself into a full-blown fright.

In a rare form of sleep disorder known as a night terror, a child awakes suddenly, but seems to be in a trance. He may stare at some unknown horror, shout in anger or sob in grief. He is unaware of a parent's efforts to comfort him. Turn on all the lights and speak to the child soothingly but do not try to talk him out of his trance. Generally, he will drift back to sleep and never recall what happened.

Disturbing as they are, such incidents do not mean that a child is mentally unbalanced. Many night terrors are triggered by a high fever or some physical or emotional shock; in a few, the cause is as simple as a child's misunderstanding of something he has overheard. One four-year-old had night terrors in which he screamed, "No wolf house! No wolf house!" Finally the parents made the connection: They had been considering buying a house owned by a family named Wolf, and their child, hearing them talking about "the Wolf house," apparently feared he was about to be taken to a den of wild wolves. Once the parents explained that no real wolves stalked the new house, the night terrors vanished.

Typically, both nightmares and night terrors disappear without treatment. If either persist for several months, however, consult a psychologist or child-guidance clinic.

Toilet training: a job of patient persuasion

Of the three major hurdles in the preschool years, toilet training most clearly represents the child's struggle to gain control over his own body. Introduced at the right time and in the right way, it can often be accomplished in a matter of days or weeks. But theories about when to start toilet training vary

These extensions of the charts on page 96 show patterns of growth between the ages of one and five years. The explosive growth rate of the first year of life drops off sharply in childhood. Between the ages of four and five, for example, typical heights increase by about 7 per cent, and weights by 12 per cent; corresponding increases for the first year are 50 and 200 per cent.

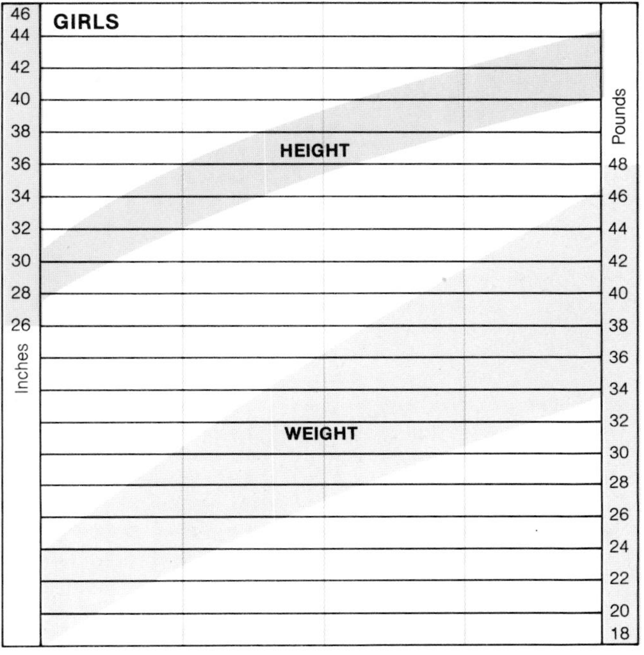

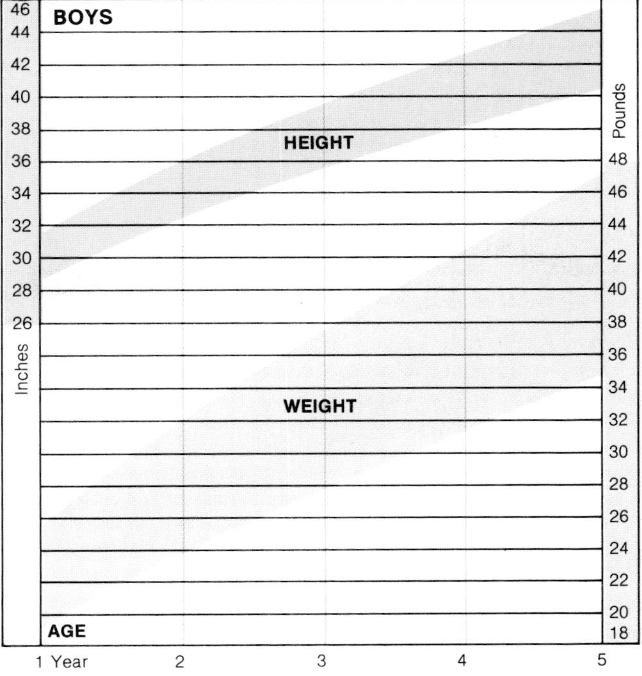

Thoroughly spattered with food, an infant girl attempts—thus far in vain—to master the art of eating with a spoon. Most babies become interested in feeding themselves between six and nine months of age; however, they generally cannot hold a spoon even in the fashion shown here before they reach 15 months, and often do not use it correctly before the age of two.

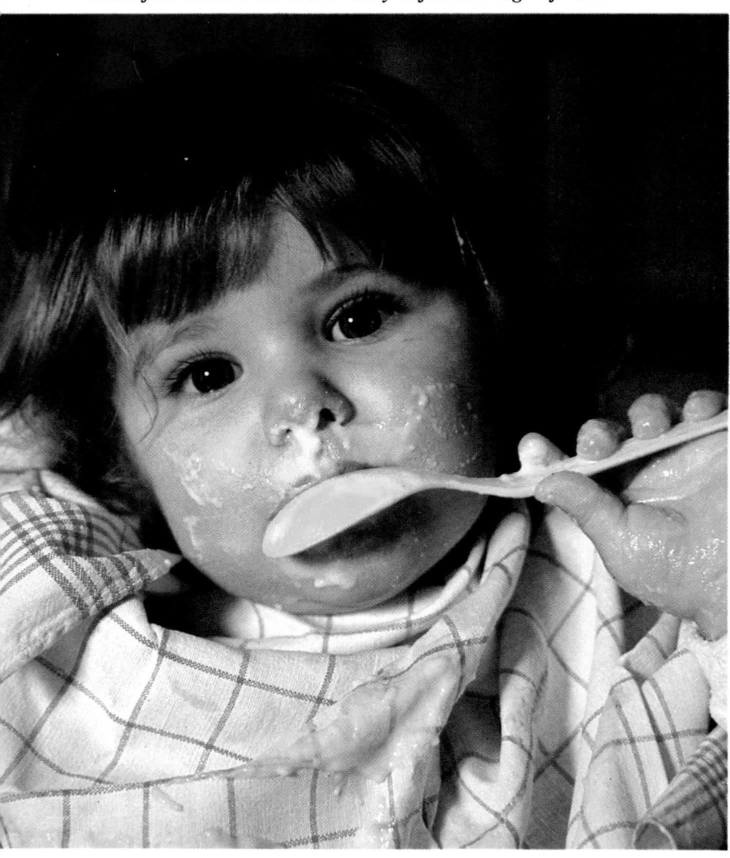

from culture to culture and decade to decade. In Europe, traditionally, parents try to train a child before his first birthday, sometimes with apparent success. But the success is deceptive; generally the mother, not the child, learns to recognize the moment when she must rush the child to a toilet or a potty. This is not true toilet training, because the child is not voluntarily controlling his own body functions.

Most authorities now agree that it is a waste of time to put much effort into toilet training until a child is two and a half. The fact of the matter is that parents do not actually toilet train a child, but merely help him master the task; even if the parents did nothing, most children would eventually train themselves. But three crucial steps in development must be achieved before a child can handle what is, after all, a fairly complex act. First, the child must be able to control his body. Before the age of 12 to 15 months, a child's nervous system is not mature enough to allow him much control over the sphincter muscles; most children only begin to acquire this control after they begin to walk well by themselves. Second, toilet training depends in part on a child's ability to talk, because he must communicate with a parent when he needs to use the potty and, if necessary, ask for assistance. Finally, the child must have the psychological maturity to understand what is being asked of him and to want to use a potty.

The most direct indication that a child is ready for toilet training is a visible awareness on his part—by facial expression, perhaps, or by the gesture of clutching himself—that he is about to have a bowel movement. He also may signal that he is uncomfortable with dirty diapers. More subtle signs of readiness include a pattern of imitating adults or older brothers and sisters, and a compulsion to put personal belongings, such as toys and clothes, in their proper place.

When the time does come to toilet train your child, you will be offered advice in plenty on how to do it. Much of the advice will be self-defeating, and some of it will be absurd. One team of psychologists, for example, devised a super-fast conditioning method in which children were rewarded with potato chips and soft drinks when they managed to stay dry—a system that, at best, creates a dietary problem where none may have existed previously.

What seems to work best is a gradual, step-by-step approach that allows children to proceed at their own rate. For the children in his own practice, Harvard pediatrician T. Berry Brazelton developed just such a system. Among 1,200 children he studied, 80 per cent quickly achieved control of both bowel and bladder at an average age of 28 months. By the age of three, they were staying dry at night.

Like most experts, Dr. Brazelton prefers to train children on a potty rather than a child's seat set over an adult toilet; the potty is more secure, and its small scale encourages the child to think of it as a piece of personal furniture. Dr. Brazelton recommends introducing the child to the potty by letting him sit on it with his clothes on, so that it is not frightening to him.

After he gets used to it, explain that the bathroom is the place where grown-ups and older children have a bowel movement. Help him make the association by placing him on the potty without clothes and diapers when he is likely to have a bowel movement or just after he has had one in his diapers. At this stage, do not flush the child's bowel movement down the toilet in his presence. To many children, the sight of part of themselves disappearing down the toilet is terrifying.

If the child seems cooperative, take him to the potty two or three times a day when he gives any signal that he has to urinate or have a bowel movement, and praise him when the maneuver is successful. Then, when you feel the child is ready for the next and final step, allow him to play for periods with no clothes on from the waist down and put the potty near him, reminding him that he might want to try going by himself. If he has an accident or seems resistant, put his diapers back on and try again a few days later. As Dr. Brazelton puts it: "He will tell you in some way when he is ready."

Many children control themselves well during the day, but continue to wet the bed until they are three or four. Do not make a fuss about it: Simply put diapers on the child at bedtime until he can do without them. If a child consistently wets the bed to the age of five and beyond, consult a pediatrician, particularly if incontinence is accompanied by pain, discolored urine or consistent day-wetting. The youngster may have a urinary-tract disease, diabetes, or an emotional disorder. In most cases, however, there is no obvious cause for extended bed-wetting. According to some theories, the problem is genetic; others suggest that it occurs more often in deep sleepers, and still others that it is the result of small bladder capacity, emotional distress or harsh toilet training. But all these theories are based on limited evidence, and doctors simply do not agree with one another.

Theories about a cure for bed-wetting are equally numerous. As recently as the 19th Century, some parents tried to solve the problem by such grotesque and semimagical methods as forcing a child to eat the petals of a chrysanthemum or the testicles of a rabbit. Today's parents often resort to giving children drugs, alarm systems that wake a child when urine trickles onto an electrically rigged bed pad, and exercises for increasing bladder capacity and control. All have their proponents, and all achieve some degree of success. Many authorities, though, consider potent drugs and frightening alarm systems unduly harsh remedies for a problem that usually vanishes on its own before a child reaches adolescence.

In any case, no method of treatment should be imposed upon an unwilling child. Parents can help most by being understanding and offering practical help such as waking the child before they go to bed to see if he needs to go to the bathroom. Above all, never shame or punish a child for wetting the bed or having an accident during the day. Think, instead, of the child's own state of mind. The Jewish Talmud specifies that a criminal who loses bowel or bladder control because of fear as he is about to be flogged should be spared the whip—the loss of control in public was thought punishment enough. Certainly, the same is true for a young child.

Discipline: learning to live by the rules

Learning self-control in the preschool years involves far more, of course, than the basic habits of eating, sleeping and toileting. A young child must also learn to control his actions and emotions, to respect the rights of others and to abide by the rules of the adult world. Children cannot learn these things by themselves; parents instill a sense of what constitutes civilized behavior, and from parental discipline evolves the child's self-discipline.

Discipline and punishment are not the same, however. Discipline establishes and enforces rules and punishment is the price the child pays for disobeying those rules. Disciplining a child can be considered an expression of concern and love, because children basically want rules and limits, and often persist in bad behavior in an attempt to provoke some parental control. Consider the case of Billy, the four-and-a-half-year-old son of parents who prided themselves on a permissive approach to child-rearing. One evening Billy entered the living room and took a peach from a bowl on the table. After taking one bite, he put the peach back, picked up a pear, and did the same thing. He repeated the procedure until he had sampled half the fruit, glancing at his parents as he put back each piece in the bowl. In effect, Billy was looking for guidance, and for some sign that his parents cared about what he did.

Disciplinary goals and practices vary considerably in different cultures. The scene in Billy's house would be unthinkable in China, where children are expected to fade quietly into the background. Similarly, and closer to home, child-rearing among Mexican Americans and Chinese Americans generally stresses obedience and respect for elders. Most children in the United States, however, grow up in child-centered homes where they are permitted—indeed, expected—to participate actively in family life.

Whatever the parents' basic philosophy, discipline should begin early, as soon as a child begins exploring his environment and testing his motor skills. A one-year-old who crawls to the television set, turns to make sure a parent is watching, and starts twiddling the knobs is clearly indicating that he needs to have limits imposed upon him. At this age, many potential conflicts can be defused by distracting the child or physically removing him from the scene. Distraction is useful, too, in avoiding arguments with the typically negative two-year-old; for example, a stream of rapid chatter can be enough to hold his attention while you dress him, even when he is in a balky mood. A four- or five-year-old is less distractible, but more responsive to verbal directions. At that age, for example, it is best to give a child absorbed in play a friendly warning that bedtime is coming up in 10 minutes and he had better think about putting his toys away.

At times, attempts at reasonable discipline seem to blow up in parents' faces. Between the ages of one and three, particularly, thwarted or overtired children are prone to uncontrollable temper tantrums, marked by fits of screaming, kicking and pounding. Sometimes a child in the throes of a tantrum will hold his breath until he turns blue and nearly loses consciousness. As frightening as these episodes may be, they are not dangerous. A child's natural reflexes will force him to take a breath long before any damage is done.

The only effective way to handle a tantrum is to refrain from reinforcing it in any way. Make sure the child does not hurt himself or anyone else, but otherwise remain calm. If he is in no danger, leave the room and return when he is finished screaming. Above all, do not give in to unreasonable demands or begin to scream back. Tantrums are rarely a sign of serious trouble. They usually disappear after the age of three when the child learns to express anger coherently.

Parents can do much to avoid tantrums and other clashes by following a few simple rules in disciplining a child:

- Be consistent. If a child gets the same reaction every time he tests a specific form of unacceptable behavior, he quickly learns the lesson you are trying to teach. Unpredictability, on the other hand, makes him feel anxious and uncertain.
- Stress the positive side of a direction or command. The word "Don't!" poses a tempting challenge to a young child. His response is likely to be better if you tell him something positive he can do—"Put your toy over there so no one trips over it"—or issue a command in the form of a question—"Where does your coat belong?"
- Explain to your child why you are telling him to do something. The explanation will help him to understand cause and effect, an important element in learning to think for himself.

Punishment as such should never take a central role in discipline. The most powerful motivating force in a young child's life is his basic desire to please his parents and make them like him. Rewarding good behavior with your approval or registering annoyance at naughtiness is usually enough to keep a child fairly well under control. But there are times when virtually all parents must resort to punishment to show that they mean what they say. Just as for discipline, there are a few clear-cut rules for effective punishment:

- Punish without delay. If a mother uses the timeworn tactic of waiting "till Daddy comes home," the child will have long forgotten what he is being punished for.
- Make the punishment fit the offense as nearly as possible. When a child rides his tricycle into the street despite repeated warnings, it is appropriate to prohibit him from riding the tricycle for an entire day—but it is irrelevant, even silly, to deny him dessert at dinner.
- Never issue threats that will not be carried out. You know, for example, that no matter how angry you are, you will not lock a child in his room for a week. Threatening to do so only confuses the child and undermines your authority.

Perhaps the most troubling question in punishment is whether it is ever appropriate to strike a child. Some authorities, including Drs. Spock and Brazelton, argue that a light spanking can sometimes clear the air and prevent parents from taking out their irritation in more destructive ways. Most child-care experts contend, however, that the bad effects of physical punishment outweigh its benefits. The most persuasive argument against it is that it can quickly get out of hand. An angry adult can easily harm a small child without intending to, and once a parent begins to use spanking, the tendency is to apply it more harshly the next time the child commits the same transgression. An additional argument against spanking is that it violates one of the cardinal rules of punishment, for it never truly fits the offense. Even if a child has hit someone else, spanking is not appropriate, for it consists of the very behavior you are telling him is unacceptable.

The formidable power and danger of TV

While discipline and punishment generally take place within the family circle, children must also cope with an onslaught of stimuli from outside the home. The major outside influence is surely television. Indeed, it is all but universal. TV sets are more common in American homes than refrigerators or indoor plumbing; among adults, TV watching consumes more time than any activity but work and sleep; the average 18-year-old has spent more hours at the set than at school; and in the preschool years, interest in television soars dramatically. A baby as young as six months will stare fixedly at a television program for a short time. By two and a half, most children start to watch in earnest, and at the age of four they are watching more than half the time the set is on, even if there are toys and other distractions in the same room.

For many reasons, however, long periods of television watching may not be good for children. Avid viewers are obviously physically inert. (One Illinois father, in a creative attempt to solve that problem, powered his set with a stationary bicycle connected to a generator. "Now," he said, "the kids can feed their television habit with their own energy.") The child watching TV is also mentally passive. Television does everything for him at the flick of a switch. Information flashes by continually, and the child has no chance to reflect on it or to create his own imagery. By contrast, a child leafing through a picture book uses his imagination to transform the static images on the page into real characters.

The worst effects of television, however, arise from the violence depicted on it—in detective shows, the Saturday morning cartoons, or the evening news. Researchers now agree that televised violence leads to increased aggressiveness among children of all ages—even preschoolers. In one

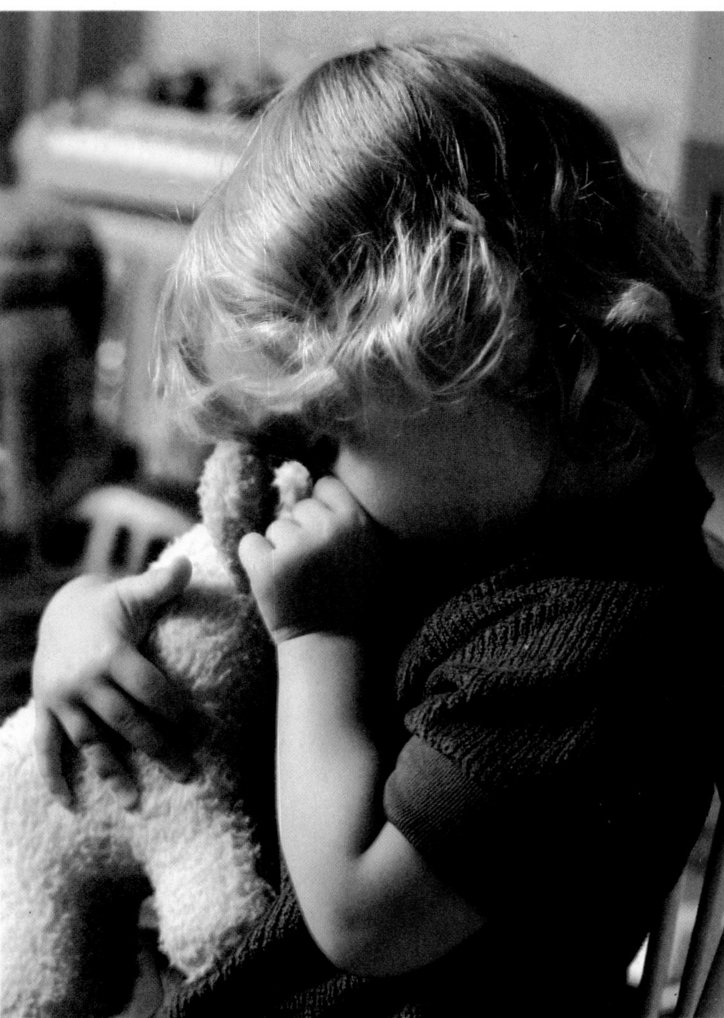

Plugged into private sources of comfort and pleasure, a toddler sucks her thumb while cuddling a favorite toy. Thumb sucking, a normal reflex exhibited by more than 85 per cent of healthy babies, need not be discouraged before the eruption of permanent teeth at the age of five or six; a child's fixation on a security toy or blanket is generally outgrown by the age of five.

typical study, conducted in 1977 by psychologists Jerome and Dorothy Singer of Yale University, trained observers watched a group of 141 three- and four-year-olds playing spontaneously at a nursery school. The observers rated the children in such areas as imaginativeness, cooperation with playmates, and aggressive acts. At the same time, the parents kept logs of the children's television viewing. The results, the Singers reported, showed "a clear linkage between parents' reports of TV viewing by the child and more 'unpleasant' behavioral patterns in the nursery school setting."

Not surprisingly, the study showed that heavy viewing of action-adventure shows was most likely to lead to overt aggression. But the Singers later found that almost all noisy, fast-paced programs—cartoons, some variety shows, the more hysterical game shows, even the educational *Sesame Street*—can arouse a child to jumpiness and aggressiveness.

It is up to parents to provide guidance in television viewing. To begin with, every parent should set definite limits to the amount of viewing. For preschoolers, one hour a day is sufficient; when the hour is up or the program is over, turn off the set. Virtually every parent needs to use the television as a babysitter at some point, but even then the time the child spends in front of the set should be limited and the parent should be familiar with the programs the child is watching. And while busy parents may not always be able to watch television with their children, they should try to join them for at least one or two full programs a week. In this way, parents get a chance to comment on violence—to express disapproval perhaps, or to point out that real violence is not funny—and to talk about the people and values depicted in the show.

Used constructively, television offers children a source of knowledge about the world around them. What is more, it can help develop the skills of communication, which equip children to learn more about that world on their own.

Mastering humanity's greatest skill—the use of language

The greatest of these skills is the mastery of language. To a large extent, this is a natural process. The baby who is spoken to and hears people talking learns to use language himself almost automatically. But parents play a major role in stimulating a child's interest in language, and in encouraging him to practice his new skills at each stage of development.

In all cultures and countries, healthy children acquire the basics of language in much the same sequence and schedule. Most begin to utter their first recognizable words around the age of one. Invariably, these first words are labels for people, animals and other important things—"Mama," "Dada," "dog," "cookie." Over the next year, the child learns to string two or three words together. The typical two-year-old talks in telegraphese—"Where ball?" for "Where is the ball?"; "Baba cry, quick!" for "The baby is crying, come quick!" By adult standards, the child's sentences are ungrammatical, his pronunciation faulty, his voice loud and poorly controlled. He may stop and start, or repeat words, but such stammering is usually temporary and does not signify a stuttering problem. Despite these speech difficulties, half of what the two-year-old says is understandable.

By the age of three, a child has a speaking vocabulary of a thousand words and understands at least twice that many. He speaks in complete sentences and within another year will have mastered all the basics of grammar. Over the next few years, the child continues to polish his verbal skills. He may not learn to make all speech sounds correctly until he is nearly eight, but by the age of five an average child is completely understandable, even to strangers.

How much and how well children talk depends largely on what they hear. Obviously, a child who is spoken to a good deal will recognize that language is important and will work hard to acquire it. But there are also specific things parents can do to help their children use language to communicate. Look at your child when you speak to him, and match your facial expressions and gestures to what you say. Describe simple actions verbally—"Up we go," for example, as you lift him—and name objects as you hand them to him. In everyday conversation, give him labels for ideas and things. If he struggles to move a new bag of sand to his sandbox, you might normally say, "Let me help you," but that sentence teaches the child little about language. If you say, "Let me help you with that bag of sand; it's heavy," he may learn at least two things: Sand in a certain type of container is a "bag of sand''; ''heavy'' is a label for the concept of weight.

Talk with a child in genuine, two-way conversations. Show him that you are really listening, and give him a chance to speak his own language without constantly correcting him or pretending that you do not understand him. With his parents' correct speech as a model, his own will gradually improve. (This fact, incidentally, makes a persuasive argument against baby talk: If you use it, so will your child.)

Each child acquires language at his own pace between the ages of one and three. One child may start talking at about a year and progress steadily; another may say little until he is two, then suddenly begin to talk in three-word sentences; still another may speak his first words at 10 months, but add few more during his entire second year. These are all normal variations. But some children lag so far behind that learning in other areas is impeded. For this reason, parents must recognize potential problems and seek help early.

If a child is not using words at all by the time he is two, consult a pediatrician or speech-language specialist; a specialist can distinguish the nonverbal two-year-old who needs help from the one who does not. Similarly, parents should be concerned about a three-year-old who seems unable to put ideas into words, or does not form the correct sounds for words, or pronounces words correctly but brings them out in jumbled order. At three, the child who cannot get his point across through language is in need of help.

In general, any speech impediment that persists beyond the stage when most other children outgrow it should also be checked out. A three-year-old who says ''wabbit'' for ''rabbit'' does not have a speech problem; in an older child, the same speech pattern is cause for concern. Stuttering may come and go in your children, but if it lasts more than four to six months, consult a professional. Delayed language development does not mean that a child is unable to learn or is intellectually inferior. In fact, children with language difficulties are sometimes above average in such areas as motor skills, coordination and visual perception.

Some language problems can be traced to poor hearing (especially after repeated middle-ear infections) or to a neurological defect; even stuttering, once thought to be psychological, may result from faulty muscle control of the vocal cords. More often, poor speech has no obvious cause; specialists know what has gone wrong, but do not know why. Nonetheless, the majority of afflicted children can be helped.

A speech-language pathologist diagnoses a child not only by applying formal tests but also by talking with parents and watching the child in a normal play situation. Once the problem is identified, treatment often takes such forms as encouraging the child to use language in a context important to him—usually in group play—rather than drilling him with lists of words. Parents can help by acting as the child's interpreter and gently telling him how to state a thought to make his point. It is important for the parents to focus on the content of what the child says rather than how he says it; constant correcting or testing will only frustrate him the more.

Where there are no such problems, a common gauge of a child's language development and general intelligence is how soon he learns to read and write. Some parents set out to develop these skills before a child enters school. Do not make that decision without careful thought. Certainly, a child who speaks and understands language well and is motivated to read should not be restrained, but no child should be pushed into reading prematurely. There is no strong evidence that children who learn to read at age four do better in school than those who wait until later, and too much formal instruction in the preschool years deprives a child of experiences essential to other kinds of learning. ''If a child spends half his time sitting at a desk learning his ABC's and how to write at age three,'' said Dr. Patricia Cole, an Austin, Texas, speech pathologist, ''he is missing out on a lot of experiential stuff going on out on the playground—things like what makes chewing gum sticky and how far can you stretch it?; how big does a box have to be before you can fit into it?; how do you argue with people and get them to do what you want?''

On balance, the most important contribution parents can make toward a child's future success in school is to instill the attitude that learning is fun. Giving the child opportunities to learn—not only through written language, but through a rich variety of childhood experiences—is the best preparation for the adventure of life. ❋

Beneath the bright leaves of their painted oak, preschoolers at the Little Acorn Patch take part in "circle time," a communal learning period. At this session, which is devoted to learning their own addresses, the children in the circle hold cutouts of houses marked with their street numbers, while a "mail carrier" delivers "letters"—usually to the correct addresses.

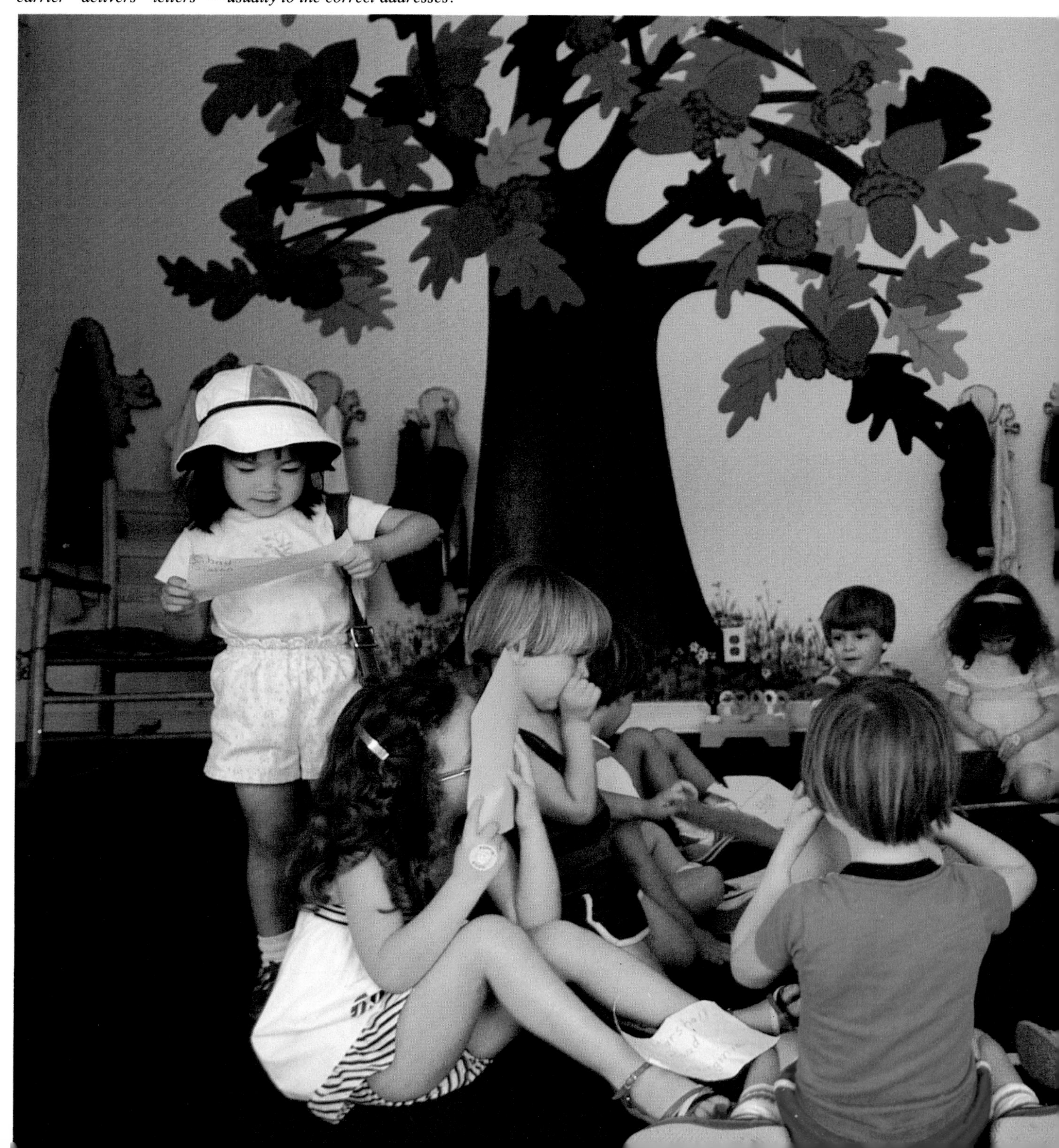

Learning together in the Little Acorn Patch

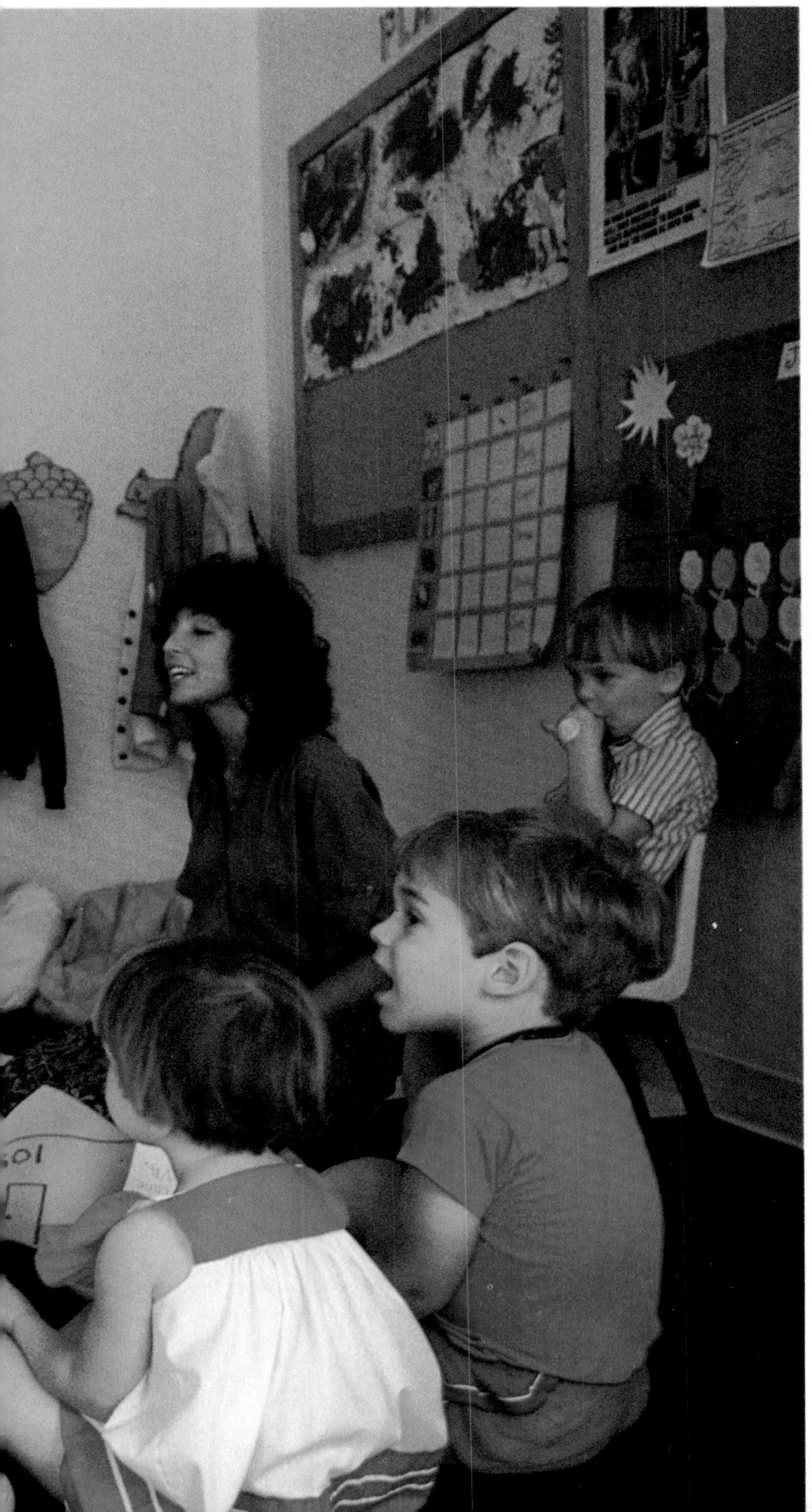

By the age of three, according to Dr. Benjamin Spock, a child "needs other children of the same age, not just to have fun with but also to learn how to get along with. This is the most important job in a child's life." Nowadays, when both of a preschooler's parents are likely to be employed, that kind of companionship develops less in neighborhood backyards than in nursery schools and the like. Increasingly, it is found in places like the Little Acorn Patch, a day-care center in the Virginia suburbs of Washington, D.C.

The Acorn Patch does not lie in a picturesque stand of oaks. It is, in fact, located in a neighborhood shopping plaza, and its most prominent tree is painted in bright reds, greens and browns on a classroom wall. Every weekday, groups of children gather beneath the branches of the painted tree for day-long education and constructive play under professional supervision.

Neither a nursery school nor a simple babysitting service, the center attempts to blend the best of both. As in a nursery school, time is programed in a variety of educational and social activities. Children learn the meanings of words, the uses of numbers, the difference between square and round. Regularly assigned chores teach responsibility. To feed the children's curiosity about their world, the Patch organizes field trips and receives classroom visits—a park naturalist, for example, brought a four-foot snake for the children to watch and touch. Practice in motor skills develops coordination in the children's arms, legs and hands, and time is set aside for group and individual play, either indoors or in a fenced-in yard. Perhaps of greatest educational importance, however, is the fact that the staff consists of professional educators, many with master's degrees.

Unlike traditional nursery schools, however, the Little Acorn Patch accepts children younger than three, and they can stay at the center all day: Parents can drop them off between 7 and 9 a.m. and pick them up from 3 p.m. until 6 in the evening. During that time, the day-care center meets all the children's physical needs for food, rest, supervision, hygiene and grooming. And because the ratio of children to staff is a desirably low 5 to 1 (ratios as high as 9 to 1 are considered acceptable by child-care experts), the youngsters get generous amounts of personal attention.

The most telling evidence of the Little Acorn Patch's success is to be found on the faces and in the attitudes of the teachers and their young charges. As the center's codirector Mary Byers says, "At the Little Acorn Patch we all have a really good time."

Mastering the movements of arms, legs and fingers

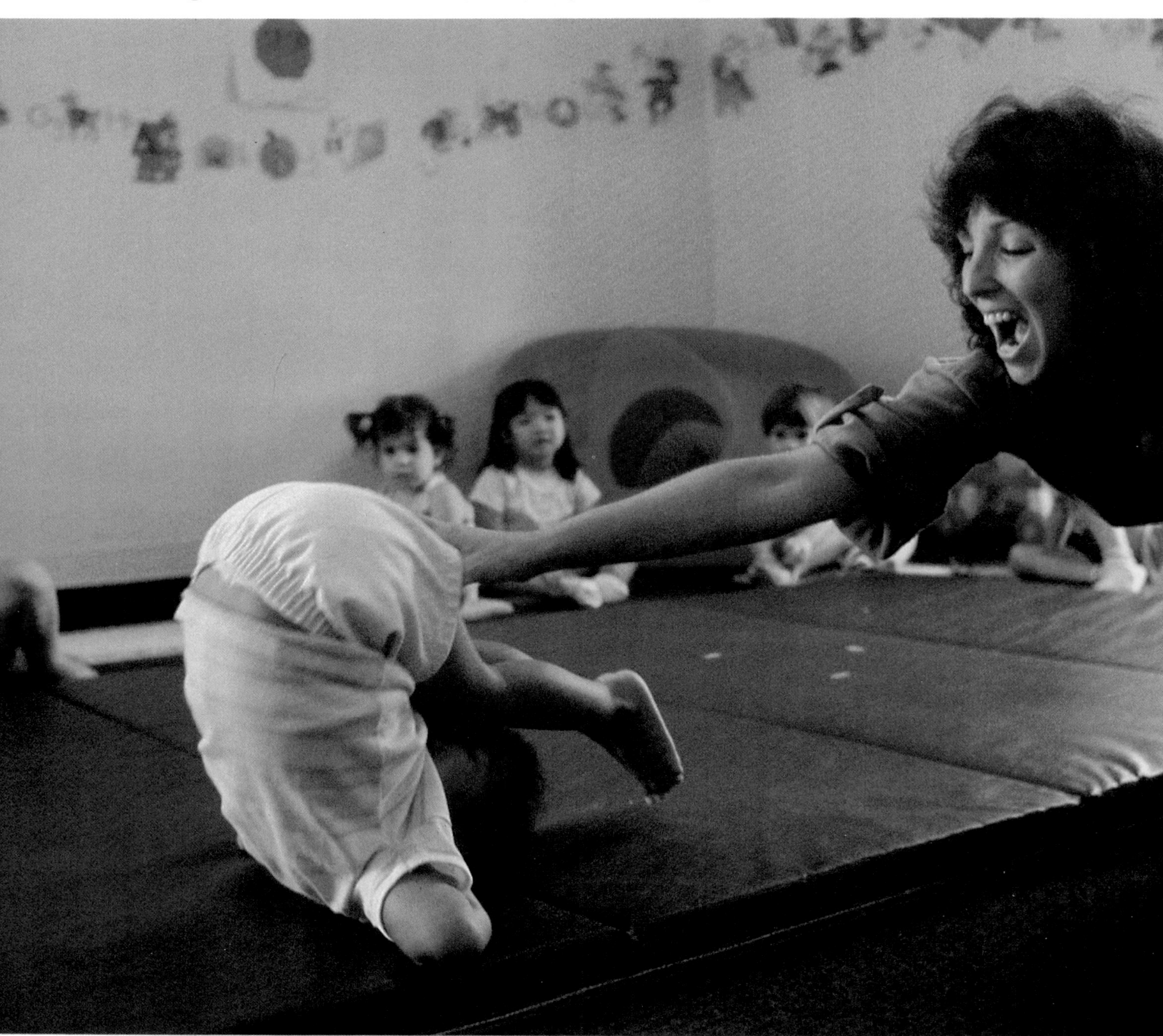

Aided by a push from teacher Doreen Fulton, a two-year-old acrobat turns a triumphant somersault on a padded mat. In this weekly gymnastics class, the children develop coordination, balance and strength in the large muscles of their arms and legs.

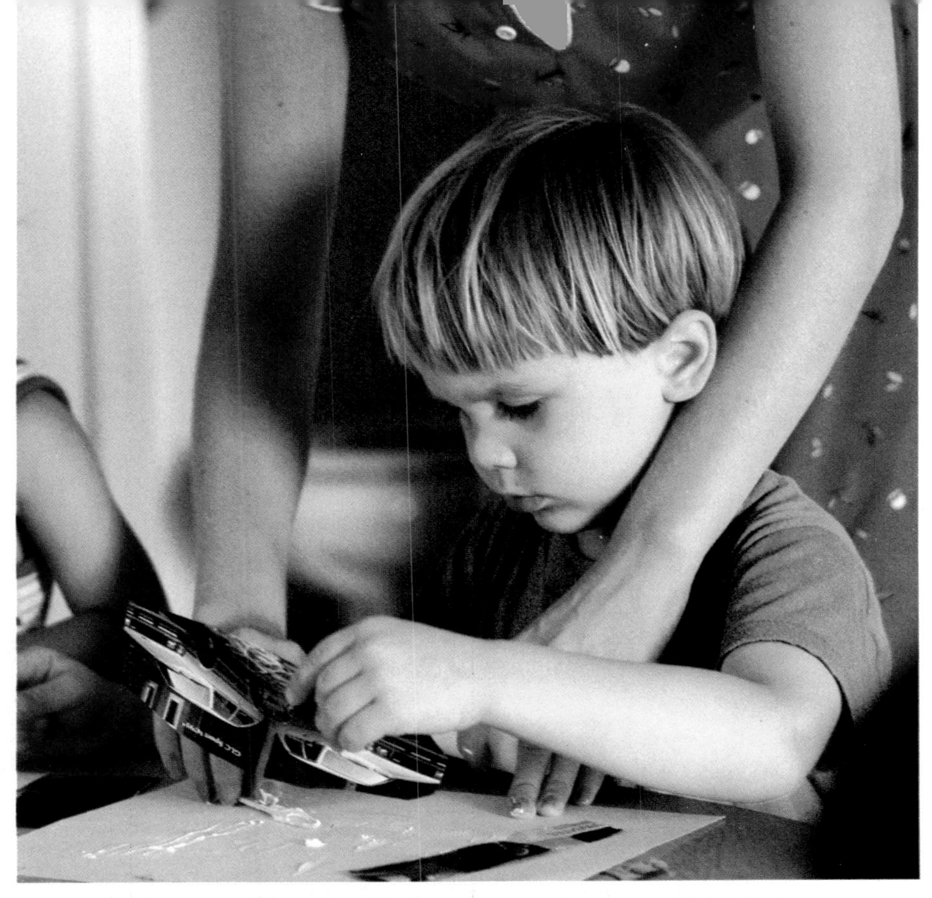

In an art class, a pupil pastes a picture of a car on a sheet of paper to create a unique Father's Day card. The activity not only fosters his emerging sense of creativity, but promotes eye-hand coordination.

Lost in an imaginary world, a budding city planner (below) builds a town out of plastic blocks. Like the supervised task shown at left, his work encourages dexterity and creativity, but it does so in a different way: Because it is solitary and self-initiated, this activity fills a private time in which the child's imagination has free rein.

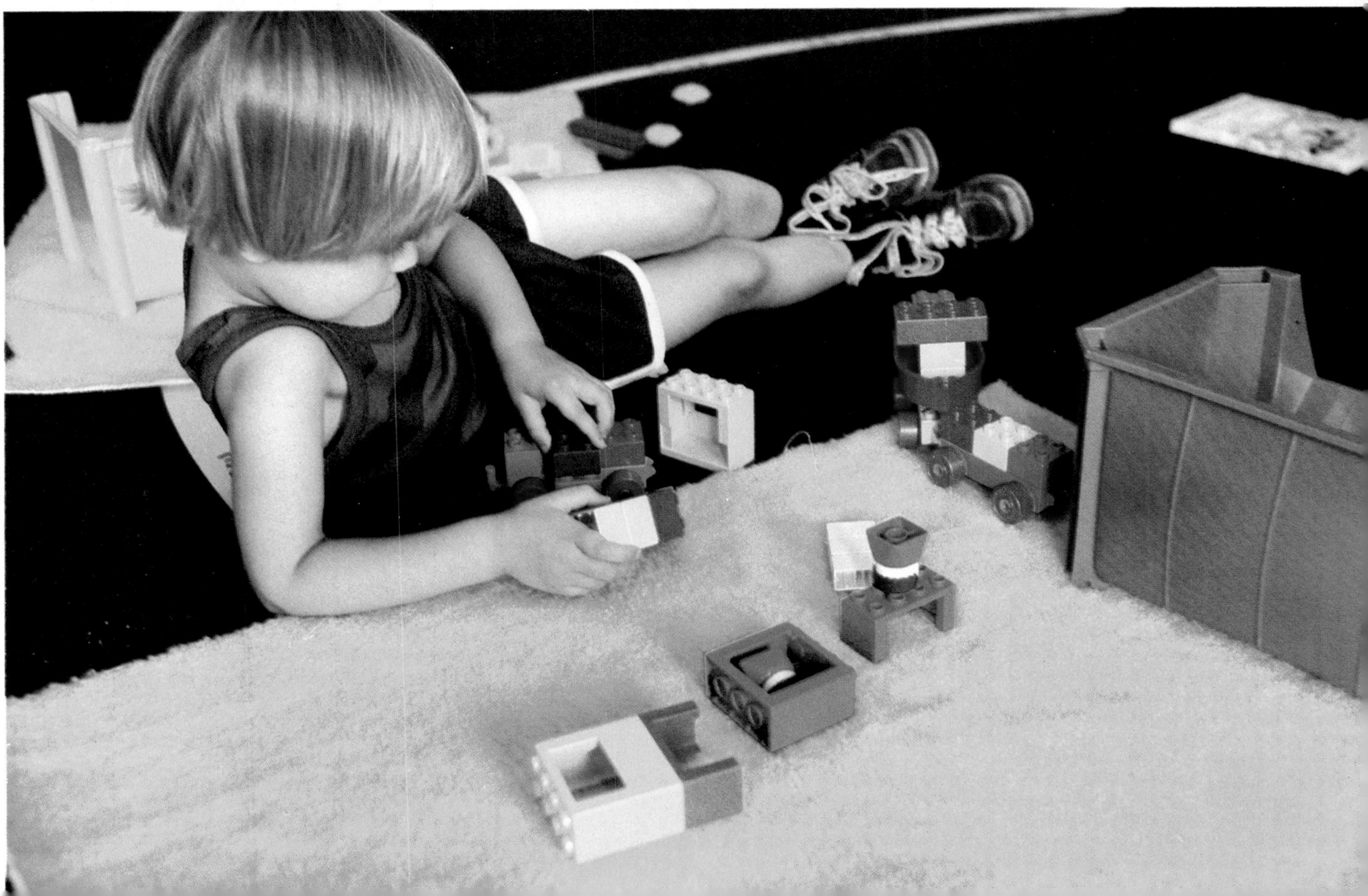

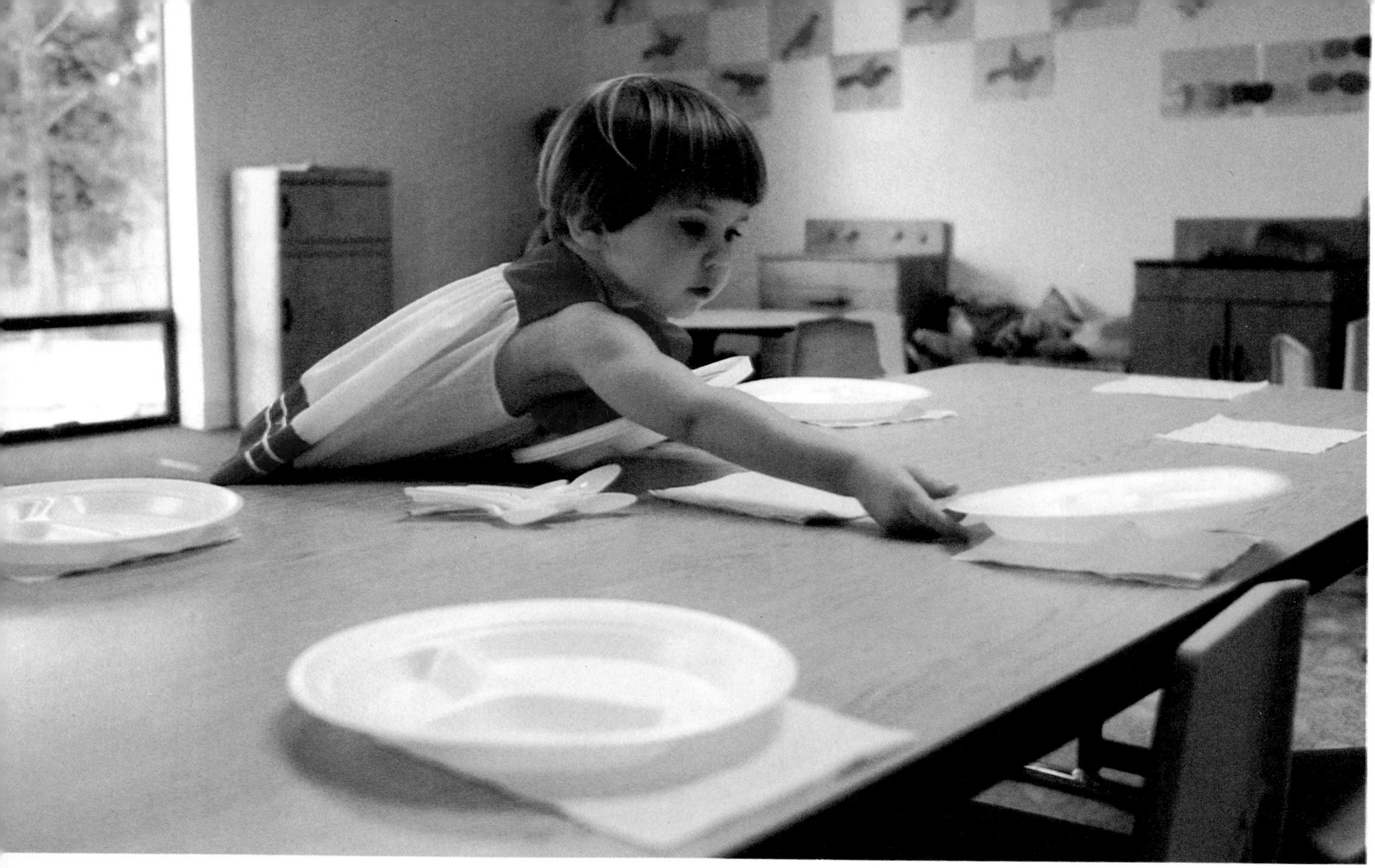

Stretching to place a plate, two-year-old Shelley helps set the table for her group. To encourage a sense of responsibility, specific tasks are assigned each morning. At lunch, for example, two children set the table; when a group enters or leaves the building, one child holds the door; and in class, a child serves as the teacher's "happy helper"—the most coveted job of all.

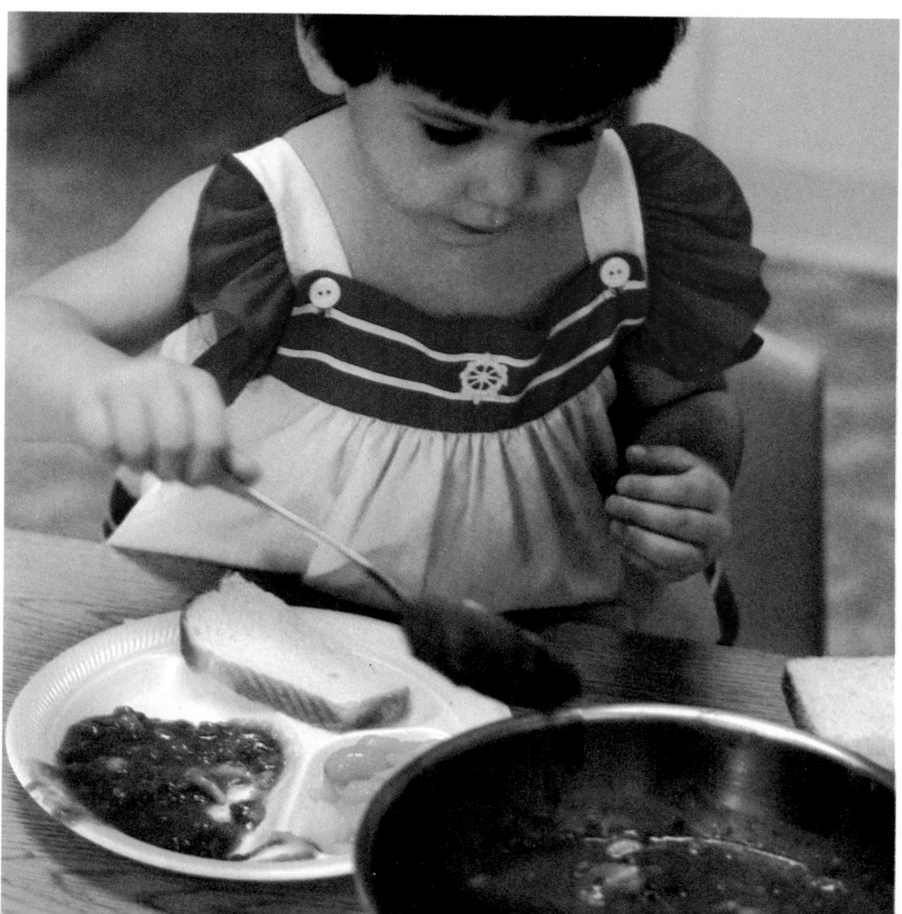

After the table is set, Shelley dips into a pot of stew. Lunch is served family style and the children help themselves, in a procedure that is sometimes messy but teaches cooperation and sharing.

Practical lessons in responsibility

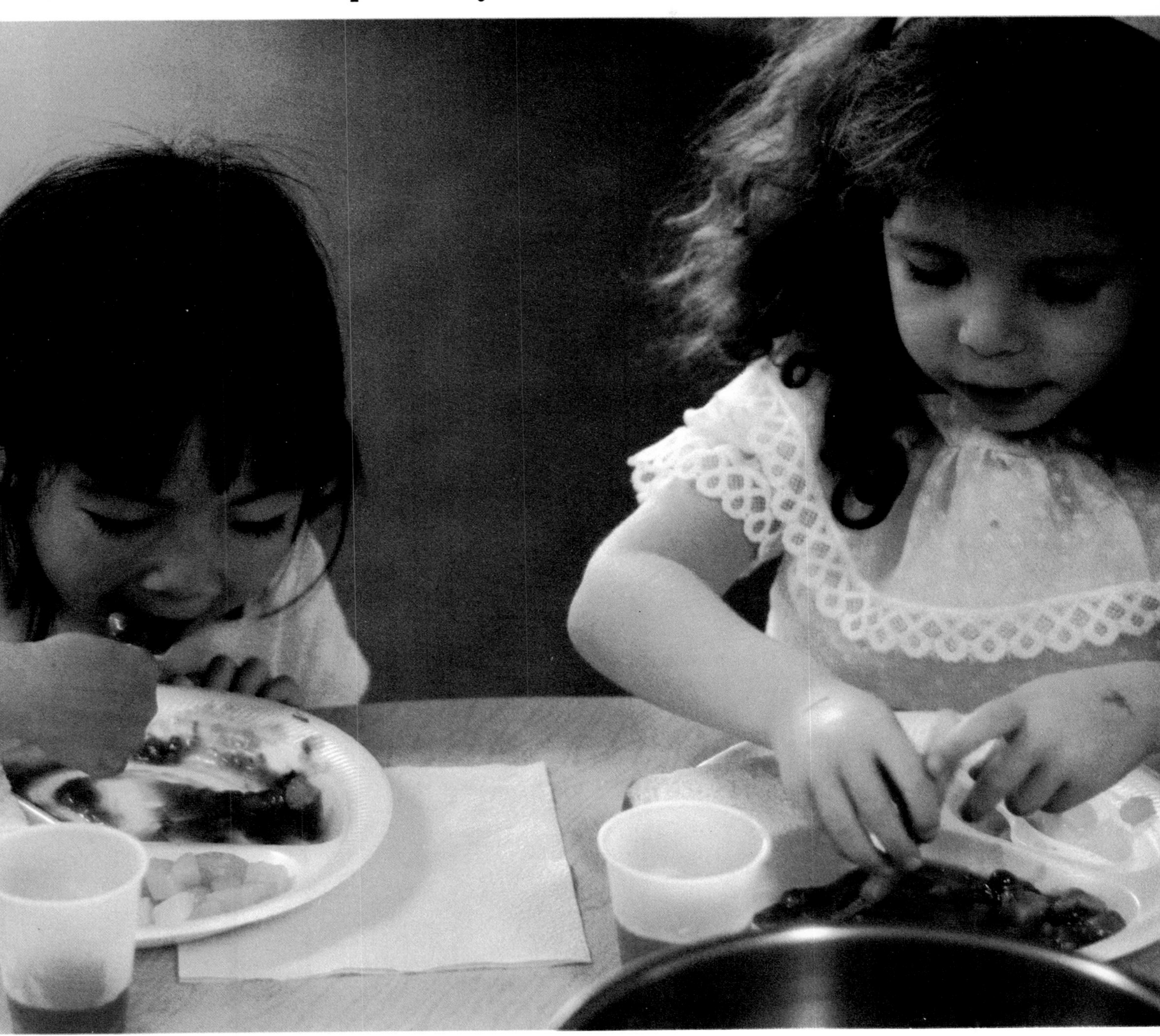

Two hungry lunchers dig into a well-balanced meal of stew, celery, fruit and bread, accompanied by a fruit drink. The children are encouraged to try everything on their plates. When they balk, teachers generally try indirect psychological persuasion, such as musing aloud on what a nice color carrots are.

A quiet time: the afternoon nap

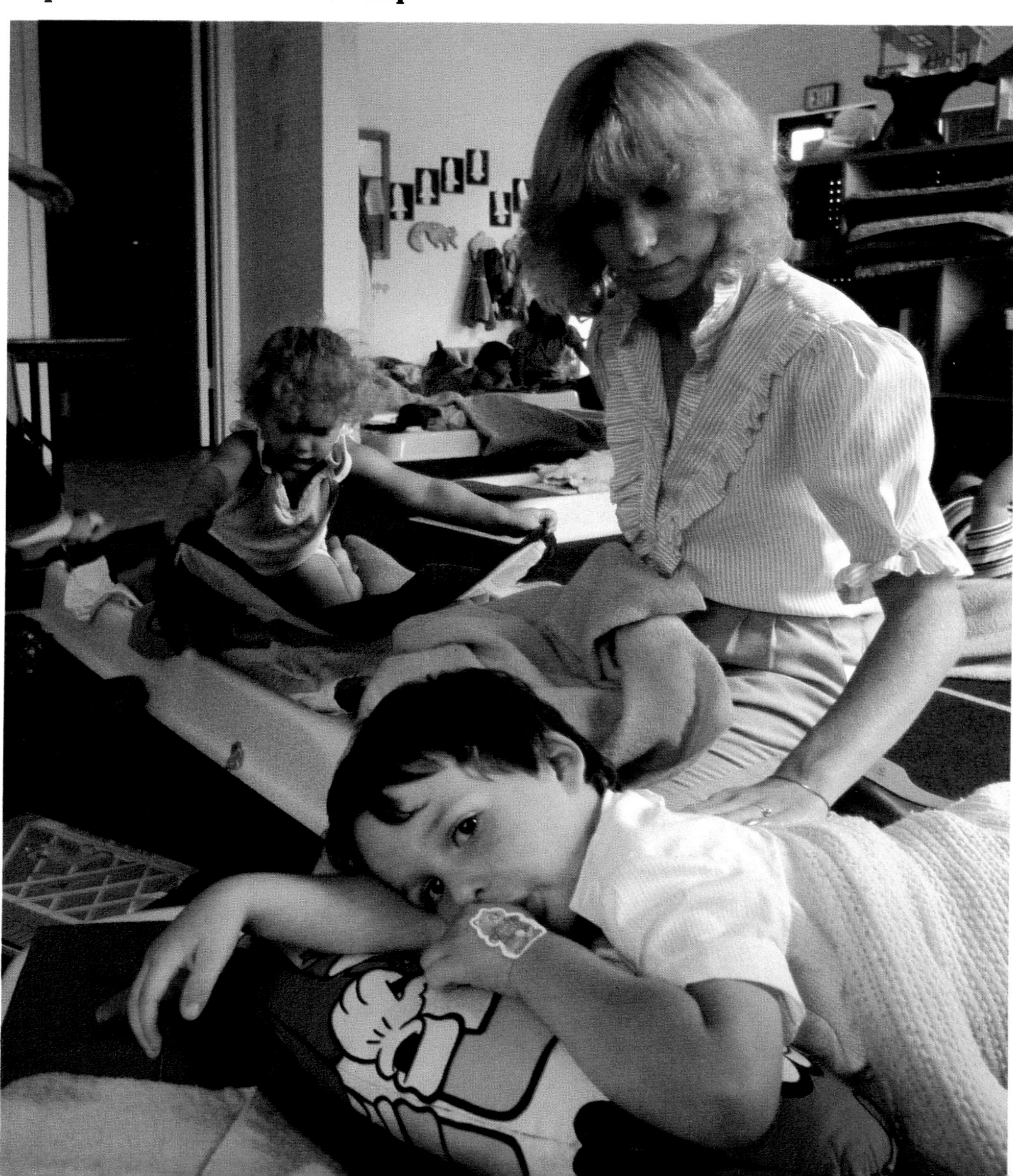

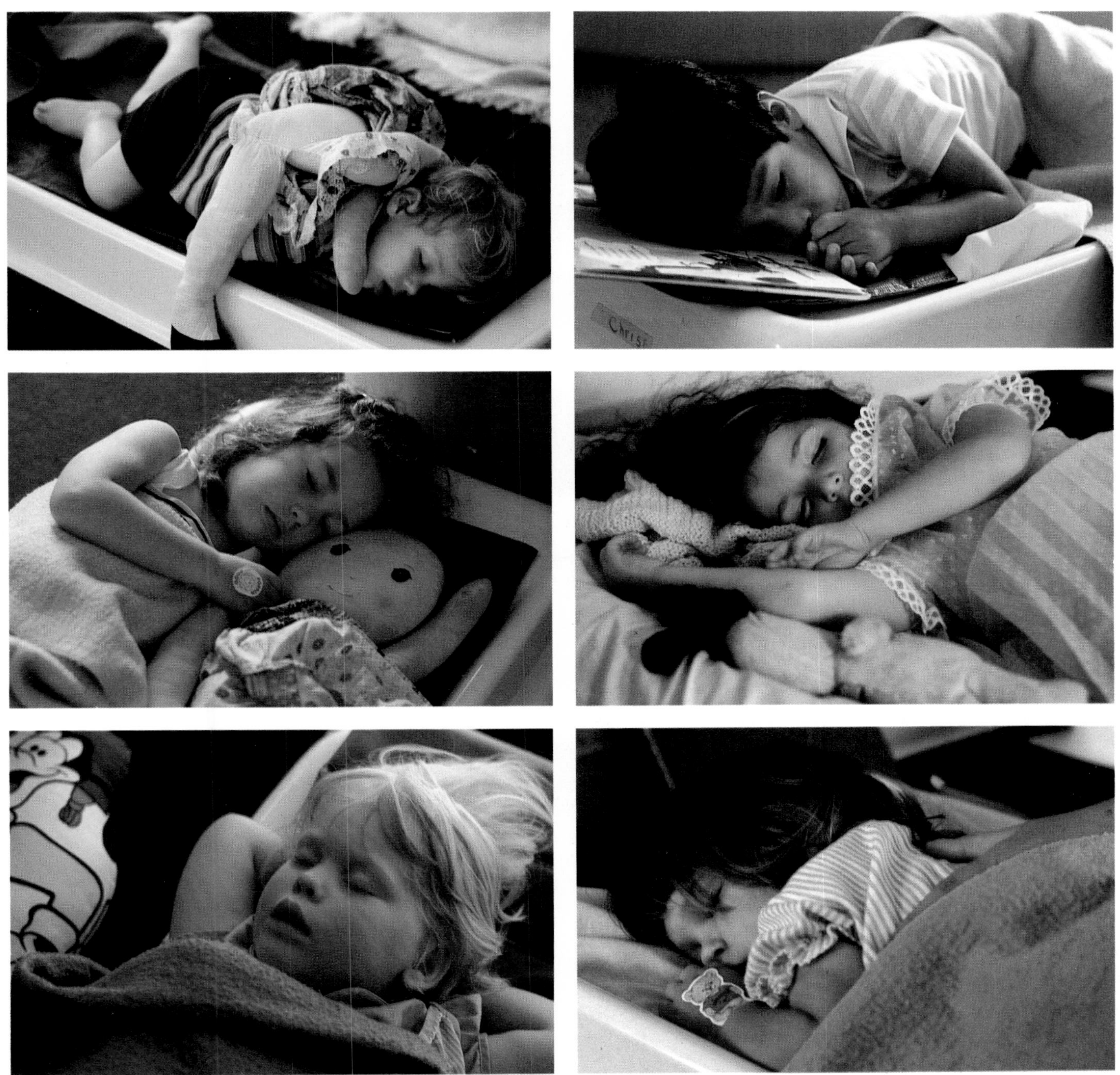

Every day from one to three in the afternoon, the children of the Little Acorn Patch nap together, each secure in his regular place with his personal blanket and plastic cot. At left, in a prenap ritual performed for every child, a teacher administers a soothing back rub. Above, the children sleep or doze in a variety of moods and postures.

Her eyes intent on the faucet, two-year-old Rachel rinses her toothbrush, normally stored along with her own toothpaste in a personal container in the bathroom. The children wash their hands before each meal and brush their teeth afterward.

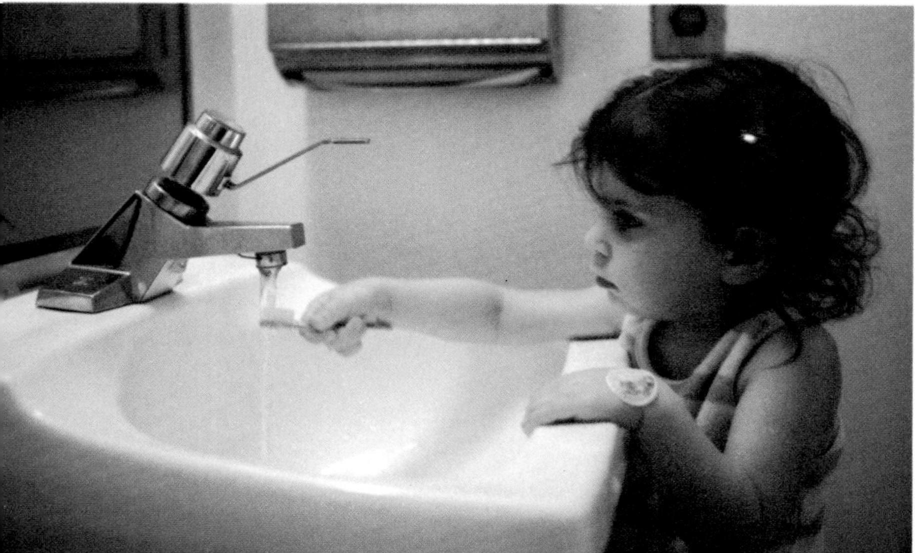

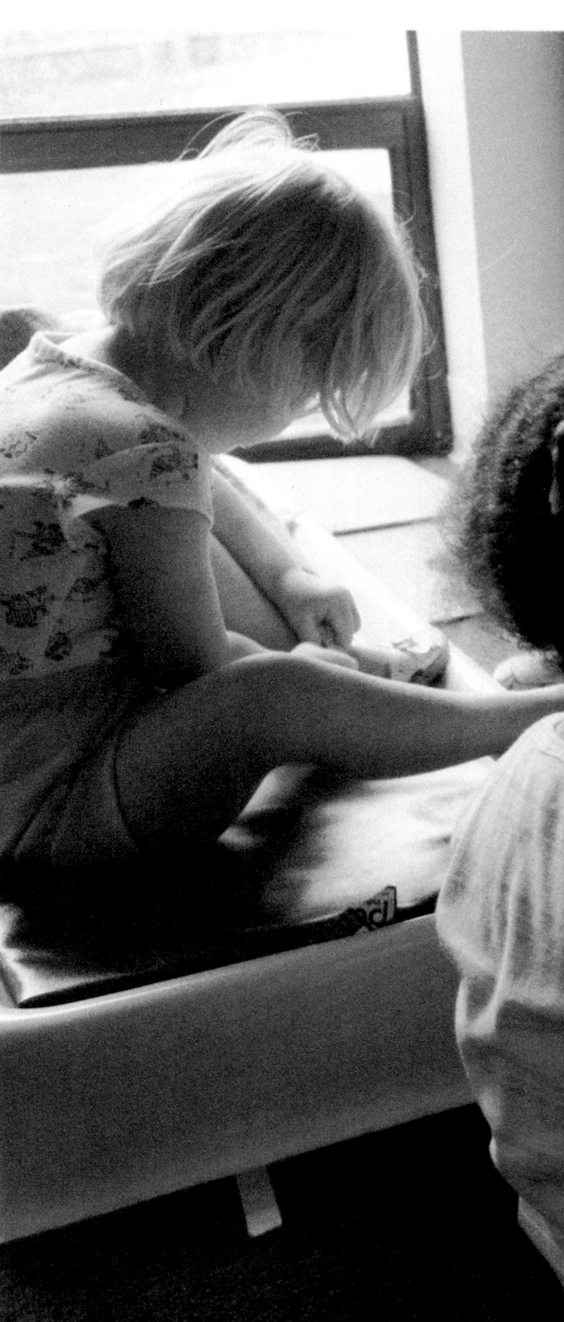

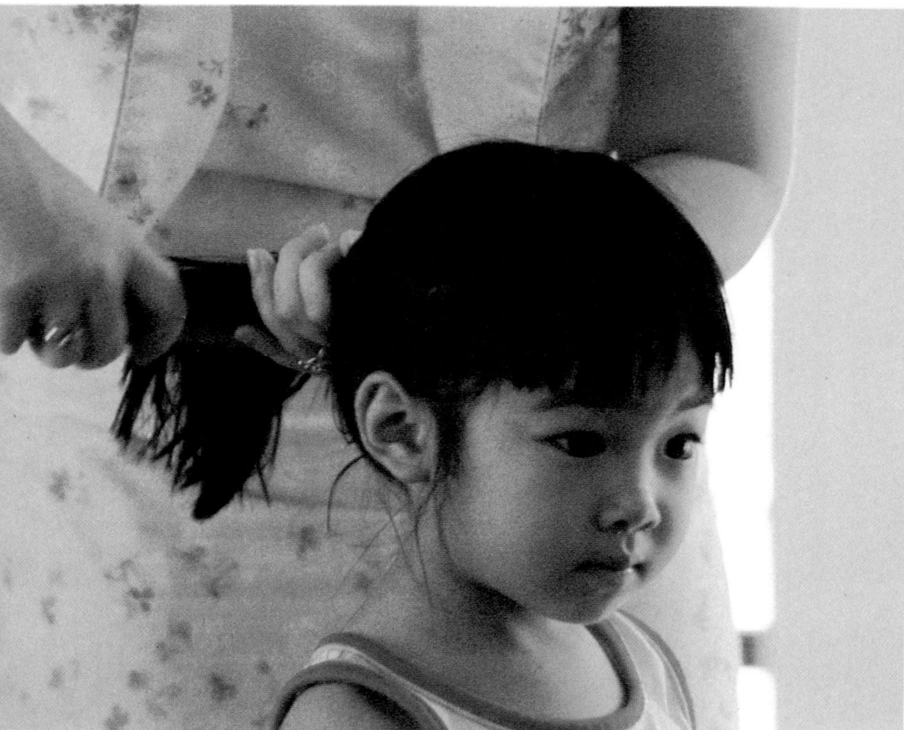

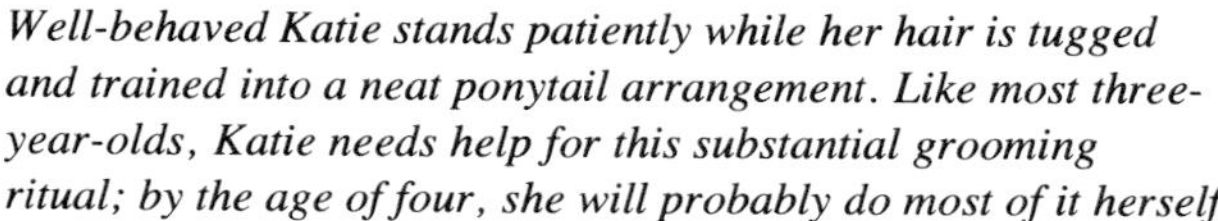

Well-behaved Katie stands patiently while her hair is tugged and trained into a neat ponytail arrangement. Like most three-year-olds, Katie needs help for this substantial grooming ritual; by the age of four, she will probably do most of it herself.

The ABCs of keeping clean and looking good

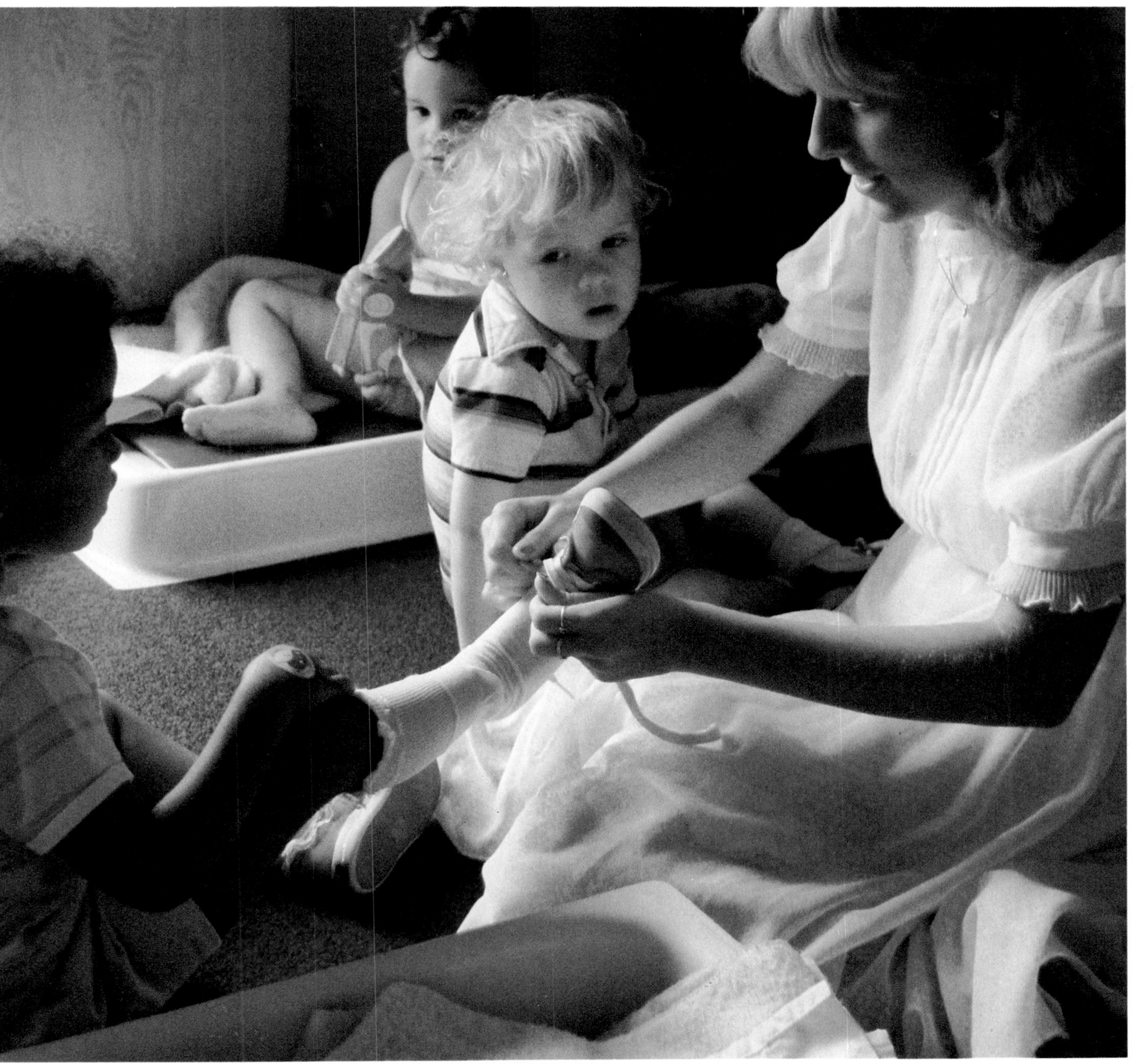

Still drowsy after their nap, four children address the job of donning shoes and socks. Most three-year-olds can put on their socks without trouble, and some can get into their sneakers—but the task of tying laces almost always calls for outside aid.

CHAPTER 6

A range of ills and remedies

How to read the meaning of a fever
Inescapable, but self-healing—the common cold
Trouble in the digestive tract
Threats to a sensitive skin
Helping the doctor to do his job

As part of their training at Duke University Medical Center, interns study photographs of a rare skin rash. The disease that causes the rash is measles—just a few decades ago an all-but-inevitable infection of childhood—and the object of the exercise is to help them to diagnose the disease if they ever encounter a case. But these interns may never have a chance to use their knowledge. Inoculation against measles is now mandated by law, and by the time the student doctors enter practice, the United States will probably have seen its last case of the disease.

The virtual elimination of measles is one of many medical success stories. In the late 19th Century, some 200 of every 1,000 American babies died before their first birthday, victims of dysentery, pneumonia, measles, diphtheria, whooping cough, and other infectious diseases. By the mid-1970s, only 15 of every 1,000 babies died during their first year, most of them in the first few days after birth. Immunizations now protect children against such once-dreaded diseases as polio, and have rendered smallpox a historical curiosity. Antibiotics have countered the threats of such bacterial illnesses as strep throat and certain forms of pneumonia.

Children still get sick, of course, sometimes seriously sick. A life-threatening disease such as cancer continues to take its toll among the young. Sudden infant death syndrome—a mysterious killer that strikes apparently healthy babies as they sleep *(page 141)*—remains a threat in the first months of life. But most childhood illnesses now inflict no lasting damage. Their effects are limited to transient discomforts—sneezing, runny nose, fever, sore throat, upset stomach, skin rash—that can usually be treated at home.

To deal with these common problems, parents must know how to recognize their signs, how to relieve the symptoms, when to consult a doctor, and how to make a sick child comfortable while he recuperates. Finally, when a child's medical needs cannot be met by home care, the parents must prepare the child psychologically for a trip to the hospital.

To be sure, these jobs alone are considerable, and sometimes seem almost unremitting. Despite the best efforts of parents and doctors, children get sick more often than adults. Frequent illnesses, in fact, are not only a normal part of childhood, but an essential part. Born with little immunity, babies build up defensive antibodies by meeting infections head on. According to pediatrician Jack Shiller: "Just as a locksmith needs the lock in order to make a key that fits, so the body needs the infection in order to produce the right pattern for the antibody that will fit it and thus fight it." As a result of childhood infections, the average adult has partial immunity against at least 60 different virus strains.

Children not only get sick more often than adults, but get sick faster, just as they do everything at a biologically faster pace. A toddler who seems fine at bedtime and goes peacefully to sleep may awaken in the middle of the night crying and clearly unwell. Fortunately, children usually recover just as suddenly as they fall ill. For parents, the problem is to recognize subtle signs of a developing illness and act quickly to minimize the misery and prevent complications.

A patient helps in an oral temperature reading by sealing her lips around a thermometer lodged under her tongue. Though often used, this method of taking temperature is relatively unreliable; most pediatricians prefer the rectal method (page 142).

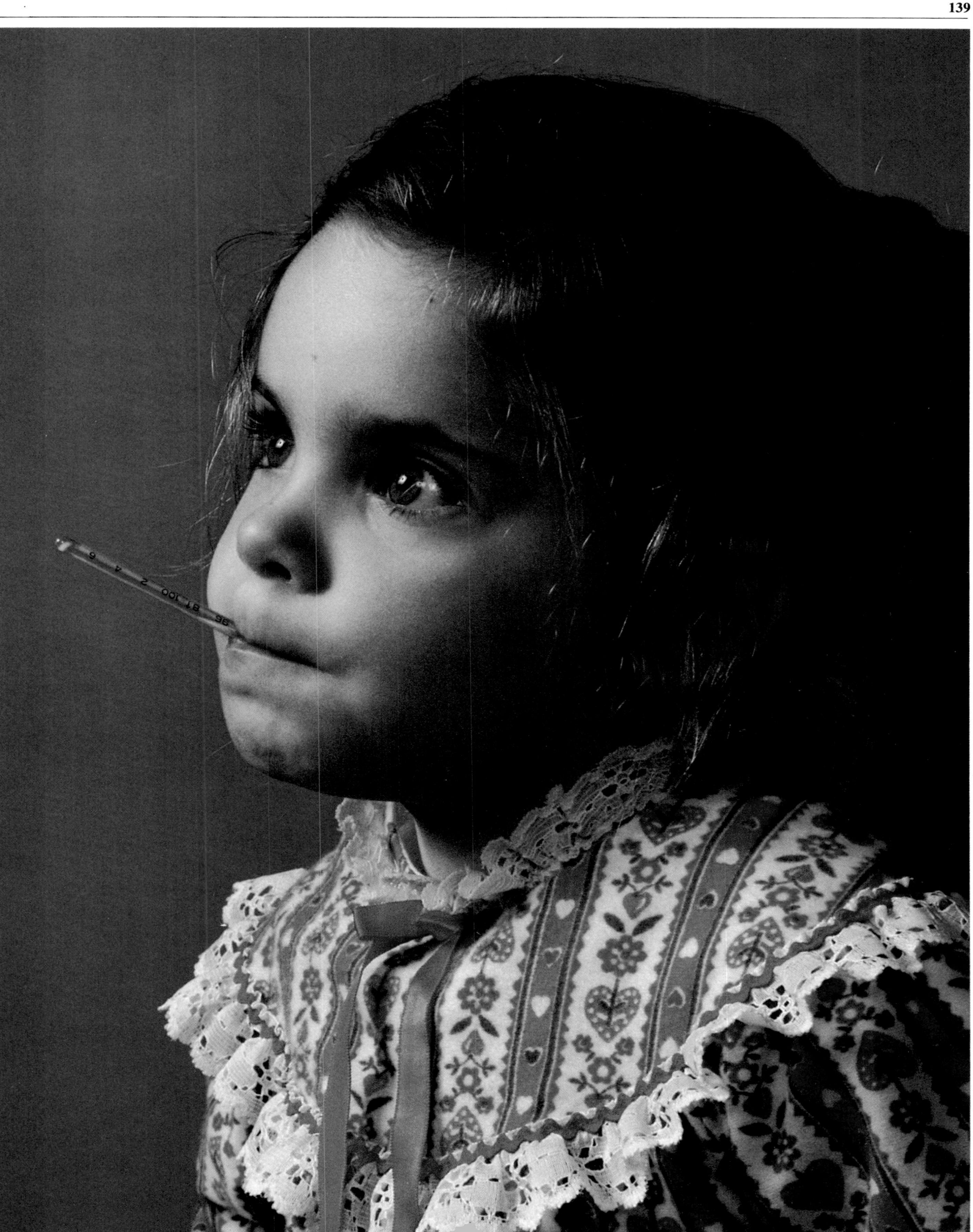

A subtle but most reliable clue that a child is sick is some change in normal behavior. The typically playful baby who is cranky and lethargic, or the irrepressible toddler who falls asleep while playing, probably does not feel well. If the child has one or more overt symptoms—chills, flushed skin, aches, sneezing or coughing, vomiting, diarrhea—watch him closely. Have him rest, take his temperature and, if the symptoms persist or are especially severe, call the doctor.

How to read the meaning of a fever

Often the very first sign of illness in a child is fever. More correctly, however, fever is a sign of active resistance to illness. For centuries, it has been recognized as an essential part of the body's defense against disease. The ancient Greeks believed that a high body temperature "cooked" unwanted body substances so that they could be easily eliminated—and there was an element of truth in the theory. Modern researchers have shown that as the body's white blood cells fight off infection, they release substances called pyrogens into the bloodstream. These pyrogens act upon a central "thermostat" in the brain, prodding the body to produce more heat, much as adjusting the thermostat in a room switches a furnace on. The extra heat, in turn, inhibits the growth and reproduction of the infecting organisms.

A child develops fever faster and more frequently than an adult. Moreover, children generally have higher body temperatures than an adult, because they are more active; for example, a perfectly healthy child may have a temperature of 100° F. after hard play. But in almost any child, a temperature of 101° signifies illness.

The level of fever above 101° F. is not a reliable gauge of the seriousness of a child's illness. Between the ages of one and five, children with a mild virus infection can easily develop fevers of 104° or 105°; by contrast, a really dangerous illness may not drive a child's temperature much beyond 101°. But any fever in an infant less than six months old can signal a serious infection that may spread to the bloodstream and brain, and a doctor should be informed at once. A fever in an older child is less ominous, but his behavior must be watched. If he is active and eating, his illness is probably minor. If he seems sleepy and apathetic or does not want to be touched, he may be seriously ill; consult a doctor immediately. Check with the doctor, too, if a fever is accompanied by pain, vomiting or diarrhea and persists for 24 hours.

Knowing the precise level and course of a fever is important for both parents and doctor. Choose for yourself among the three ways of taking a youngster's temperature—rectally, orally, or in the armpit. Most pediatricians recommend the rectal method because it is fastest, most accurate and perfectly safe when correctly executed *(page 142)*. An oral reading is sometimes difficult to obtain because the thermometer must be kept in a child's closed mouth for three minutes; it is virtually worthless if the child has a stuffy nose and breathes through his mouth. Armpit readings are preferable to rectal when a child has diarrhea.

In general, a child's temperature should be kept under 104°; high fever can make a youngster trembly, jumpy, even delirious. Even though a feverish child will often feel chilly, dress or cover him lightly—bundling him up will only drive up the fever. Urge the child to drink plenty of liquids. Overheating and increased sweating can soon lead to dehydration.

The most direct way to bring a fever down is sponging the skin with tepid water, which produces rapid cooling through evaporation. Never use cold water or alcohol because sudden chilling is not only uncomfortable but may trigger a spell of shivering that actually increases body temperature.

Slower than sponging but just as reliable are the two common fever-reducing drugs, aspirin and acetaminophen. Both work by altering the brain's response to pyrogens, and both are equally effective in lowering a fever. But important considerations of safety affect the choice between them. Statistical evidence links aspirin with Reye's syndrome—a rare disease that strikes children recovering from viral infections, particularly influenza and chicken pox. First recognized in the early 1960s, the disease starts with fever, vomiting and headaches, but progresses rapidly to convulsions and coma. It is fatal in about 25 per cent of cases and causes permanent brain damage in many more. Some scientists speculate that aspirin contributes to the disease by interfering with a child's natural defenses against viral infection.

The enigma of sudden infant death

The leading cause of death among children between one month and one year old is a baffling phenomenon called sudden infant death syndrome (SIDS). Commonly known as crib death, the malady strikes about two infants in every thousand in the United States, most often in the third, fourth or fifth month of life. In a typical case, an apparently healthy child is put to bed and, hours later, is found dead. No unusual sounds mark the onset of death, and there are only occasional signs of struggle.

Scores of theories have been advanced to explain the perplexing deaths. Some proposed causes, such as suffocation and an allergy to cow's milk, have been eliminated. Others, such as botulism infection and apnea, a brief stoppage of breathing, seem to be involved in some cases, but not in most. Many scientists now suspect that SIDS results from a mix of factors, and that the victims may not be as healthy as they seem. For example, a metabolic defect or a subtle impairment of the nervous system may predispose a child to SIDS, and death may occur when the child is exposed to some precipitating factor, such as a viral infection. In fact, about half of all SIDS victims are in the midst of or have recently had a slight cold or other mild respiratory problem.

While researchers hunt for the causes of crib death, practical measures for preventing it are being developed. In one promising program, apnea—the probable cause of some deaths—is electronically monitored for immediate action *(below)*.

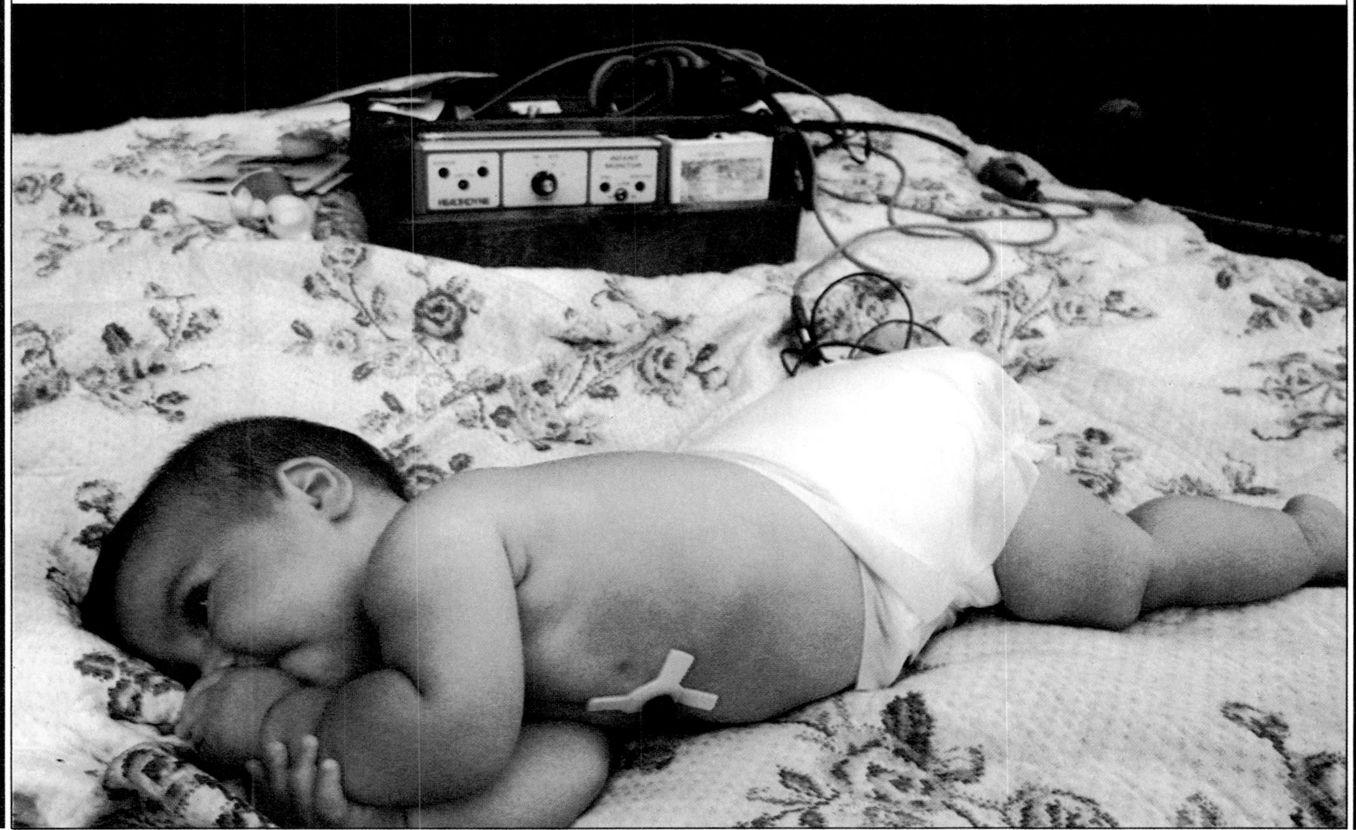

In a program offered by Boston's Massachusetts General Hospital, an infant prone to interruptions in breathing is wired to an electronic monitor that keeps a running check on her breathing and heartbeat. If either rate drops below a preset level for as long as 20 seconds, her parents, trained in resuscitation methods, are alerted by a loud beeper.

To measure a baby's rectal temperature, lay the child across your lap; place one hand under his chin to support his upper body. Coat the end of the thermometer with lubricating jelly, grasp its tube firmly between two fingers of the other hand, and insert it about one half inch into the rectum. Press the child's buttocks together, and hold the thermometer in place one minute.

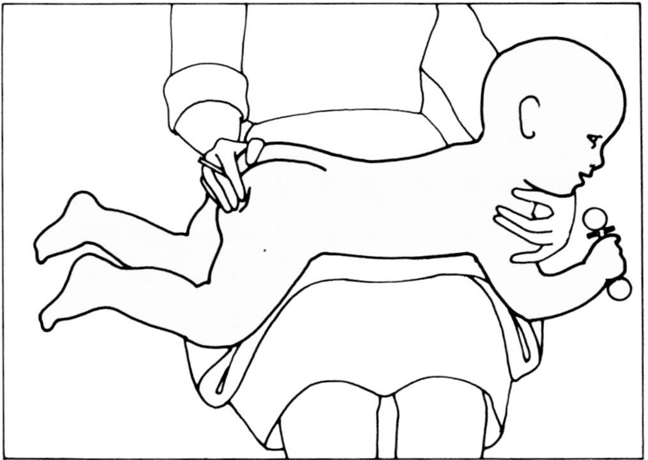

Whatever the specific effect, the evidence against aspirin is now all but conclusive. The U.S. Department of Health and Human Services and the American Academy of Pediatrics strongly advise against giving aspirin to any child suffering from flu or chicken pox. In these cases, control a fever with acetaminophen or such nondrug remedies as sponging.

While drugs can complicate a fever, fever itself can have frightening complications. The threat of convulsions, also called febrile seizures, is a compelling reason for keeping a child's fever low. In such a seizure, the child may collapse, or his entire body may stiffen. His eyes may roll backward, and his head begin to jerk. Extremities often twitch, and bladder or bowel control may be lost. Fever-induced convulsions occur in 3 to 5 per cent of normal children, usually during a rapid upswing in temperature. They are most common between the ages of three months and five years.

A seizure is sure to strike terror in any parent who has never witnessed one, but it is not especially dangerous and almost always subsides in a few minutes. While a child is in its grip, try to remain calm and follow a few simple rules:

- Protect the child from falling or hitting his head. Ease him to the floor or place him on a bed.
- Make sure the child's breathing passage is open. Clear any vomit or frothy material from his nose and throat, and pull his head backward slightly to maintain a clear airway.
- Do not jam a spoon or other object into the child's mouth to protect his tongue. He is not likely to bite or swallow his tongue, and forcing something into his mouth can do more harm than good.
- When the attack subsides, take immediate steps to reduce the fever. The child may be extremely weak and groggy and may fall into a deep sleep; there is no need to arouse him.
- Finally, call the doctor. Though convulsions rarely cause lasting damage, each episode should be studied to be sure it was not triggered by some underlying problem such as meningitis—an infection of the lining of the brain or spinal cord.

Any seizure is bound to stir fears of epilepsy. The fact is that a simple fever-related convulsion neither causes epilepsy nor signals its onset. The vast majority of children who experience febrile seizures enjoy normal health, and more than half the children who have one seizure never have another.

Inescapable, but self-healing—the common cold

The illness most likely to produce a fever in a small child is an upper-respiratory infection—the common cold. Most children get 10 times as many colds as all other illnesses combined; an average child under five may have as many as eight or 10 a year. Some are brief and mild, but the typical cold lasts a week or two, and is accompanied by sneezing, stuffy nose, cough and scratchy throat. Some victims may vomit up swallowed mucus or develop diarrhea or constipation; most become cranky and lose their interest in food.

It is all but impossible to prevent successive colds, even in the healthiest child. Colds are caused by several hundred different agents, and one infection provides little immunity against the next to come along. Thus children often catch one cold after another. They cannot, however, contract a "chronic" or constant cold. There is no such thing. A child with a perpetually runny nose is probably suffering from an allergy.

The agents that cause colds are viruses; antibiotics, which act upon the larger organisms called bacteria, have no effect on viruses. Therefore, giving antibiotics to a child with an uncomplicated cold is worthless in itself; what is more, it puts him at needless risk of an allergic reaction, and fosters the development of antibiotic-resistant strains of bacteria. In fact, all drugs should be kept to a minimum during a cold. The goal is to alleviate discomfort while allowing the body's healing mechanisms to operate. Sneezing, coughing and a runny nose, for example, can be relieved by commercial decongestants if they become insupportable; otherwise, they are actually valuable to the sufferer, because they clear mucus from the respiratory tract. Your child should learn to blow his nose at as early an age as possible; teach him to exhale gently through both nostrils, so that he does not force infected mucus back into his nose.

An infant with a stuffy nose is at a special disadvantage, particularly at feeding time, because he cannot suck and breathe through his mouth at the same time. One way to relieve the obstruction calls for a nasal syringe, a simple rubber bulb with a plastic tip. Compress the bulb, insert the nozzle into the baby's nostril, and slowly release the bulb; suction pulls the mucus into the bulb. Babies are not fond of the procedure, but it is safe even for the tiniest infants. If the mucus is thick and sticky, as it often is in the late stages of a cold, loosen it with a few drops of salt solution (about one level teaspoon of salt to a quart of water).

In lieu of medicines, certain simple remedies help relieve coughing and stuffiness. Ordinary fluids, given in quantity, help loosen mucus, soothe a sore throat and replenish water lost because of fever. Water and juices are good, but milk is not; it can stimulate mucus production. To prevent mucus from dripping down the throat (a common cause of coughing at night) prop a baby on his side or place a pillow under the mattress at the head of a child's bed to raise him slightly.

The dangers of a cold's complications

Throughout the course of a child's cold, be alert for signs of complications. A cold virus lowers a child's resistance to other viruses and to bacteria, permitting more serious infections. If a high fever recurs several days after the cold's onset, or if the child develops a persistent cough, particularly during the day, consult a doctor. Labored breathing and a painful, mucus-producing cough may indicate bronchitis or pneumonia. If a child sneezes up yellow or bloody mucus after most other cold symptoms have passed, his sinuses may be infected. Drowsiness or lethargy, especially if accompanied by a high fever and stiff neck, can signal meningitis. All these conditions require prompt medical attention. Many are of bacterial origin and respond quickly to antibiotics.

One of the most frightening respiratory infections in young children is croup, a severe form of laryngitis marked by swelling, spasms and mucus in the airways—mucus so thick it threatens suffocation. Typically, a child suffering from a mild cold wakes suddenly in the night, gasping for air and coughing with a high-pitched sound that has been likened to the barking of a seal. These symptoms call for fast action: Take the child to the bathroom and turn on a hot shower to produce thick clouds of moist air, which reduce the swelling and thin the secretions. If breathing does not improve within 10 minutes, get the child to a hospital immediately.

By far the most frequent complication of a childhood cold is a middle-ear infection. Almost every child has at least one earache during the preschool years; many have one or two a year. An ear infection occurs when a Eustachian tube (the tube between an ear and the upper throat) becomes swollen, blocking the normal drainage of fluid from the ear. The accumulated fluid provides a growth medium for bacteria migrating up the tube from the top of the throat. As the pressure of infection builds, the eardrum becomes inflamed and bulges outward, causing severe pain and impaired hearing.

Signs of an ear infection in an infant include tugging at the ear and crying when swallowing. The child may cry at night but stop when he is picked up, because the pain lessens when his head is erect. An unmistakable sign of infection is a white or yellow discharge from the ear, released through an eardrum that has been ruptured by pressure.

Contrary to popular belief, a ruptured or perforated eardrum usually heals in a few days, with no lasting effect on hearing. But there is no reason to let things get to this point. Ear infections respond to antibiotics, and prompt medical treatment spares a child both excruciating pain and the risk of recurring infection that can permanently damage the ear. If hours must pass before you can see a doctor, you can relieve some of the child's pain by giving him aspirin or acetaminophen, placing a warm heating pad or water bottle against the inflamed ear, and having him sit up rather than lie down.

Persistent soreness in the throat, as in the ears, calls for professional attention. A slight sore throat often accompanies the early stages of a cold or flu, but one kind of sore throat, called strep throat because it is caused by streptococcus bacteria, is potentially dangerous. If untreated, it can lead to inflammation of the kidneys or to rheumatic fever, which can permanently damage the heart.

It is impossible to distinguish a strep throat from a viral throat infection on the basis of physical symptoms alone. Consult a doctor about any sore throat that lasts longer than 24 hours, even if the child has only mild pain or fever, or slightly swollen glands under the jaw. To make a definite diagnosis, the doctor will take a culture by swabbing the throat with a piece of sterile cotton on the end of a stick—a procedure that some pediatricians are now teaching parents to do at home. The swab is then sent to a laboratory, where it is smeared onto a nutritive medium in which germs multiply rapidly. Within about 24 hours, the colony of germs will be large enough for the infecting organisms to be identified.

If the culture is positive—that is, if it shows a strep infection—the doctor will prescribe an antibiotic, usually penicillin. If the culture reveals a viral infection, drugs are useless, and you must wait for the infection to run its course. In either case, ease the child's discomfort by giving him plenty of liquids and having him gargle with warm water.

Years ago, the blame for recurrent colds, sore throats and ear infections was often placed on the tonsils, two lumps of spongy tissue located at the sides of the throat near the base of the tongue; and on the adenoids, a mass of similar tissue on the roof of the throat. In fact, the tonsils and adenoids were largely misunderstood. Among doctors, part of the misunderstanding stemmed from the large size of these organs in young children. If the tonsils and adenoids were so big, the reasoning went, they must be diseased, and removal by the age of five was almost mandatory.

Today physicians believe that these tissues, far from being useless obstructions, are an important first-line defense against invading bacteria and viruses. They store the white blood cells that fight foreign invaders, and stimulate the production of antibodies—and they are large in early childhood simply because there are so many infections to fight. As the child's immune system becomes more efficient, their role and size diminish. If left alone, they generally start to shrink by age 12, and by adulthood they virtually disappear.

Most pediatricians now recommend removing these natural protectors only if they are repeatedly infected or become so large that they interfere with swallowing or breathing. Exceptionally noisy breathing is sometimes a clue. One mother recalled that she always knew when her three-year-old daughter was asleep by the sound of snoring, which carried easily through closed doors. "I thought this was normal," the mother said, "until another child slept over and breathed so silently that I had to watch her chest move to reassure myself she was alive!"

The only sign of illness in the young snorer consisted of painful earaches every time she got a cold. During one of these bouts, her pediatrician saw that her tonsils were so large that they almost met in the middle of her throat; her adenoids, he found, were just as huge. No doubt the organs were blocking both the nasal passages and the Eustachian tubes. For this child, the penalties of tonsils and adenoids clearly outweighed their benefits, and the tissues were removed. In the majority of youngsters, though, problems are not this severe. Occasional tonsillitis and slight snoring at night are a normal part of childhood and do not justify surgery.

Trouble in the digestive tract

Like the respiratory tract, the digestive system is a prime target for childhood disorders. The single most common complaint is a stomach-ache—a problem with causes so varied that parents can rarely hope to pin them down. A sound rule of thumb is to call the doctor if pain is severe or persists for two or three hours, or if milder but chronic stomach-aches interfere with eating or sleeping.

A stomach-ache may be a prelude to the most obvious signs of digestive-tract distress—vomiting and diarrhea, usually symptoms of inflammation in the stomach and intestinal walls. The most common cause is a viral infection, and the symptoms are part of the body's attempt to get rid of the infection. In addition, an inflamed intestine is less able to absorb food and liquids: It leaks fluid and passes its contents out of the body more frequently than normal.

Both vomiting and diarrhea are potentially dangerous in a young child because an excessive loss of body fluids can rapidly lead to dehydration—a condition that, if untreated, can be fatal. To prevent dehydration, replenish lost fluids as quickly as possible. When a child has diarrhea, give him clear liquids. If he has vomited, give him nothing at all for an hour or two, then try having him suck on ice chips or take a sip of water every 10 or 15 minutes. If he holds down the water, offer tablespoonfuls of other clear liquids. Cold drinks are better than warm ones; fruit-flavored popsicles or ice-cold soft drinks that have been allowed to go flat are among the best. Milk is the worst. It is one of the hardest liquids to keep down, and if the child has diarrhea, the enzyme lactase, needed to digest milk, has probably been lost from his intestines. Keep the child on liquids for about 24 hours to allow his system to settle. Do not give him antidiarrheal or anti-vomiting medicines without a doctor's approval.

A child who suffers from both vomiting and diarrhea, as in many digestive-tract infections, is at double risk of dehydration. Early clues to advanced dehydration include deep-yellow urine, infrequent urination and listlessness. The child may produce few tears when he cries. Further warning signs are a dry mouth, sunken eyes, and skin that feels either doughlike or papery and dry. If any of these symptoms appear, consult a doctor immediately. The younger the child, the greater the threat. Infants can become seriously dehydrated in less than a day because they require more water per pound than older children and their fluid reserves are smaller.

Though less serious than diarrhea, constipation is also fairly common among young children. But a failure to have a bowel movement every day does not in itself mean constipation. A youngster is constipated only if the stools are hard, dry, and difficult or painful to pass. A vicious cycle of constipation usually begins when a child voluntarily withholds a movement—perhaps because a previous one was painful, or he is too busy playing or is asserting his control during a struggle over toilet training. As the restrained stool builds up, it loses moisture and becomes harder to pass, causing the child to withhold even more.

Treating constipation through a change in diet is always preferable to giving a child laxatives. Give the child plenty of fluids—including the traditional stand-by, prune juice—raw fruits, vegetables, and whole-grain breads and cereals. For an infant, use a mixture of one tablespoonful of corn syrup to four ounces of water or milk.

Aside from infection, one of the most common causes of digestive upset is the motion of riding in a car, an airplane or a boat. This is an age-old problem; the very term "nausea" comes from the Greek word for "ship." Humans are not alone in their misery; studies show that monkeys, birds and even some fishes suffer from motion sickness. Among children, the ailment rarely strikes youngsters under two; middle childhood, however, is a particularly vulnerable time.

A few children take motion sickness in stride. For one six-year-old who loved to fish, nausea was almost a part of the sport; he would vomit over the side of the boat and quietly go back to his pole. For most of the afflicted, though, the experience is something to be avoided. Simple precautions can help: Never start a trip just after a heavy meal or on an empty stomach; keep a car window open and distract a child with games. For those susceptible, the front seat of a car is preferable to the back. In a plane, a seat over the wing is the most stable location. When nausea strikes, have the child lie down on his back, if possible. For severe cases, over-the-counter drugs can make a long trip more bearable.

Threats to a sensitive skin

Not all childhood health problems are internal; some common afflictions strike the outside of the body. A child's skin, like an adult's, may overreact to stimuli, fall prey to invasion by bacteria, fungi and viruses or, through a defect of the immune system, develop chronic disorders marked by itching or scaling. Other disorders are less serious, but especially common in children. The skin of an infant or a toddler is extremely sensitive, because the outer barrier layer characteristic of adult skin is not yet fully developed; therefore, the child's skin is easily burned by sunlight or hot water, and easily irritated by harsh soaps, medicines or dirty diapers.

Whatever their age, children with light skin and blue eyes are especially vulnerable to the ultraviolet rays of the sun. The cute freckles they develop are actually signs of a desperate attempt by pigment cells to form a layer of protection against the sun. Limit children's exposure to the sun between the hours of 10 a.m. and 2 p.m., when ultraviolet intensity is greatest, and protect their skin with sunbonnets or visored caps, loose-fitting clothing and such traditional stand-bys as a parasol or canopy affixed to a carriage or stroller. If exposure to the sun is unavoidable and protracted, use a sunscreen lotion, which absorbs the most dangerous rays.

Despite all safeguards, a few sunburns are inevitable. Cool compresses and cool baths with baking soda will soothe tender skin. Lubricating oils and such salves as petroleum jelly retain heat, and should not be used until the discomfort of the burn eases off; commercial medicines containing benzocaine should not be used at all: They can irritate the skin. Consult a doctor immediately if a sunburn causes extensive blistering, nausea, chills, fever or vision problems.

As the body's shield, the skin endures all sorts of minor assaults that invite infection. Superficial burns, scrapes and cuts usually mend quickly and cause no problem unless overzealous treatment interferes with the healing process. If the skin is injured but not broken, as in a blister, leave it alone; puncturing the skin increases the risk of infection. When skin has been scraped or cut, rinse the wound thoroughly. Do not bandage a slight wound; the dark, moist environment under the bandage is perfect for bacterial growth.

Skin rashes, ubiquitous in children, may represent nothing more than a response to the environment—the heat and humidity of summer, for example, can lead to blockage of the sweat glands. A few rashes are symptoms of such diseases as chicken pox. Others follow no typical pattern, but are part of a viral infection of the respiratory or digestive system.

Periodic outbreaks of a rash without an accompanying illness are often the result of allergic reactions. One of the most common agents is poison ivy, which triggers a reaction in seven out of 10 people. Exposure results not only from touching the plant, but from contact with its oils, which may cling to clothing or the fur of a pet. If your child has been exposed to poison ivy, scrub his skin with soap and water for 15 minutes as soon as possible, and wash or clean all his clothes and shoes. If a rash does occur, ease the itching with calamine lotion or with cool compresses soaked in Burow's solution or salt water. For extreme cases apply a .5 per cent solution of hydrocortisone, but do not continue this more than seven days without consulting a doctor.

One of the most mysterious and agonizing of skin rashes is eczema, a skin disorder that usually first appears in infancy or childhood. The name comes from the Greek word for "bubbling over": The rash begins as tiny, itchy blisters or bubbles. Its probable cause is an immune-system defect.

The hallmark of eczema is a maddening tendency to itch at a slight provocation. Heat, cold, low humidity, tight or coarse clothing, soap, spicy food, physical exercise, fatigue and stress—all can trigger the intolerable itching. Scratching produces open, oozing areas on the skin, which may become infected by bacteria and turn into thickened, cracked patches.

At present, the disorder cannot be cured but often disappears by age five; treatment is designed to relieve discomfort and prevent itching. Avoid frequent baths, which can dry a child's skin, and heavy clothing (especially wool), which irritates the skin. And keep the child's nails trimmed short to minimize the damage from scratching. If home treatment fails, a doctor may prescribe antihistamines, hydrocortisone or coal-tar compounds to reduce the itching.

Helping the doctor to do his job

Many childhood afflictions do not fall neatly into the categories of respiratory, digestive or skin disorders; viral infections, for example, often produce a multitude of symptoms that can affect the entire body. The result is usually a very sick child—one who requires a doctor's care.

It is the parent's job to act as the child's interpreter, relaying the details of his condition. The doctor will want to know when and how the illness started, in what order the symptoms appeared, and whether the child has been in contact with people who have a similar problem. The symptoms must be described precisely. It is not enough to say that Johnny has a

How to give medicines to infants and children

Like adults, babies and children have a natural resistance to the intrusion of foreign substances into their bodies, especially when the substances threaten to burn, sting, tickle or just taste bad. Unlike most adults, however, children may grow extremely upset at the sight of a medicine bottle, or be unable to understand or follow verbal directions. Under these circumstances, the job of administering a medicine correctly can be messy and difficult.

The techniques illustrated below and on the following pages, based on practices used and taught by pediatric nurses, offer safe and effective ways of administering medicines in five different forms. Though firm measures may be needed to restrain any child who is squirming or trying to push the medicine aside, a toddler can cooperate in ways an infant cannot; therefore, one method is generally shown for treating younger children and another for older children. In the drawing below, for example, the baby receiving eye drops is swaddled to keep his arms and legs out of the way; with an older child, a steadying arm or hand would suffice.

Approach medicine-giving in a positive, no-nonsense manner, without threats or bribes; let the child know that he has no choice but to take the medicine. Your candor and honesty are crucial to getting his cooperation in the future; do not pretend that a medicine will taste or feel better than it actually does.

Before administering a medicine, set the container in a convenient location, then wash your hands thoroughly. Never use more than the prescribed dosage. Children are especially susceptible to the side effects of medicines, and an overdosage that would have little or no effect upon an adult can seriously harm them. For the same reason, take special care to follow the physician's instructions exactly, and read the label of an over-the-counter medicine for specific references to children. After administering the medicine, return a dropper to its bottle immediately, and promptly recap a bottle, box or tube.

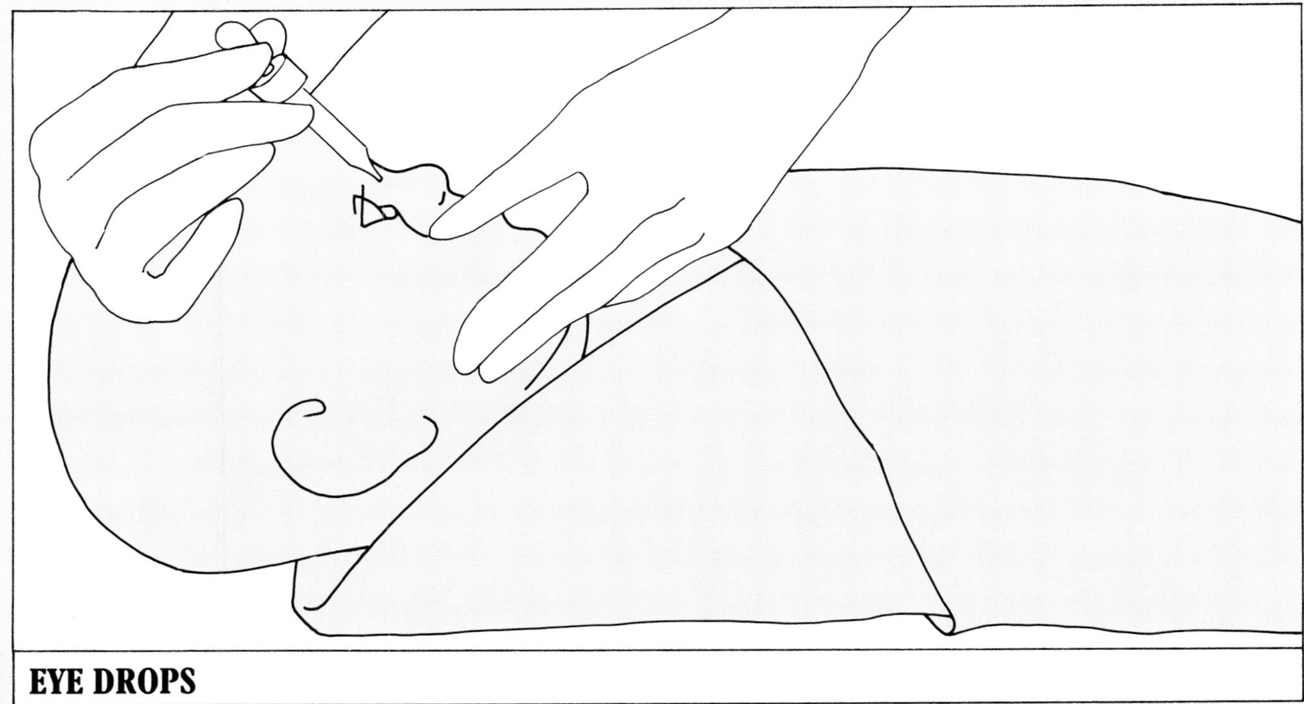

EYE DROPS

Press the cheek to open a pouch between the lower lid and the eyeball. While steadying the child's head with the hand holding the dropper, place drops into this pouch. Never touch the dropper to the eye or eyelid, and do not put drops directly on the eyeball; blinking will spread the medicine over the cornea.

Use a dropper to give oral medicines to a baby. Protect your clothing with a cloth. Hold the baby snugly against your body, grasping his outside leg and arm in your hand and raising the baby's head to reduce the risk of choking. Slowly squeeze medicine from the dropper into the corner of the baby's mouth.

A toddler can take liquids from a hollow medicine spoon (below) or an ordinary teaspoon. Circle the child's shoulders with one arm to keep him still, and gently squeeze his cheeks to hold his head still. The child may cooperate more readily if he is offered a chaser of water or juice, or allowed to hold the spoon himself.

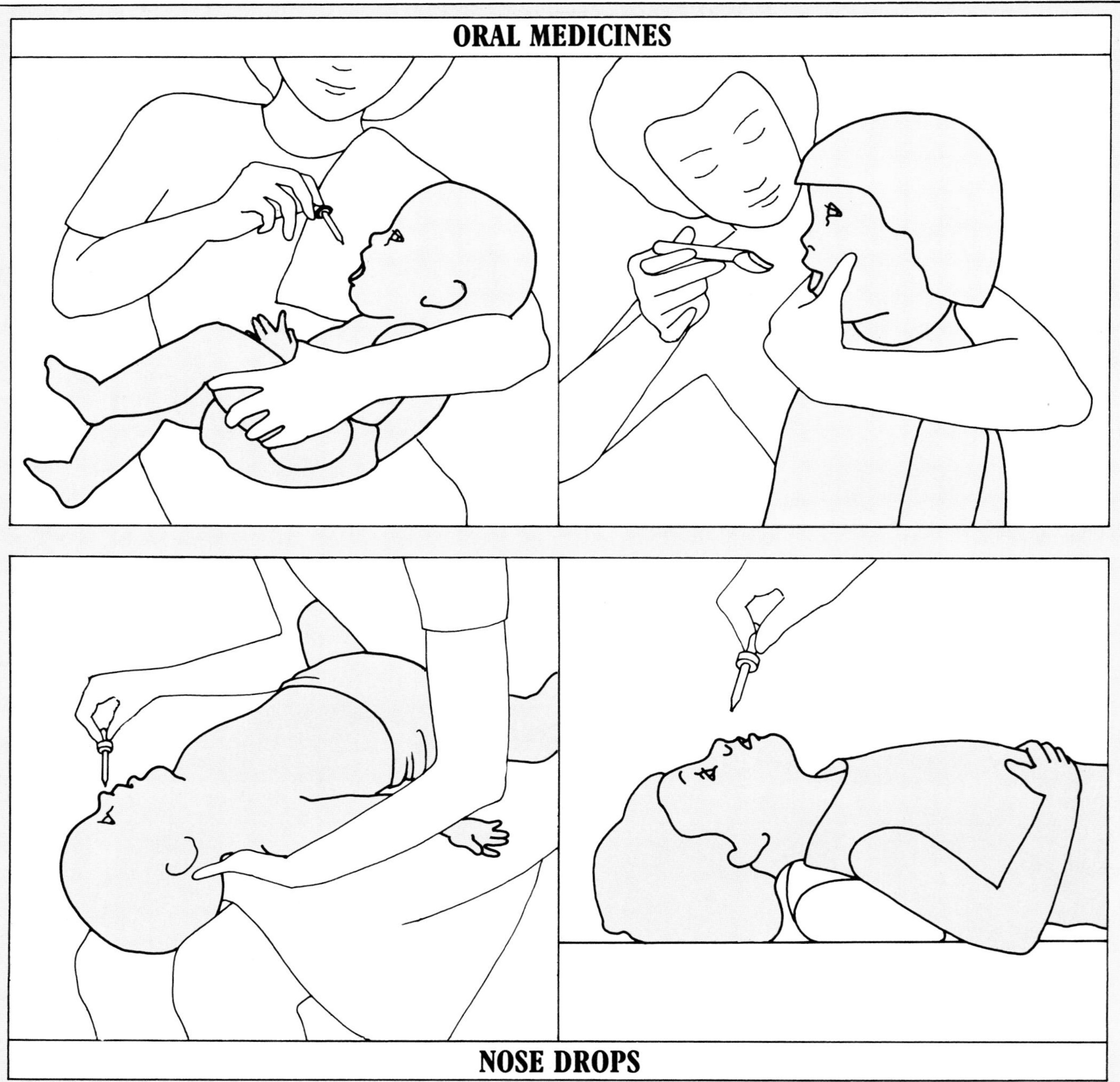

Set a baby on your lap, restraining his limbs with your arms, and angle his head down and back; this position allows the drops to flow into the folds of the nasal passages. If the baby's nose is completely blocked, suction some mucus out with a bulb beforehand; loosened mucus can be suctioned out afterward.

An older child can take nose drops in the usual adult position, lying on a bed or couch; prop a pillow under his shoulders to tilt the head rather than letting it hang over the side or end. After you have administered the drops, ask the child to sniff them in, then keep him in position for at least a full minute.

Lay the child on his side or back, and steady his head with the hand holding the dropper. For babies and children less than three years old, pull the ear flap down and back (arrow) before depositing the drops; this maneuver straightens the upward-curving ear canal, creating a clear path to the eardrum.

By the age of three a child's ear canal has assumed the adult shape, curving slightly downward; pull the ear flap up and back (arrow). After administering the drops, keep the child's head in position for a minute or two to make sure that the medicine completely fills the ear canal.

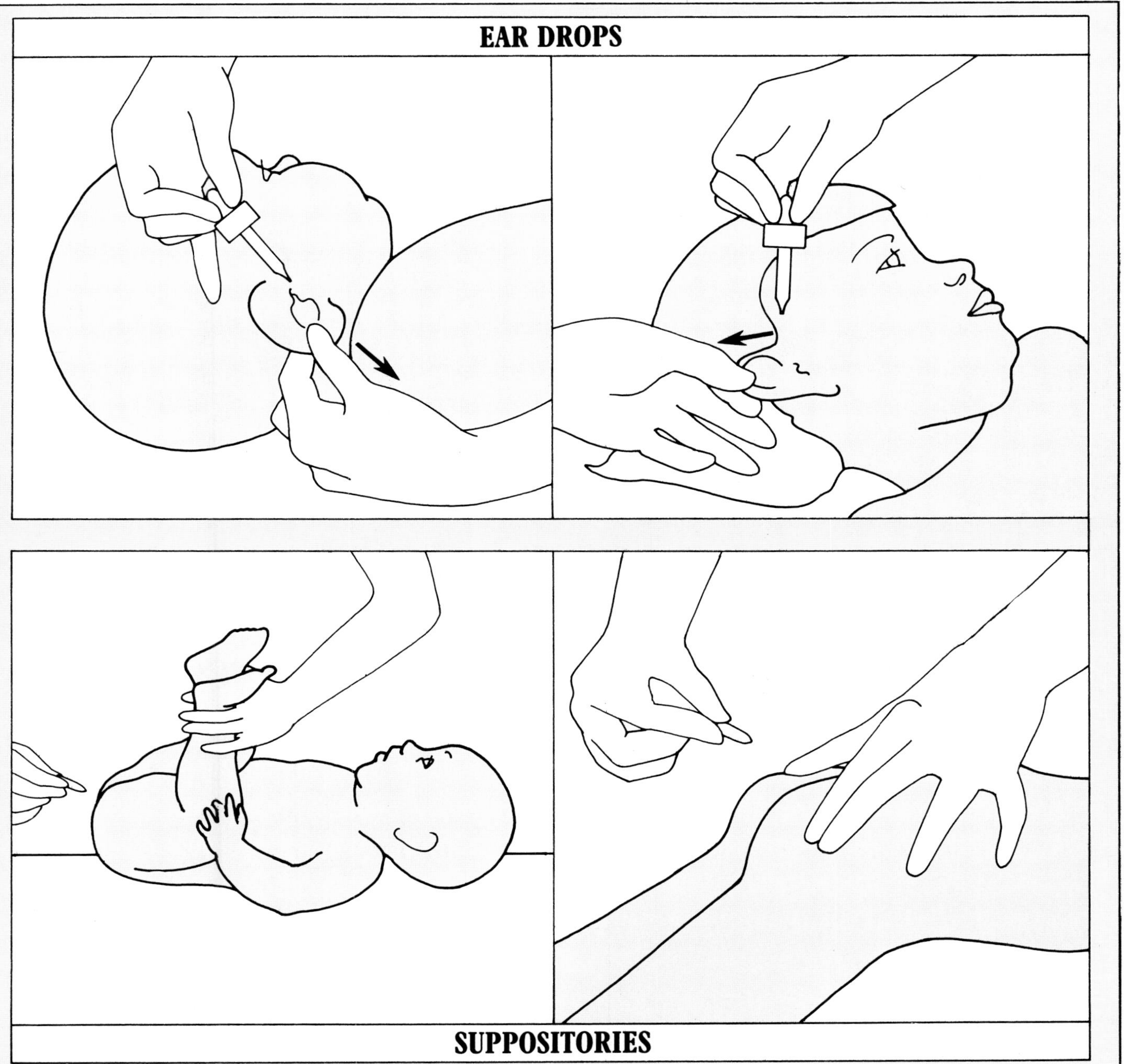

Position an infant by pulling his ankles up and back with one hand; then, using the little finger of the other hand, push the suppository quickly but gently past the tight sphincter muscle and into the rectum. Press the baby's buttocks together and hold him still for about five minutes while the pellet melts.

An older child may be positioned on his stomach to receive a suppository; spread his buttocks apart and push the pellet past the sphincter muscle, then hold his buttocks together to prevent premature expulsion. If a stool is blocking the anus, encourage the child to move his bowels, then insert another pellet.

pain in the abdomen; the doctor needs to know where it is in the abdomen, if it is continuous or intermittent, and whether there are other symptoms such as fever or diarrhea. Keep notes as the symptoms progress. Whenever you take your child's temperature, for example, jot down the reading and the time. When the child has severe diarrhea, keep a record of the number of bowel movements, the appearance of the stools, and how much and what kind of fluid the child drinks. When you talk to the doctor, write down his instructions on medicines or the reporting of symptoms.

Prepare the child for a visit to a doctor's office with a brief, simple account of what is likely to happen there. To diagnose a vague, feverish illness, for example, the doctor will surely take the child's temperature, and may weigh him to make sure that dehydration has not caused a sudden weight loss. The doctor will check the likely sites of infection—throat, ears, chest, and lymph nodes. He may take a throat culture, or probe the abdomen for an enlarged liver and spleen or an inflamed appendix. Be honest with the child; never tell him that a procedure "won't hurt a bit" if you think it might.

Illnesses severe enough to require a doctor's care will also require a period of rest and recuperation at home, and this can be trying for parents and child alike. But there are ways of getting through an illness with a minimum of tears on a child's part and only a few frayed nerves on yours. The first hurdle is persuading the child to take the prescribed medicines. Many parents can appreciate comedian Sam Levenson's story of the youngster who resists his parents' most ingenious efforts to get him to take two pills. At last, in despair, they hurl the tablets to the floor and stamp out of the room—whereupon the child promptly picks up the pills and eats them. Fortunately, there are more reliable techniques for getting medicine into a young child effectively and with little fuss *(pages 147-149)*. But whatever approach you use, always tell the child it is medicine. And for obvious reasons, never describe a medicine as something good to eat.

Medicine-giving is struggle enough. There is no point in doing battle over food as well. A child's appetite naturally falls off when he feels ill, but a few days with little food will not hurt as long as he gets plenty of fluids. Forget the usual rules about diet and proper mealtimes. Give the child whatever he wants, whenever he wants it, so long as it stays down and does not make him sicker. This is one time when even doctors and nutritionists believe that soft drinks are fine. Entice the child to keep drinking by varying the menu. Make ice-tray popsicles from fruit juices or dissolved gelatin. Give the child a lollipop or cracker—both will make him thirsty.

When a child has a fever, replace calories as well as fluids by offering him fruit drinks or sweetened tea. If he has diarrhea, carrot soup made with one jar of commercial baby food and one jar of water replaces both fluids and minerals. As the illness subsides, introduce bland foods, such as custard, gelatin, cereal or soft-boiled eggs. Fruits, sherbets and sweet but nutritious concoctions whipped up in the blender make appealing snacks. A good postdiarrhea menu is the so-called BRAT diet—named not for a child, but for the initials of its components: bananas, rice, applesauce and toast. These foods are all slightly constipating, and they restore such minerals as sodium and potassium. Never force a sick child to eat; doing so can provoke vomiting or turn the child against a specific food for years to come. Once their systems are back to normal, children tend to replenish their stores by eating ravenously for a week or two.

Keeping a sick child quiet and amused, as well as nourished, can test the limits of the most patient and resourceful parent. Fortunately, few illnesses require that a child be confined to bed all the time. If staying in bed makes him unhappy and increases his demands for attention, move him to a more convenient spot—a sofa, perhaps, or a lounge chair. Indeed, if he feels well enough, he can play quietly anywhere in the house, or even in the backyard when the weather is warm.

In the sickroom itself, time can be saved with a little planning. Set up a table for food, drinks and toys, place a box of tissues and a wastebasket nearby and leave a glass of fluid that the child can sip at will. Keep him busy with activities he can do alone and objects he can watch—balloons, mobiles or a bowl of goldfish are good diversions. A special "surprise and comfort bag" of small toys, trinkets, a flashlight, a magnifying glass and household discards such as coin purses and thread spools can provide many hours of enjoyment.

No matter how many diversions you provide, caring for a sick child will be time-consuming—and indeed, it should be. The child needs extra love and attention and as much of your time as you can offer. Be patient if he regresses and seems more immature; he will soon return to normal when he recovers. This does not mean you should let him become a tyrant, or make being sick so attractive that he learns to enjoy it. Dr. Spock sums up the objectives this way: "Let the child lead just as normal a life as is possible under the circumstances, expect reasonable behavior from him toward the rest of the family, and avoid worried talk, looks, and thoughts."

Handling a visit to the hospital

Of all the experiences a sick child may face, hospitalization requires the most preparation and understanding. He will be away from home and parents—perhaps for the first time—in a setting where strangers will do unusual and painful things to him for reasons he cannot understand. Although your child's medical treatment will be out of your hands, what you say and do will greatly affect how he reacts to treatment, and may shape his attitude toward medical care for years to come.

To begin with, find out as much as you can about the child's health problems, how long he will have to stay in the hospital, what tests or procedures will be necessary and, if surgery is planned, what type of anesthesia will be used and how it will be administered. Inquire about the hospital's routines and its policies on bringing personal items, such as toys and pajamas, from home. Find out whether you will be able to sleep over in the child's room; for surgery, ask whether you can be present in the operating room before he is anesthetized and in the recovery room when he wakes up.

Just what you tell the child depends partly on his age. Tell a very young child exactly when you will be with him, and stress that people you trust will be caring for him when you cannot be present. The child may view being sent to the hospital as a punishment. Assure him that this is not the case—that he must go only because neither you nor the doctor can fix what is wrong without the hospital's help. Promise that you will bring him home as soon as he is well.

Older children worry that they may suffer harm in the hospital, and that they will permanently lose some part of themselves or come out looking different than when they went in. They may find it hard to understand why a doctor must inflict pain when he is supposed to be making them feel better. To help the child understand, give him a full account of the steps of his treatment, and explain that a brief period of pain may be necessary in order for him to get well.

As you give these explanations, remember that a child's fertile imagination can conjure up misconceptions about what may happen to him. Children commonly believe that "taking blood" will drain them dry or that being "put to sleep" will have the same finality it did for the family dog; a simple word like "cut" can conjure up images of gruesome mutilation. Choose words carefully, but be honest. Now more than ever, the child needs to know he can trust you. If he will feel sore after surgery or if you know a test will hurt, tell him so, reminding him that the pain will soon go away.

Some hospitals have programs to prepare youngsters for hospitalization. Inquire about such programs, and use them if they are available. At Children's Hospital National Medical Center in Washington, D.C., for example, children can go to a get-acquainted puppet show featuring "Clipper the Clown." After the show, which tells the story of a little girl who has her tonsils removed, each child receives a coloring book that explains what will happen after he enters the hospital. Similarly, before surgery at California's Stanford University Medical Center, pediatric play specialists use a slide show and a miniature hospital to show children the kind of bed they will sleep in, the mask they will wear when going to sleep in the operating room, and the recovery room where they will wake up. Said one child: "It's not that bad things don't happen here, but at least there are no bad surprises."

Finally, in dealing with sick children—as in all aspects of child care—it helps to keep things in perspective. Remember that children are remarkably resilient. According to an old medical-school dictum, nine out of 10 patients get well regardless of what the doctor does. The adage applies in many ways to child care. Despite the inevitable uncertainties that parents experience, the vast majority of youngsters grow up to be healthy, well-adjusted adults. ❋

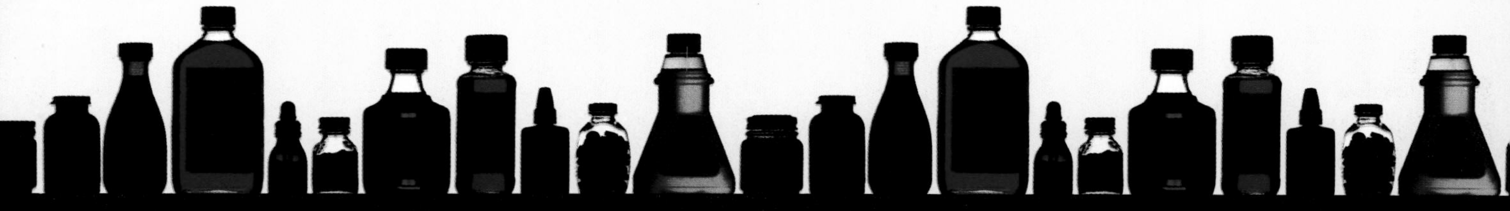

Drugs for a diversity of patients

A list of specialized drugs is generally designed for a patient suffering from a single type of disorder—digestive, respiratory, or the like. By contrast, reproduction, birth and early childhood create no fewer than three different kinds of patient, each with unique needs and problems. An adult man or woman may require drugs to treat sexual disorders or infections, or to encourage conception. A pregnant woman requires special care throughout her pregnancy, during labor and delivery, and into the days that follow. And an infant or young child is subject to a host of illnesses characteristic of the first five years of life.

The table below, prepared with the help of Christopher S. Conner, Director of the Rocky Mountain Drug Consultation Center, gives a representative sampling of the drugs used for all three types of patient. Each drug is listed by its generic chemical name, generally followed by its most common trade names. The insignia *Rx* identifies a drug that requires a prescription; an asterisk marks those containing more than one active ingredient.

The treatment of pregnant women, mothers and children presents unique problems. During pregnancy and nursing, drugs taken by the mother can harm the child; therefore, pregnant women and nursing mothers should consult a doctor before taking any drug. Infants and children are especially prone to side effects. Always follow a doctor's directions when administering a prescription drug to a child; when giving an over-the-counter drug, look for label instructions for children or consult a pediatrician.

In using any drug, observe these basic cautions: Anyone taking a drug that causes drowsiness should avoid alcohol or other depressants, and should not drive a car or operate heavy machinery. Consult a doctor if a condition worsens or does not improve, or if serious side effects or unusual symptoms appear.

DRUG	Intended effect	Minor side effects	Serious side effects	Special cautions
ACETAMINOPHEN **DATRIL** **NEBS** **TYLENOL**	Treats headache in pregnancy; relieves post-partum and episiotomy pain; treats pain in infants and children	Dizziness; upset stomach	Liver damage with overdose in adults; reduced blood-cell counts	Consult doctor before taking if you have liver disease. Inform doctor of sore throat, bruising or bleeding—signs of reduced blood-cell counts.
ACYCLOVIR (Rx) **ZOVIRAX**	Treats genital herpes infections	Transient burning or stinging; itching; rash	None	Avoid use in the eye. Apply as directed for seven days. This drug cannot prevent recurrences.
ALPROSTIDIL (Rx) **PROSTIN VR PEDIATRIC**	Stabilizes abnormal heart arteries in newborn infants with heart defects	Flushing; diarrhea	Fever; convulsions; slow heartbeat; fluid retention; bleeding	None
AMOXICILLIN (Rx) **AMOXIL**	Treats urinary infections and gonorrhea in adults; treats infections in infants and children	Nausea; diarrhea; vomiting	Allergic reactions, such as skin rash, itching or wheezing; inflammation of the colon (colitis)	Take as directed until drug is gone. Consult doctor before taking if you have any allergies, particularly to penicillin, or if you have kidney disease. Inform doctor of severe or persistent diarrhea, a sign of colitis.
AMPICILLIN (Rx)	All effects similar to AMOXICILLIN			
ASPIRIN **MANY BRAND NAMES**	Treats headache in first six months of pregnancy; relieves post-partum pain; relieves pain and fever in infants and young children	Upset stomach; ringing in ears	Severe nausea or vomiting; bleeding or erosion of stomach lining (ulcer) with prolonged use; hearing loss; allergic reactions, such as wheezing; slowed blood clotting; may be linked with development of Reye's syndrome	Consult doctor before taking if you have allergies or asthma. Consult doctor before taking if you have bleeding disorders, are taking drugs to prevent blood clots, have an ulcer or a liver disease, or are pregnant. Do not use for acute influenza-like illness or viral infections in infants and children. Avoid use in last trimester of pregnancy. Stop taking one week before surgery. Discard tablets that smell like vinegar. Do not take more than 10 tablets in 24 hours. Protect stomach by taking with a glass of milk or water. Inform doctor of bloody or black, tarry stools.

*Combination drug. Refer also to other active ingredients on label.

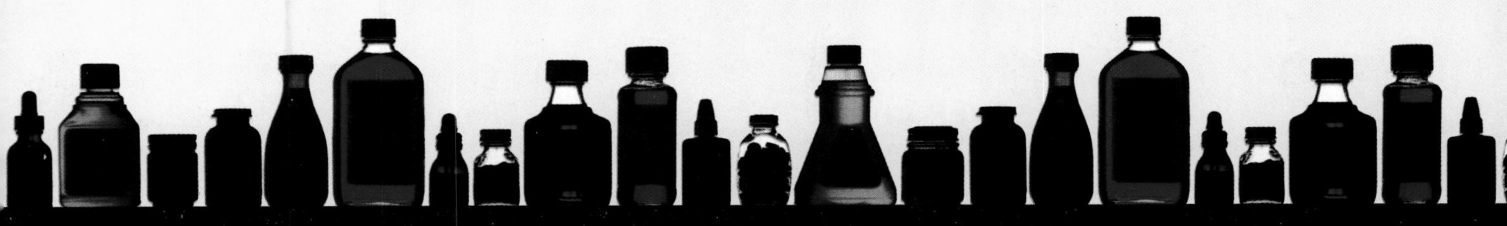

DRUG	Intended effect	Minor side effects	Serious side effects	Special cautions
BROMOCRIPTINE (Rx) **PARLODEL**	Treats infertility; suppresses post-partum lactation	Nausea; vomiting; dizziness; constipation; blurred vision	Liver disease; decreased blood pressure; irregular heartbeat; confusion; hallucinations; abnormal body movements	Consult doctor before taking if you have liver disease. Inform doctor of yellowing of the whites of the eyes or of the skin—signs of liver damage. Take with food or antacids to reduce stomach upset.
BROMPHENIRAMINE **DIMETANE** **DIMETANE EXPECTORANT* (Rx)** **MIDATANE (Rx)**	Treats allergies, skin rashes and symptoms of colds in infants and young children	Drowsiness; dry mouth; dizziness; blurred vision; nervousness	Irregular heartbeat; hallucinations or delirium; confusion	Consult doctor before administering if child has heart disease, high blood pressure or urinary obstruction. Extreme drowsiness can occur if this drug is taken with other antihistamines or depressant drugs.
BUPIVACAINE (Rx) **MARCAINE**	Acts as nerve-block anesthesia during labor	Nervousness; nausea; vomiting; chills	Decreased blood pressure; decreased heart rate; ringing in ears; tremors; convulsions; with central nervous system block (epidural, spinal), decreased blood pressure, urinary retention, severe headache, paralysis, backache; allergic reactions, such as wheezing, tightness in chest, skin rash	Consult doctor before taking if you have liver disease, heart disease, neurological disease, or any medication allergies, particularly to local anesthetics.
CARBOPROST (Rx) **PROSTIN/M 15**	Induces abortion between 13th and 20th week of pregnancy	Diarrhea; vomiting; nausea	Fever; shivering; wheezing or difficulty in breathing; abdominal pain	Consult doctor before taking if you have pelvic inflammatory, liver, kidney, heart or lung disease, high blood pressure, diabetes, epilepsy or anemia, or if you have had uterine surgery. Fever may occur after injection but temperature returns to normal after treatment.
CEFACLOR (Rx) **CECLOR**	Treats urinary-tract infections in adults and inflammation of the middle ear (otitis media) and other infections in infants and children	Nausea; diarrhea; vomiting	Allergic reactions such as wheezing, itching, skin rash	Consult doctor before taking if you have allergies, particularly to any type of penicillin. Take with food if upset stomach occurs. Take as directed until drug is gone, even if you feel better in a few days. Inform doctor if symptoms worsen, or do not improve in a few days.
CHLORPHENIRAMINE **CHLOR-TRIMETON**	All effects similar to BROMPHENIRAMINE			
CLOMIPHENE (Rx) **CLOMID**	Treats infertility in females and males	Nausea; vomiting; hot flashes	Ovarian enlargement and cyst formation; blurred vision; sensitivity of eyes to light; vision reduction; liver damage	Consult doctor before taking if you have abnormal vaginal bleeding, uterine tumors, liver disease, mental depression or cysts of the ovary. Inform doctor of yellowing of the whites of the eyes or of the skin—signs of liver damage.
CLOTRIMAZOLE (Rx) **GYNE-LOTRIMIN** **LOTRIMIN** **MYCELEX**	Treats fungal infection of the vagina (candidiasis)	Stinging; itching; rash; frequent urination	Severe vaginal irritation or burning	Inform doctor if vaginal irritation becomes severe. Take as directed until drug is gone.

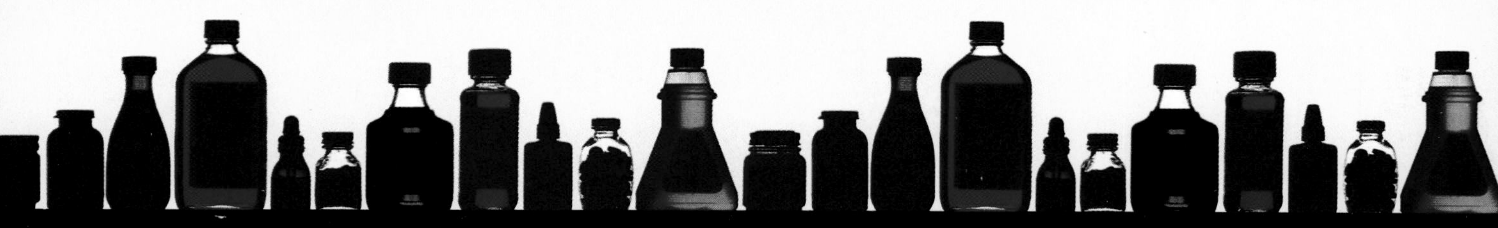

DRUG	Intended effect	Minor side effects	Serious side effects	Special cautions
CONJUGATED ESTROGENS (Rx) **PREMARIN**	Relieves menopausal symptoms; controls menstrual cycle; treats uterine bleeding	Abdominal cramps; nausea; fluid retention and swelling; loss of appetite; diarrhea; loss of some scalp hair	High blood pressure; depression; changes in vaginal bleeding; liver damage; breast tenderness; endometrial cancer; blood clots	Consult doctor before taking if you have migraine headaches, blood-clotting disorders, liver disease, breast cancer, vaginal bleeding or gall-bladder disease. Inform doctor of yellowing of the whites of the eyes or of the skin. Inform doctor of severe headaches, loss of coordination or leg or chest pain. Discontinue and consult doctor immediately if you think you are pregnant.
CORTISOL	See HYDROCORTISONE			
CYPROHEPTADINE (Rx) **PERIACTIN**	Treats allergies, such as hay fever, skin rash and itching in infants and young children	Dizziness; drowsiness; dry mouth; constipation; difficulty in urination	Allergic reactions, such as difficulty in breathing, skin rash, itching; delirium; confusion	Consult doctor before administering if child has high blood pressure, thyroid disease or urinary obstruction. Can cause extreme drowsiness if taken with other antihistamines or depressant drugs.
DANAZOL (Rx) **DANOCRINE**	Treats occurrence of excess uterine tissue (endometriosis)	Skin flushing; nervousness; sweating; vaginal itching or dryness	Fluid retention; weight gain; swelling of legs or feet; acne; liver disease; growth of body and facial hair	Consult doctor before taking if you have heart disease, high blood pressure, liver disease or kidney disease. Inform doctor of yellowing of the whites of the eyes or of the skin—signs of liver damage.
DIAZEPAM (Rx) **VALIUM**	Relieves apprehension and anxiety in labor	Drowsiness; slurred speech; weakness; clumsiness	Excited or agitated behavior; confusion; difficulty in breathing	Consult doctor before taking if you have lung, liver or kidney disease.
DIETHYLSTILBESTROL (DES) (Rx) **STILBESTROL**	Relieves menopausal symptoms; treats estrogen deficiency	Abdominal cramps; nausea; fluid retention and swelling; loss of appetite; diarrhea; loss of some scalp hair	High blood pressure; depression; changes in vaginal bleeding; liver damage; breast tenderness; endometrial cancer; blood clots	Consult doctor before taking if you have migraine headaches, blood-clotting disorders, liver disease, breast cancer, vaginal bleeding or gall-bladder disease. Inform doctor of yellowing of the whites of the eyes or of the skin. Inform doctor of severe headaches, loss of coordination or leg or chest pain. Discontinue and consult doctor immediately if you think you are pregnant.
DIPHENHYDRAMINE **BENADRYL (Rx)** **BENYLIN**	Relieves allergies, hay fever and skin problems in infants and young children; produces mild sedation in children	Drowsiness; dizziness; dry mouth; difficulty in urination	Irregular heartbeat; hallucinations; confusion; delirium	Consult doctor before administering if child has heart disease, high blood pressure or urinary obstruction.
DIPHENOXYLATE (Rx) **COLONIL*** **LOMOTIL***	Relieves diarrhea and abdominal cramps in young children	Drowsiness; constipation; dizziness; headache	Intestinal obstruction; difficulty in breathing with overdose	Consult doctor before administering if child has liver disease or inflammation of the colon (colitis). This drug can cause dependence with extended use in high doses.
DOXYLAMINE (Rx) **BENDECTIN***	Controls morning sickness in early pregnancy	Drowsiness; dry mouth; difficulty in urination	Irregular heartbeat; hallucinations; confusion; delirium	Consult doctor before taking if you have urinary obstruction, heart disease, high blood pressure, thyroid disease or glaucoma. Recent studies have reported this drug is safe for administration in early pregnancy.
EPINEPHRINE **ADRENALIN (Rx)** **MICRONEFRIN (Rx)** **SUS-PHRINE (Rx)**	Relieves acute asthmatic attacks and other allergic disorders in infants and young children	Headache; fast heartbeat; nervousness; nausea; dizziness; tremors	Irregular heartbeat; chest pain; increase in blood pressure	Consult doctor before administering if child has diabetes, high blood pressure, heart disease, thyroid disease or any type of neurological disease. Do not use solution if it is cloudy or pink-brown.

*Combination drug. Refer also to other active ingredients on label.

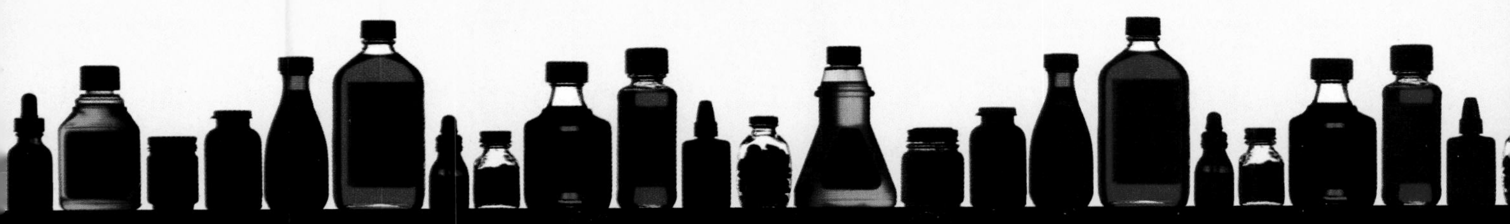

DRUG	Intended effect	Minor side effects	Serious side effects	Special cautions
ERGONOVINE (Rx) **ERGOTRATE** **MALEATE**	Decreases uterine bleeding and increases strength of uterine contractions following childbirth	Nausea; vomiting; cramps; diarrhea	Allergic reactions; high blood pressure; convulsions; severe headache	Consult doctor before taking if you have liver disease, kidney disease, vascular disease or heart disease.
ERYTHROMYCIN (Rx) **E-MYCIN** **ERYTHROCIN** **ILOSONE** **PEDIAMYCIN**	Treats syphilis in adults with penicillin allergy; treats infections in infants and young children	Diarrhea; nausea; vomiting	Liver damage (with Ilosone)	Consult doctor before taking if liver disease has been diagnosed. Take as directed until drug is gone. Inform doctor if symptoms become worse, or do not improve in a few days. This drug may enhance side effects of theophylline, a drug used for asthma. Take with a full glass of water on an empty stomach.
ETHINYL ESTRADIOL (Rx) **ESTINYL** **FEMINONE** **NORLESTRIN***	Relieves menopausal symptoms	Abdominal cramps; nausea; fluid retention and swelling; loss of appetite; diarrhea; loss of some scalp hair; skin rash; menstrual irregularities	High blood pressure; depression; changes in vaginal bleeding; liver damage; breast tenderness or enlargement; endometrial cancer; blood clots	Consult doctor before taking if you have migraine headaches, blood-clotting disorders, liver disease, breast cancer, vaginal bleeding, kidney disease, heart disease, asthma, epilepsy, depression, or gall-bladder disease. Inform doctor of yellowing of the whites of the eyes or of the skin—signs of liver damage. Inform doctor of severe headaches, loss of coordination or leg or chest pain—signs of blood clots. Discontinue and consult doctor immediately if you think you are pregnant.
FERROUS SULFATE **FEOSOL** **FERO-GRADUMET** **MOL-IRON**	Treats anemia of pregnancy	Nausea; constipation; appetite loss	Severe stomach pain; in overdose, vomiting, severe diarrhea, decreased blood pressure, erosion of stomach lining and shock	Consult doctor before taking if you have anemia, a deposition of iron in the tissues (hemochromatosis), liver disease (cirrhosis), ulcers or inflammation of the colon (colitis). Take with food to minimize stomach upset. Avoid concurrent use with antacids or tetracycline—take at least 2 hours apart.
FLUOCINOLONE (TOPICAL) (Rx) **FLUONID** **SYNALAR**	Treats skin irritation and rash in young children	Irritation; dryness; itching	Aggravation of local infection; skin eruptions; blistering of the skin; with prolonged use, suppression of adrenal-gland function	Avoid use in chicken pox. Consult doctor before administering if child has an infection of the skin. Avoid eye contact. Avoid plastic pants or tight-fitting diapers on the areas being treated. Do not apply to areas of the skin other than those requiring treatment.
HUMAN CHORIONIC GONADOTROPIN (HCG) (Rx) **A.P.L. SECULES** **ANTUITRIN-S**	Treats infertility in men and women	Headache; irritability; restlessness	Fluid retention; breast enlargement; mental depression	Consult doctor before taking if you have epilepsy, migraine headache, asthma, heart disease, kidney disease or any tumor, particularly of the prostate.
HYDROCORTISONE (TOPICAL) **CALDECORT** **CORTAID** **HYTONE (Rx)**	All effects similar to FLUOCINOLONE			
HYDROXYZINE (Rx) **ATARAX** **VISTARIL**	Sedative in first stages of labor; treats allergies in infants and young children	Dry mouth; drowsiness	Skin rash; tremor; convulsions (rare)	None

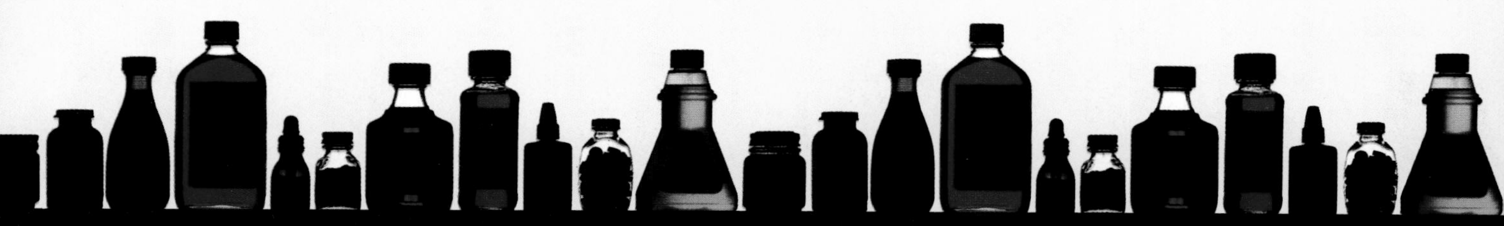

DRUG	Intended effect	Minor side effects	Serious side effects	Special cautions
IBUPROFEN (Rx) **MOTRIN**	Treats pain during menstruation (dysmenorrhea)	Diarrhea; nausea; dizziness	Ringing in ears; fluid retention; ulcers; vision disturbances; skin rash; kidney damage; reduced blood-cell count	Consult doctor before taking if you have ulcers, or have had unusual reactions to drugs used to treat inflammation. Take with food or milk. Inform doctor of bloody or black, tarry stools—signs of stomach bleeding. Inform doctor of swelling of legs or feet—signs of fluid retention. Inform doctor of pain during urination or blood in urine—signs of kidney damage. Risk of ulcers is increased if taken with other anti-inflammatory drugs or with alcohol or aspirin. Inform doctor of sore throat or fever—signs of reduced blood-cell count.
LIDOCAINE (Rx)	All effects similar to BUPIVACAINE			
MAGNESIUM SULFATE (Rx)	Prevents and treats convulsions in pregnancy	Flushing; increased sweating	Decreased blood pressure; depression of respiration; depressed reflexes; paralysis	Consult doctor before taking if you have kidney or heart disease, or if you are taking digitalis, a drug to maintain regular heartbeat.
MEDROXYPRO-GESTERONE (Rx) **CURRETAB** **DEPO-PROVERA** **PROVERA**	Regulates menstruation; treats uterine bleeding; treats occurrence of excess uterine tissue (endometriosis)	Menstrual irregularities; weight loss or gain; nausea; dizziness; weakness; acne; increase in body or facial hair	Changes in vaginal bleeding; blood clots (thrombosis); mental depression; liver damage	Consult doctor before taking if you have liver, kidney or gall-bladder disease, vaginal bleeding, phlebitis or clotting disorders, breast cancer or depression. Avoid use if you are pregnant. Inform doctor of severe headache, loss of coordination, leg or chest pain, changes in vision or shortness of breath—signs of possible thrombosis. Inform doctor of yellowing of the whites of the eyes or of the skin—signs of liver damage.
MENOTROPINS (Rx) **PERGONAL**	Treats infertility in males and females	Abdominal discomfort	Ovarian enlargement and hyperstimulation, with symptoms of weight gain, fluid accumulation in the abdomen, decreased kidney function; multiple pregnancy	Consult doctor before taking if you have abnormal bleeding, ovarian cysts, thyroid or adrenal abnormalities. This drug should be avoided in pregnancy.
MEPERIDINE (Rx) **DEMEROL** **DEMEROL APAP***	Relieves labor pain	Dizziness; drowsiness; flushing; nausea; constipation; vomiting	Difficulty in breathing; slowed heartbeat	Consult doctor before taking if you have liver, kidney, lung or heart disease.
MEPIVACAINE (Rx)	All effects similar to BUPIVACAINE			
METAPROTERENOL(Rx)	All effects similar to ISOPROTERENOL			
METHYLERGONOVINE (Rx)	All effects similar to ERGONOVINE			
METHYL-TESTOSTERONE (Rx) **METANDREN** **ORETON METHYL**	Treats hormone deficiency in males; treats infertility in males	Acne; hair growth; skin flushing; insomnia	Liver damage; testicular atrophy; impotence; breast enlargement; fluid retention	Avoid this drug if you have prostate or breast cancer. Consult doctor before taking if you have heart, liver or kidney disease, increased calcium levels or prostatic enlargement. Inform doctor of yellowing of the whites of the eyes or of the skin—signs of liver damage. This drug may enhance the effects of warfarin, a blood-thinner.

*Combination drug. Refer also to other active ingredients on label.

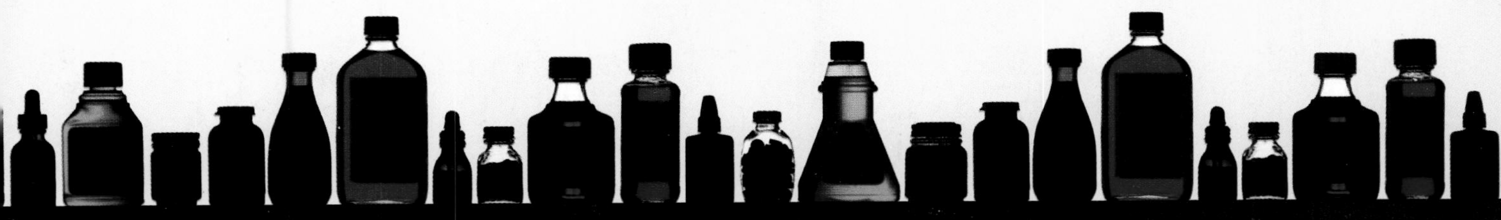

DRUG	Intended effect	Minor side effects	Serious side effects	Special cautions
METRONIDAZOLE (Rx) **FLAGYL**	Treats trichomoniasis, a venereal disease in males and females; treats protozoal infections (giardiasis) and other infections in young children	Nausea; vomiting; diarrhea; metallic taste	Sore mouth or tongue; inflammation of nerves (neuritis); skin rash; decreased blood-cell counts; confusion or depression	Consult doctor before taking if you have any neurological disease or blood disorders, or are pregnant or breast-feeding. Take medication as directed until the drug is gone. Consult doctor if symptoms worsen, or do not improve in a few days. When the drug is used for trichomoniasis, sexual partners should also be treated with it. Inform doctor of sore throat or fever—signs of decreased blood-cell counts. Take with food to minimize stomach upset. Inform doctor of numbness of hands or feet—signs of neuritis. Drug may cause darkening of the urine, which is harmless. Avoid alcoholic beverages. This drug may increase the effects of warfarin, a blood-thinner.
NAPROXEN (Rx) **NAPROSYN**	All effects similar to IBUPROFEN			
NYSTATIN (Rx) **MYCOSTATIN** **NILSTAT**	Treats vaginal fungal infection (candidiasis)	Vaginal irritation or burning	None	Use as directed until drug is gone. Insert tablets high into vagina. Use continuously, even during menstruation. Sexual partner should use a condom to avoid reinfection.
OXYMETAZOLINE **AFRIN** **ST. JOSEPH DECONGESTANT FOR CHILDREN**	Relieves nasal congestion in young children	Sneezing; burning sensation	Rebound nasal congestion; lightheadedness; headache; excitability; nervousness; insomnia; irregular heartbeat; tremors; increased blood pressure	Consult doctor before administering if child has heart disease, diabetes, high blood pressure or thyroid disease. Do not exceed recommended doses and avoid prolonged use, which may result in rebound congestion and swelling of nasal mucosa.
OXYTOCIN (Rx) **PITOCIN** **SYNTOCINON**	Induces labor; controls post-partum bleeding	Nausea; vomiting	Allergic reactions, such as difficulty in breathing and shock; irregular heartbeat; slowed heartbeat in fetus; uterine spasm or rupture; uterine bleeding; convulsions and coma	This drug is indicated to achieve early vaginal delivery to relieve or avoid medical complications, not for the convenience of a more rapid delivery.
PAREGORIC (Rx)	Relieves diarrhea in young children	Nausea; drowsiness; constipation; dizziness	Appetite loss; persistent vomiting; abdominal pain; shortness of breath or difficulty in breathing; severe nausea; reduced blood pressure	Consult doctor before administering if child has inflammation of the colon (colitis), or liver, kidney, lung or heart disease. This drug contains morphine and may cause dependence with prolonged use. Give with food to minimize stomach upset. Inform doctor if fever develops.
PHENYLEPHRINE	All effects similar to OXYMETAZOLINE			
PHENYLPRO-PANOLAMINE **PROPADRINE**	Treats nasal congestion due to colds or allergies in young children	Nausea; restlessness; nervousness; difficulty in sleeping; headache; sweating; vomiting	Increased blood pressure; rapid or irregular heartbeat; chest tightness; hallucinations; severe behavioral disturbances	Consult doctor before administering if child has heart disease, diabetes, high blood pressure or thyroid disease, or is about to undergo surgery. Inform doctor if symptoms do not improve within seven days or if a fever is present. Administer several hours prior to bedtime. Avoid high doses for prolonged periods—may cause mental changes resembling psychosis.

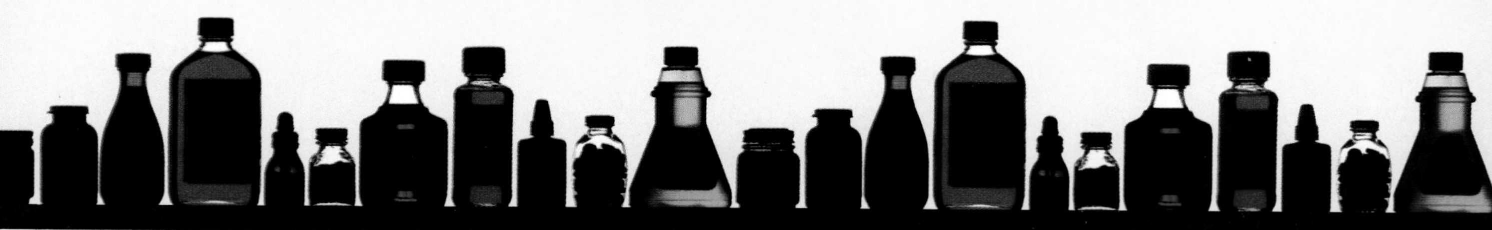

DRUG	Intended effect	Minor side effects	Serious side effects	Special cautions
PREDNISONE (Rx) **DELTASONE** **ORASONE** **PARACORT**	Treats asthma and other inflammatory conditions in infants and young children	Indigestion; nausea; muscle cramps; weight gain; insomnia	Depression or emotional disturbances; potassium loss; acne; increased blood pressure; ulcers; inflammation of the pancreas; bone disease; increased pressure in the eye (aggravated glaucoma); impaired immune response; increased glucose levels in blood (diabetes)	Adhere to a low-salt diet as outlined by doctor. Inform doctor of black, tarry stools or persistent stomach pain—signs of stomach bleeding. Inform doctor of persistent muscle cramps or unusual tiredness—signs of potassium loss. Do not discontinue abruptly after prolonged use—adverse reactions can occur, such as fever, weakness and decreased blood pressure. Avoid any vaccinations or skin tests without consulting doctor. Take with food or milk to lessen stomach upset. Risk of ulcers is increased if drug is taken with aspirin. May interfere with effects of drugs to treat diabetes.
PROCAINE PENICILLIN G (Rx) **CRYSTICILLIN A.S.** **DURACILLIN A.S.** **WYCILLIN**	Treats syphilis and gonorrhea in adults	Nausea; pain or irritation at injection site	Allergic reactions, such as wheezing, itching or skin rash; kidney damage; anxiety; confusion; agitation; depression; hallucinations; convulsions	Consult doctor before taking if you have kidney disease or any allergies, particularly to penicillins or to local anesthetics.
PSEUDOEPHEDRINE	All effects similar to PHENYLPROPANOLAMINE			
QUINACRINE (Rx) **ATABRINE**	Treats protozoal infection (giardiasis) in young children	Nausea; appetite loss; headache; dizziness	Skin rash; nervousness; irritability; psychotic-type reactions; convulsions; changes in the cornea of the eye with long-term administration	Consult doctor before administering if child has porphyria (a disorder of metabolism), liver disease or mental disorders. This drug may give the urine and skin a yellowish color, which is not harmful. Discontinue if changes in mental state occur such as irritability, nervousness, or difficulty in sleeping.
QUINESTROL (Rx)	All effects similar to CONJUGATED ESTROGENS			
RH_0 (D) IMMUNE GLOBULIN (Rx) **GAMULIN Rh** **HypRho-D** **RhoGAM**	Prevents a blood disorder characterized by breakdown of red blood cells (erythroblastosis fetalis) in second and subsequent newborns	Irritation at injection site; mild fever	None	This drug is given in the hospital within 72 hours after delivery where there is Rh blood-factor incompatibility between mother and infant.
RITODRINE (Rx) **YUTOPAR**	Inhibits contractility of uterus and premature labor (given by injection, followed by oral administration)	After injection, increased heart rate, increased blood glucose, nausea, vomiting, tremors. After oral administration, increased heart rate, palpitations, nausea, tremors	After injection, persistent increases in heart rate, decreased blood pressure, chest pain, irregular heartbeat, shock. After oral administration, irregular heartbeat, decreased blood pressure	Consult doctor before taking if you have high blood pressure, heart disease, thyroid disease or diabetes. Propranolol, a drug used for high blood pressure, can inhibit the effects of ritodrine.
SILVER NITRATE (Rx) **SILVER NITRATE OPHTHALMIC**	Prevents and treats gonorrheal eye infection in newborns (ophthalmia neonatorum); given as eye drops at birth	Local irritation; conjunctivitis	None	To be used only by a physician, and never in eyes other than those of newborns.

*Combination drug. Refer also to other active ingredients on label.

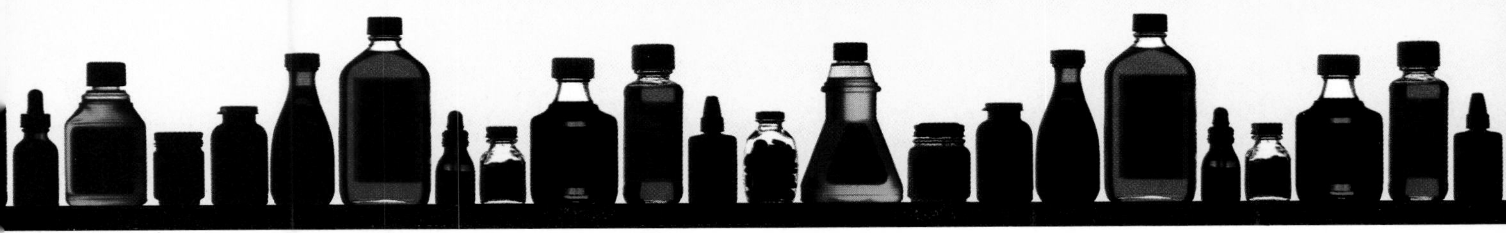

DRUG	Intended effect	Minor side effects	Serious side effects	Special cautions
SULFAMETHOXAZOLE (Rx) **GANTANOL**	Treats urinary infections in adults and inflammation of the middle ear (otitis media) and other infections in infants and young children	Nausea; vomiting; diarrhea; headache; loss of appetite; light sensitivity	Allergic reactions, such as wheezing, itching or skin rash; reduced blood-cell counts; severe skin reactions; liver or kidney damage; muscle aches and pains	Consult doctor before taking or administering if you or your child has liver or kidney disease, or porphyria (a disorder of metabolism), or if you are pregnant. Take as directed until drug is gone. Drink plenty of fluids while taking this drug. Avoid in infants under one month of age. Inform doctor if you develop weakness, sore throat, or unusual bleeding or bruising—signs of decreased blood-cell counts. Inform doctor of low-back pain, pain on urination or blood in urine—signs of kidney damage; inform doctor of yellowing of the whites of the eyes or of the skin—signs of liver damage. Inform doctor if symptoms worsen, or do not improve, in a few days.
SULFISOXAZOLE (Rx) **GANTRISIN**	All effects similar to SULFAMETHOXAZOLE			
TETRACYCLINE (Rx) **ACHROMYCIN** **SUMYCIN**	Treats inflammation of the prostate (prostatitis), urinary-tract infection, gonorrhea, syphilis and inflammation of the urinary tubes (urethritis) in adults	Nausea; diarrhea; stomach cramps; heartburn; sensitivity to sunlight	Allergic reactions, such as wheezing, skin rash and hives; inflammation of the colon (colitis); decreased blood-cell counts; severe headache and blurring of vision	Consult doctor before taking if you are pregnant or breast-feeding, or if you have kidney or liver disease, or any allergies. Discard preparations older than 3 months—they can cause kidney damage. Take as directed until drug is gone. Consult doctor if symptoms become worse, or do not improve in a few days. Inform doctor of persistent or severe diarrhea—signs of colitis. Avoid taking concurrently with antacids, dairy products or iron preparations, and space doses at least two hours apart.
TETRAHYDROZOLINE (Rx) **TYZINE**	All effects similar to OXYMETAZOLINE			
THEOPHYLLINE (Rx) **ELIXOPHYLLIN** **SLO-PHYLLIN** **THEO-DUR**	Prevents and treats asthmatic symptoms in infants and young children	Nausea; vomiting; nervousness; diarrhea; insomnia; headaches	Irregular heartbeat; confusion; persistent vomiting; tremors; convulsions	Consult doctor before administering if child has heart, liver, thyroid or kidney disease. Inform doctor if child vomits blood or material resembling coffee grounds, or experiences any serious side effects. If breathing does not improve, do not increase dose without consulting doctor. Restrict caffeine-containing beverages. Administer with food.
TRIMETHOPRIM AND SULFAMETHOXAZOLE (Rx) **BACTRIM** **SEPTRA**	Treats inflammation of the prostate (prostatitis); treats urinary-tract infections in adults and inflammation of the middle ear (otitis media) and other infections in infants and young children	Diarrhea; nausea; vomiting	Allergic reactions, such as wheezing, skin rash, itching; muscle aches and pains; reduced blood-cell counts, severe skin reactions; liver damage; disturbed kidney function	Consult doctor before taking if you have kidney disease, liver disease, or any allergies, particularly to sulfa drugs, or if you are pregnant or breast-feeding. Drink at least three 8-ounce glasses of water daily while taking this drug. Take as directed until drug is gone. Inform doctor of weakness, sore throat, or unusual bleeding or bruising—signs of reduced blood-cell counts.
VITAMIN K (Rx) **AQUAMEPHYTON**	Treats and prevents a bleeding disorder (hemorrhagic disease) in newborn infants	Pain or swelling at injection site; flushing; sweating	Allergic reactions, such as difficulty in breathing and skin rash; increased blood pressure; increased bilirubin level in newborn (kernicterus)	None

An encyclopedia of symptoms

Starting and raising a family involves innumerable challenges and changes, including a dramatic increase in the number and kinds of ailments to which a household is vulnerable. The sexual activity of the parents, the nine months of a mother's pregnancy and the first five years of a child's life—each is subject to specific patterns of symptoms and disorders. Moreover, many diseases exhibit different degrees of severity and call for different treatment according to the age and sex of the patient. Diarrhea can be a devastating ailment for a newborn but a mere annoyance to an adult male; with mumps, the opposite holds true. German measles, easily weathered by a youngster, can cause serious damage to a fetus.

The most common complaints of childhood, of maternity and of the adult reproductive systems are described below, grouped alphabetically. In each entry, the symptoms for each type of potential patient are discussed separately; for example, the entry dealing with BREATHING DIFFICULTY treats this problem first in pregnant women, then in infants and children. The disorders that cause each symptom appear in small capital letters. Always consult a doctor if the seriousness of any symptom is in doubt.

ABDOMINAL PAIN. Most abdominal pains are short-lived and inconsequential, caused by INDIGESTION. The solution is to avoid foods that produce the symptoms.

- **Abdominal pain in women of childbearing age** is often a result of normal functioning of the female body.

If lower-abdomen pain recurs each month, about two weeks before menstruation, it is likely to be the sign of ovulation called MITTELSCHMERZ, irritation of the lining of the abdomen caused by release of the egg cell from the ovary. There is no treatment, but aspirin or acetaminophen eases the pain, which should pass within a day or so.

If menstruation causes lower-abdomen pain and cramps, they may simply be uterine muscle spasms or obstruction of the cervix due to menstrual clots. But if pain is more intense than usual and recurs for several months, it can suggest ENDOMETRIOSIS, abnormal growth of tissue within the abdomen. Consult a physician if the character of menstrual periods changes.

If abdominal pain occurs suddenly on one side of the lower abdomen, it can be a sign of an OVARIAN CYST, a noncancerous growth of the ovary. Consult a physician within a day or so.

If one-sided lower-abdomen pain is associated with vaginal bleeding in a woman of childbearing age who has missed periods or had lighter periods in preceding months, it may indicate ECTOPIC PREGNANCY, growth of the fertilized egg in a location outside the uterus, such as the Fallopian tube. Consult a physician immediately.

If right-sided lower-abdomen pain is associated with fever, nausea, vomiting or loss of appetite, the cause may be APPENDICITIS, obstruction and infection of a section of the intestine. Consult a physician for any steady abdominal pain that persists for more than four to six hours.

If abdominal pain is accompanied by fever, chills and vaginal discharge in a sexually active woman, it can suggest PELVIC INFLAMMATORY DISEASE, an infection of the genital system, usually the Fallopian tubes. Consult a physician within several hours.

- **Abdominal pains in a pregnant woman**—the normal sign of the beginning of the birth process when they occur late in pregnancy—are common during earlier months and can generally be relieved by rest or diet, but in some cases they warn that some part of the complex development process has gone wrong.

If abdominal pain in a pregnant woman occurs after the ingestion of a large meal, fatty or gas-forming foods or chilled beverages, they may signal INDIGESTION. This is a common complaint during pregnancy because digestive action in the stomach is slowed down and also because the enlarged uterus displaces and compresses the bowel, interfering with intestinal action. To avoid the problem, avoid the offending dishes, chew foods thoroughly and eat several small meals a day instead of a few large ones.

If abdominal pain feels like heaviness or sagging in the pelvic area, it may be due to the increasing weight of the uterus. A maternity girdle and frequent rest periods—lying on the back or side—should provide relief.

If abdominal pain is accompanied by contractions of the uterus, its importance depends on the frequency and force of the contractions and the stage of pregnancy during which they occur. If brief, infrequent and only mildly uncomfortable, they are called BRAXTON-HICKS CONTRACTIONS. Pains and forceful contractions during the first 20 weeks of pregnancy, especially when accompanied by vaginal bleeding, may be MISCARRIAGE, premature release of the developing fetus; consult a physician immediately. Pain and forceful contractions from the 20th to the 37th week may be PREMATURE LABOR; consult a physician immediately.

- **Abdominal pains, irregular brief contractions and mild back pains in late pregnancy** may be FALSE LABOR. The contractions do not increase in intensity and do not cause the cervix to dilate. The discomfort may be relieved by walking, but consult a physician if you are unsure whether the labor is false or true. True labor in late pregnancy is signaled by abdominal contractions that increase in duration, frequency and intensity; call physician when pains are five minutes apart. If there is leakage of clear, thin, watery fluid from the vagina, this may mean that the membranes enclosing the baby have ruptured. In that case, call the physician immediately and start for the hospital.

• **Abdominal pain in children** often results from overeating, but it can also be prompted by stress, such as going to school. If your child has no associated symptoms such as fever, vomiting or diarrhea, the stomach-ache is likely to be emotional and will disappear when the stress does.

If a child's abdominal pain is associated with fever, vomiting or diarrhea, the cause may be GASTROENTERITIS, an intestinal infection. Symptoms generally pass within a day or so. Such symptoms in an infant require a doctor's care, but older children can generally be treated with home remedies: Give clear liquids such as water, tea, bouillon or ginger ale, and keep the child in bed. Consult a physician if vomiting lasts for more than 24 hours or if steady abdominal pain persists or worsens over four to six hours.

APPETITE LOSS. Loss of desire to eat is usually temporary and related to stress or minor illness. If accompanied by withdrawal, feelings of hopelessness and helplessness, and sleep disturbances, it may indicate DEPRESSION. The depression called POST-PARTUM BLUES afflicts many new mothers, bringing lack of interest in the baby, but the symptoms generally disappear with extra rest and reassurance from family and friends. If loss of appetite lasts for more than a few days and causes weight loss, consult a physician.

BAD BREATH. Bad breath is most often caused by foods or the use of alcohol or tobacco and is generally eliminated by frequent, careful tooth brushing. But, particularly in children, bad breath can be an early sign of illness.

If a child's bad breath is accompanied by mouth-breathing, it may be due to LARGE ADENOIDS, NASAL POLYPS, SINUSITIS or a foreign body in the nose. A child who continually breathes through the mouth should be examined by an otolaryngologist.

If a child's bad breath is accompanied by fever, crying or complaints of pain, it may indicate infections of the mouth, VIRAL SORE THROAT or STREP THROAT. Consult a physician if symptoms persist for 24 hours, or sooner if symptoms are severe.

If the breath of a child or an adult has a sweetish odor and is accompanied by excessive thirst, urination, hunger and weight loss, it may be a symptom of DIABETES. Consult a physician within a day or so.

BACKACHE. Backache is one of the most common complaints of adult life. Most often, the cause is poor muscle tone, resulting from inadequate exercise, from overweight, or from the extra burden on the back during the later stages of pregnancy. But it can also warn of disease.

To reduce back pain during pregnancy, exercise to strengthen back and abdominal muscles *(pages 44-49);* sleep on a firm mattress; wear low-heeled shoes; apply a heating pad and massage the affected area.

• **Backache in a young or middle-aged woman** may indicate one of several gynecologic disorders such as an OVARIAN CYST, a noncancerous growth on the ovary; or a TIPPED UTERUS, a womb that leans backward. Consult a physician if the pain persists or recurs frequently.

• **Backache in a postmenopausal woman** can be a sign of OSTEOPOROSIS, thinning and weakening of the bones, due to loss of calcium; this may be brought on by hormonal changes, lack of exercise and insufficient calcium in the diet. To prevent this disease, exercise and eat calcium-rich foods, such as milk and other dairy products, while limiting your consumption of phosphorous-containing foods, such as processed foods and soft drinks. Some doctors may recommend vitamin and mineral pills. If back pain suggests osteoporosis, consult a physician within several days.

• **Backache in a man older than 50** may indicate OSTEOPOROSIS, but it can occasionally signal PROSTATIC CANCER, a tumor that has spread to the spine from the prostate gland. Consult a physician within a few days.

BED WETTING. Until they are more than five years old, many children urinate while sleeping. Nighttime toilet training takes longer than daytime training, and accidents must be expected. When they occur, patience and reassurance are important steps toward limiting the child's already strong feelings of guilt.

If a child takes longer than most to develop bladder control, be patient. Most often this is not the result of laziness or an uncaring attitude but a physical inability that will be outgrown.

If a previously dry child suddenly begins to wet the bed, and there are no accompanying physical symptoms, the cause may be emotional, especially if daytime function remains normal. Seemingly minor upsets such as the arrival of a new baby or even moving to a new home can result in a temporary reversion to earlier behavior. Spend extra time with the child and provide assurance that all is well.

If a previously dry child suddenly becomes incontinent and also complains of painful urination, the cause may be CYSTITIS, a bladder infection that is more common among girls than boys. Consult a physician within several hours.

BLOODY URINE. Bloody urine is always a serious symptom, and should be reported to a physician within 24 hours. It usually indicates a disorder of the kidney or bladder or of the tubes that connect those organs.

If bloody urine is associated with painful, burning and frequent urination, it may suggest CYSTITIS, a bladder infection that is more common among females than males. Urine may be dark, turbid or foul-smelling. In women, the infection can often follow sexual intercourse and has been called HONEYMOON CYSTITIS. Drink lots of water, cranberry juice and other fluids—at least 10 glasses a day—avoid coffee, tea, alcohol and spices, and consult a physician within several hours.

If bloody urine is associated with sudden, severe pain in the belly or flank, it may be an indication of KIDNEY STONES, hardened mineral deposits in the urinary tubes. Consult a physician within several hours.

If bloody urine occurs suddenly and painlessly in an adult, the cause may be a urethral, bladder or kidney tumor. Consult a physician within one day.

• **Bloody, smoky or dark urine that occurs suddenly in a child or adult** about two weeks after a sore throat may indicate ACUTE GLOMERULONEPHRITIS, inflammation of the kidney stimulated by streptococcus bacteria. Headache, fatigue, fever and swelling around the face may also be present. Consult a physician within several hours.

BREAST TENDERNESS OR SWELLING. Many women's breasts swell or become tender for a few days during the week prior to menstruation. This normal effect is also one of the first signs of pregnancy, and continues until the baby is born. A brassière that provides extra support eases discomfort. However, localized tenderness may warn of disease.

• **A localized zone of breast tenderness and redness in a pregnant or nursing woman** may be a symptom of MASTITIS, a bacterial infection that also causes chills and fever. Consult a doctor at once.

• **Localized zones of breast swelling or firmness—lumps—**are extremely common in women between the ages of 30 and 50. Most are FIBROUS CYSTS, areas of noncancerous tissue that become more prominent around the time of menstruation. But lumps can be the first warning sign of BREAST CANCER, revealing its presence during the early, curable stage. For this reason, women should examine their breasts once each month, at the end of the menstrual period, using the technique illustrated in many books and pamphlets. If an unusual or previously unnoticed lump is detected, it should be reported to a physician within a day.

BREATHING DIFFICULTY. The feeling of being unable to breathe properly is an extremely uncomfortable one. It can be produced by disorders of the throat, lungs or heart, but is generally of minor importance in adults. It is a frequent complaint of pregnant women and often seriously troubles young children, in whom it can lead to suffocation.

• **Shortness of breath during the last months of pregnancy,** particularly when lying down, most often results from pressure of the enlarged uterus on the diaphragm and lungs. Propping the head on several pillows at night may help.

• **Breathing difficulty in a child** may simply be due to the nasal congestion of a cold. Infants normally breathe only through the nose, and accumulated mucus can easily block that passage. Gently suction mucus out of one nostril at a time with a rubber bulb aspirator. For all children, use a room vaporizer to increase humidity, and have them drink more fluid to help liquefy mucus. Consult a physician if breathing becomes noticeably labored.

If a child's breathing difficulty is associated with a barking cough, hoarseness and choking spasms, the cause may be either CROUP, a viral infection; or EPIGLOTTITIS, a more serious, bacterial infection. Epiglottitis also causes fever and painful swallowing, and requires medical treatment. Consult a physician immediately. In viral croup the child's small airway can quickly become blocked entirely. If this occurs, immediate action is necessary. Take the child to the bathroom, open all the hot-water taps and keep the door closed to trap the steam, which will generally help air get past the inflamed tissues. Keep the child calm; contact a physician as soon as possible. If breathing is not improved within 10 minutes, take the child to a hospital emergency room.

If a child's breathing difficulty is associated with sore throat, fever and swallowing difficulty, the cause may be DIPHTHERIA, a bacterial infection that can occur if a child has not been immunized with DTP (diphtheria, tetanus and pertussis immunizations). Consult a physician immediately.

If a child less than two years old who has not been immunized with DTP has breathing difficulty together with repeated, violent coughing that is followed by a deep, high-pitched gasping breath, the cause may be WHOOPING COUGH, a bacterial infection also called PERTUSSIS. Early symptoms are those of a cold, including sneezing and a runny or stuffed-up nose, 10 to 14 days before the onset of the unusual cough. Consult a physician immediately.

If a child's breathing difficulty is associated with fever and a cough producing thick green or yellow sputum, the cause may be PNEUMONIA, a viral or bacterial lung infection. Consult a physician within a few hours.

• **A child suffering recurrent attacks of breathing difficulty** that are accompanied by coughing or wheezing may have the allergic disorder called BRONCHIAL ASTHMA. Consult a physician immediately if symptoms are severe; otherwise, within several hours.

• **An infant who suddenly stops breathing** may be having an episode of the rare disorder called APNEA, the failure of the brain to signal breathing muscles to act. You can usually reinitiate breathing by vigorously arousing the baby or by starting mouth-to-mouth resuscitation. Consult a physician promptly. Apnea can cause SUDDEN INFANT DEATH SYNDROME, also called SIDS or CRIB DEATH, and children subject to it should be fitted with a device called an apnea monitor, which will sound an alarm if the breathing falls below a certain rate. Consult a clinic specializing in the treatment of apnea. The disorder is usually outgrown by the age of one year.

BRUISING. A bruise, the black-and-blue mark created by a zone of bleeding under the skin, is usually the result of a bump or fall and requires no treatment beyond an ice pack during the first 24 hours. But bruises that seem to arise very easily, even in the absence of injury, may indicate a serious disorder of the blood system.

- **Easy bruising associated with fatigue and loss of appetite** may suggest LEUKEMIA, a cancer of the blood-forming organs that often strikes children. Consult a physician within a day.
- **Children who bruise easily, suffer prolonged nosebleeds and are slow to stop bleeding if cut** may be victims of either of two very rare ailments: HEMOPHILIA, a genetic blood disease that runs in families and affects boys only; or VON WILLEBRAND'S DISEASE, another clotting disorder that resembles hemophilia and can affect both sexes. Consult a physician about any signs of easy bruising.

CONSTIPATION. Occasional bowel irregularity is common and normal. Even infants may defecate only once in several days, and they normally strain, grunt and even turn red in the face when moving their bowels, regardless of the frequency.

If bowel movements are infrequent and the stool is very hard or causes pain, increase fluid and fiber in the diet to keep stools soft. Fresh fruits and bran cereals are good sources of fiber. Do not give laxatives or enemas to children without consulting a doctor.

If constipation in an adult is accompanied by painful defecation or rectal bleeding, the cause may be HEMORRHOIDS, dilated rectal and anal veins. They are particularly common during pregnancy, when the enlarged uterus presses against the large veins in the abdomen. Keep stools soft by increasing dietary fluid and fiber; keep the anal area clean and dry; use hot sitz baths if there is pain, and consult a physician if symptoms are severe or if bleeding occurs.

CONVULSIONS. Convulsions often run in families but they can occur even when there is no genetic history of seizures. To help a victim during a convulsion, clear the mouth and guard against falls. After regaining consciousness, the victim is often drowsy and disoriented, and may complain of a headache.

- **In children less than five years old, a rapid rise in fever** can precipitate a FEBRILE CONVULSION, a brief seizure that is alarming but seldom leaves permanent damage. An attack does not necessarily indicate susceptibility to further seizures. Consult a physician immediately, however, to determine the cause of both the fever and the convulsion.
- **A brief loss of muscle activity in a child,** accompanied by a vacant expression, can be PETIT MAL EPILEPSY, in which a child momentarily loses consciousness. Such seizures occur suddenly, last a short time, end abruptly and often go unnoticed. They can be treated with drugs. Consult a physician within a day about any such unusual behavior.
- **Convulsions in a woman during the late stages of pregnancy** may be ECLAMPSIA, a condition associated with a dangerous elevation of blood pressure. This is an emergency. Obtain medical treatment immediately. Among the earlier signs of eclampsia are weight gain, headaches and visual disturbances.

COUGHING. Coughing, one of the respiratory system's mechanisms for ridding itself of irritations and obstructions, accompanies a number of disorders especially common among children.

- **A nonproductive cough,** or one that brings up little material, is generally a sign of either a common cold or INFLUENZA, both viral illnesses. Use acetaminophen to relieve aches and fever, give lozenges and extra fluids to keep the throat moist, and set up a room vaporizer to increase the moisture in the air. Consult a physician if the cough becomes productive of mucus, if symptoms worsen and the child appears very ill, or if fever goes above 103° F.

If a nonproductive, hacking cough is associated with nasal congestion and sore throat as well as with fever, runny eyes, white spots inside the cheeks and a red rash, the cause may be MEASLES, a viral illness that is known to be a cause of serious, permanent damage. Children should be immunized against it. Symptoms of a cold appear first, followed after two days by spots in the cheeks and two days later by the rash. Keep the child in bed until the fever subsides, and isolated for a week after the rash appears. Consult a physician if symptoms are severe or if fever goes above 103° F. Certain types of measles are a severe hazard to the unborn baby of a pregnant woman; if the mother of a child with measles is—or even suspects she is—pregnant, she should call her doctor at once.

- **A productive cough generally requires a doctor's care.**

If a productive cough is associated with fever and breathing difficulty, the cause may be either BRONCHITIS or PNEUMONIA, two infections that may be either viral or bacterial. Consult a physician within 24 hours.

If violent, repetitive coughing is followed by a deep, high-pitched, gasping breath, it may be a symptom of WHOOPING

COUGH, also called PERTUSSIS, a bacterial infection that generally attacks children less than two years old. Most children are immunized against it. The coughing fits are preceded by one or two weeks of cold symptoms. Consult a physician immediately.

• **A recurrent cough that brings up thick mucus and is accompanied by wheezing and breathing difficulty** may be a sign of ASTHMA, an allergic disorder. If the child cannot get his breath, take him to a hospital emergency room; otherwise, consult a physician within a few hours.

DIARRHEA. The frequent passage of extremely loose and watery stools can be caused by tension, food intolerance or allergy, but it is more often the result of an infection of the large intestine. It is serious if it strikes infants, who are severely affected by the loss of large amounts of fluid. Withhold solid foods but provide extra fluids—clear liquids such as water, tea, bouillon or ginger ale. Consult a physician immediately for any case of diarrhea in an infant less than six months old. Older children and adults can be treated with home remedies and nonprescription medicines containing kaolin and pectin, unless the condition persists more than a few days or there is blood, pus or mucus in the stool.

DIZZINESS. Faintness often results from standing up quickly, which momentarily reduces the flow of blood to the brain. This can happen to children and adults and it is especially common during pregnancy. When dizziness strikes, sit down immediately and place the head between the legs until the feeling passes.

If dizziness during the later stages of pregnancy recurs frequently and is associated with headache, weight gain or swelling of the legs or face, it may be PRE-ECLAMPSIA, a condition associated with an abnormal elevation of blood pressure and requiring immediate medical treatment. Consult a doctor at once.

• **Dizziness accompanied by nausea while in a moving vehicle** suggests MOTION SICKNESS, caused by oversensitivity of the balance system; it often plagues children on car trips. Resolutely keeping the eyes fixed on the horizon or playing some distracting game may help prevent attacks. If these methods fail to work, consult a physician, who may prescribe antihistamines.

EARACHE. One of the most common childhood ailments, an earache generally signals an ear infection caused by a cold. Very young children may not complain of an earache but they will exhibit other signs such as fever, vomiting, diarrhea, fatigue, listlessness, irritability, or refusal to eat; on occasion they tug at or motion toward the ear. Because childhood infections can lead to loss of hearing, any infection-related earache calls for examination by a physician.

If a child's earache is associated with hearing loss along with fever, headache, nausea, vomiting or even diarrhea, the cause may be OTITIS MEDIA, a bacterial infection of the middle ear. Consult a physician within a few hours. If there is sudden drainage from the ear, it may signal a PERFORATED EARDRUM. Perforation often relieves pain quickly and it usually heals of its own accord, but a doctor's advice is still necessary.

If a child's earache is associated with marked pain when the earlobe is touched but occurs without other associated symptoms, it suggests OTITIS EXTERNA, an outer-ear infection often called SWIMMER'S EAR. There may be a crusty or scaly drainage from the ear canal, which can also show a zone of redness. Consult a physician within 24 hours.

If a child's earache is associated with hearing loss but not with fever or other symptoms, the cause may be obstruction by a foreign object or by earwax. If the foreign object is an insect—its buzzing audible to others—fill the ear canal with clean mineral oil. The oil should kill the insect and float it out. If the home remedies do not work, consult a physician; never try to probe or clean inside the ear with a swab or any other instrument.

FATIGUE. The physical stresses of pregnancy and of caring for a newborn baby can be expected to be tiring. Many women find that they require more sleep when they are pregnant and, later, a nap when the baby naps. However, unusual fatigue associated with other symptoms—in anyone, but particularly in children—may warn of an underlying disorder.

• **Fatigue accompanied by feelings of sadness and disinterest** can signal depression, such as the POST-PARTUM BLUES that trouble many mothers in the first weeks after childbirth. Rest and reassurance by family usually speed recovery from this depression, but a low emotional state that persists requires professional attention.

• **Fatigue during the week before menstruation** can indicate PREMENSTRUAL SYNDROME, the name given an agglomeration of discomforts including headache, irritability, swollen or tender breasts, weight gain, and swelling of the legs or face. Rest, relaxation and a low-salt diet (which counters the swelling) may help.

• **Fatigue accompanied by weight loss or pallor** may be due to ANEMIA, a deficiency of iron, but it may also be an indication of LEUKEMIA, a cancer of the blood-forming organs. Consult a physician within a few days.

FEVER. Young children readily develop fevers, often high and often for unfathomable reasons. In an infant less than six months old, any sustained rise in temperature above the normal 98.6° F., as measured with a rectal thermometer, should be reported to a physician. In older children, a doctor's attention is necessary only if required by other symptoms—nausea, pain, coughing—or if the rectal temperature exceeds 103° F. Because fever seems to help the body fight off disease, many doctors recommend that a temperature below the danger point be allowed to run its course unless it causes serious discomfort. If the temperature must be reduced, sponge the body with lukewarm water—not alcohol, which can make things worse by inducing chills. Acetaminophen will also reduce fever; aspirin is not recommended for children because of its suspected link with a serious brain ailment, Reye's syndrome.

GENITAL DISCHARGE. Secretions different from those normally produced by sexual excitement are often normal in women, but generally indicate infection in men. Men and women should consult a physician within 24 hours if genital discharge is thick or foul-smelling, or if it is accompanied by burning, itching or pain.

• **Discharge from the penis that is first watery or milky** but after one to three days is creamy and yellow may suggest GONORRHEA, a bacterial infection of the urinary tract, particularly if the discharge is accompanied by painful urination. This infection is contagious, spread almost always by sexual intercourse. A physician should be consulted within 24 hours and sexual contact must be avoided until after treatment.

If penile discharge is associated with painful urination, fever, and pain in the region between the anus and penis, it may indicate PROSTATITIS, an infection of the prostate gland. Consult a physician within 24 hours.

• **Vaginal discharge that is thick,** cheesy or foul-smelling, or is associated with itching, burning, pain or redness of the vaginal tissues may represent a form of VAGINITIS, any of several infections of the vagina that can be difficult to tell apart. Two of the most common infections are TRICHOMONIASIS, caused by a protozoan organism, and CANDIDIASIS, a yeastlike infection. All require medical treatment; consult a physician within 24 hours.

GLAND SWELLING AND TENDERNESS. Gland connections, called lymph nodes, in the front of the neck and under the lower jaw are often made swollen and tender by respiratory infection. Such swelling, frequently accompanied by sore throat, is a normal response of the body's disease-fighting system, especially in children, but it may signal serious disorders.

• **Swollen and tender glands at the angle of the jaw,** just below the ears, accompanied by fever, earache and headache, may indicate MUMPS, a viral infection of the salivary glands. Isolate the child until the swelling subsides and keep him in bed until the fever passes. Give acetaminophen for pain but consult a physician if symptoms are severe. If an adult male or teenage boy in the household has not gained immunity to the disease during his own childhood, consult a physician immediately—mumps is very painful in men, and it can cause sterility.

• **Swollen and tender glands in the neck, accompanied by fever,** sore throat, fatigue or nausea, may suggest STREP THROAT, a serious bacterial infection that can lead to heart or kidney disease if it is not treated. Consult a physician within 24 hours. Give acetaminophen if necessary to reduce pain and fever; use lozenges and saltwater gargles (¼ teaspoon salt in one cup warm water) to ease the pain of swallowing.

• **Swollen glands in the neck, groin or armpit or just above the collarbone,** particularly if accompanied by fatigue and loss of weight, may be caused by either LEUKEMIA, a cancer of the blood-forming organs; or HODGKIN'S DISEASE, a cancer of the lymph system. Consult a physician immediately.

GROIN ITCH. If groin itching, burning or tingling occurs and is followed by sores that become painful fluid-filled blisters that break and scab over, the cause may be GENITAL HERPES, a disease that is usually sexually transmitted and is triggered by the herpes simplex virus.

Once a person has contracted genital herpes, the sores can erupt again during times of physical or emotional stress. Genital herpes is very contagious. It can spread from the time the early symptoms appear until the sores are completely healed. A physician should be consulted within 24 hours for correct diagnosis, and sexual contact must be avoided during an attack.

• **Groin itch that is accompanied by a red, sometimes flaky rash** and ring-shaped markings in the groin area and inner upper thigh may be caused by a fungus infection that is commonly referred to as jock itch. Nonprescription medicines that contain micronazole nitrate or tolnaftate can eliminate this condition. Tight clothing should be avoided. Consult a dermatologist if the condition persists.

If groin itching is accompanied by excessive thirst, urination, hunger or loss of weight, the cause may be DIABETES. Consult a physician promptly.

HEADACHE. Headaches are very common in adults and are generally relieved by aspirin or acetaminophen. Children are less often afflicted. When they are, the head pain is usually accompanied by other symptoms that suggest the underlying cause.

• **Headache in a child, occurring with fever,** fatigue, muscle aches, sore throat and cough, is often due to INFLUENZA, a viral illness. Give fluids. Consult a physician if symptoms are severe or if the fever goes above 103° F.

• **Headache in a child, occurring with a skin rash,** can signal one of several disorders.

If a child's headache is associated with an itchy rash on the face, scalp and trunk, the cause may be CHICKEN POX, a viral infection that also causes mild fever and fatigue. Tub baths with baking soda or oatmeal may reduce itching. Consult a physician if symptoms are severe.

If a child's headache is associated with a red rash that is most intense in the groin and armpits, and is accompanied by fever and sore throat, the illness is called SCARLET FEVER but the cause is the same as that of STREP THROAT: the streptococcus bacteria. Scarlet fever is readily treated with antibiotics. Consult a physician within several hours.

If a child's headache is associated with a rash that looks like pinpoint bruises, the cause may be MENINGITIS, a dangerous infection of the outer lining of the brain and spinal cord. Other symptoms include fever, neck stiffness and vomiting. Consult a physician immediately.

HOT FLASHES. Waves of heat, sudden perspiration, flushing and night sweats are the most common symptoms of MENOPAUSE, the gradual change of ovarian function that ends female fertility in middle age. The discomforts, which generally disappear within six months to three years, are produced by periodic dilation of blood vessels, itself the effect of decreasing estrogen levels brought on by the change of life. Hot flashes are extremely common, affecting nearly three out of four women. Consult a physician if the flashes cause unusual problems.

IRRITABILITY. In children and especially in infants, irritability may be an early signal of illness; consult a physician about any sudden change in an infant's behavior. In women, irritability frequently is associated with the hormonal changes that precede each menstrual period and, in middle age, with the hormonal shifts that initiate the change of life called MENOPAUSE; consult a physician if symptoms are particularly bothersome.

ITCHING. Most often caused by allergy, insect bites or nervous reactions, itching can have special significance if it occurs in children or pregnant women.

• **During pregnancy,** itching may be caused by stretching of the skin around the abdomen, breasts and vulva or by the hormonal changes that occur. The application of lanolin, cocoa butter or baby oil to the affected area may provide relief. Consult a physician if the symptoms are severe or do not respond to home treatment.

• **Itching, particularly in children, that is accompanied by redness, swelling and clusters or streaks of blisters** may be caused by POISON IVY, POISON OAK or POISON SUMAC. Wash thoroughly with strong soap to rid the skin of the irritating plant secretion and prevent spread of the ailment on the body of the victim; the rash itself will not spread from person to person. Wash all contaminated clothing. Apply cool compresses containing Burow's solution, available without a prescription. A hot bath or shower may also give relief from the itching. Consult a physician if home treatment does not alleviate itching or if the rash does not disappear in a week or so.

If itching in schoolchildren is severe, accompanied by tiny red marks and occasionally by swollen neck glands, suspect LICE. All bedding and clothing must be washed. Every member of the family should be checked and treated. Consult a physician for a prescription for a medicated soap, usually one containing gamma benzene hexachloride.

If itching is accompanied by enlarged but painless neck glands, night sweats and loss of weight, it may be caused by HODGKIN'S DISEASE or LYMPHOMA, cancers of the lymph system. Consult a physician immediately.

JOINT SWELLING. The most common cause of a swollen joint is injury to its ligaments, but the swelling may warn of serious illness in a child if it arises without prior injury.

If joint swelling begins a week or two after a child has suffered a sore throat, the cause may be RHEUMATIC FEVER, a disorder of the immune system that can also cause chest pain, shortness of breath, a skin rash or small lumps under the skin. Swelling, redness, tenderness, warmth and limitation of movement begin in one joint but then move to another as the first returns to normal. This disease can damage the heart. Consult a physician within 24 hours.

If joint swelling is associated with a rash or high fever in a child, it may suggest JUVENILE RHEUMATOID ARTHRITIS, a disorder of the immune system that often attacks the joints of the spinal neck bones, the fingers and the jaws, causing stiffness. Consult a physician within 24 hours.

LEG SWELLING. Swelling of the lower legs and feet is a sign of an accumulation of fluid in the tissues beneath the skin. It can warn of heart disease but is also a normal result of standing in one place for long periods. Resting with feet elevated or exercising generally will relieve the condition. It may affect women particularly before menstruation and during pregnancy.

• **Swelling of the legs, hands or face** during the week before

MENSTRUATION is a normal reaction. Counter it by eating a low-salt diet (which reduces fluid accumulation) and wearing support stockings.

If leg swelling in late pregnancy is associated with rapid weight gain, headache or dizziness, the cause may be PRE-ECLAMPSIA, a condition characterized by abnormally elevated blood pressure. Consult a physician immediately.

If the veins beneath the skin of the legs become swollen during pregnancy, the cause is most likely VARICOSE VEINS, blood vessels dilated by pressure of the enlarged uterus. Support stockings or elastic bandages around the legs may help. So will exercise—especially walking—and frequent rests with feet elevated. Avoid crossing the legs when sitting.

MENSTRUAL IRREGULARITIES. During their three or four childbearing decades, most women experience at least one menstrual disorder: unusually painful periods, missed periods or periods with heavy flow. Most difficulties are temporary and cause no lasting harm, but any sudden change in the normal pattern of menstrual function, particularly one that has no ready explanation, should be reported to a doctor.

If menstrual periods start to be painful, after some years of relatively painless menstruations, the cramps, called SECONDARY DYSMENORRHEA, may result from ENDOMETRIOSIS, the growth of tissue in areas outside the uterus. Such tissue is not cancerous, but it is a common cause of infertility. Consult a doctor if menstrual periods become increasingly painful over several months.

- **Missed periods or scanty flow** are the normal signs of pregnancy and menopause, but can also be due to stress, excessive weight loss or gain, vigorous exercise or certain medicines—especially birth-control pills. If pregnancy is the cause, there may also be swollen breasts, nausea or frequent urination; if menopause, the most common symptom is the hot flash. Consult a physician if medication may be to blame or if there is no ready explanation for a sudden change in the usual cycle.
- **Heavy menstrual flow** is normal for many women and is especially common around the age of 40, as subtle hormonal changes herald the onset of MENOPAUSE. Heavy flow can involve significant blood loss and pills providing extra iron may be needed. Consult a physician about any sudden change in menstrual pattern.

MOUTH SORENESS. This common complaint is usually caused by infections that heal themselves but may take as long as two weeks to go away. However, a sore that persists may be a cancer. Any mouth soreness that does not disappear after two weeks should be reported to a physician.

If a sore in the mouth or on the lip starts as a blister, ruptures to form an open sore and then forms a crust, it is probably a COLD SORE, caused by the herpes simplex virus. No drug will speed healing, but nonprescription medicines containing benzocaine or hydrogen peroxide and glycerine relieve pain.

If a sore in the mouth or on the lip resembles a cold sore (above) but follows an injury—from dental work or an accidental bite inside the mouth—it is probably a CANKER SORE. Treat it as you would treat a cold sore.

If a child suffers from large white spots on the roof of the mouth, the cause may be THRUSH, a yeast infection. Consult a physician within a day.

MUSCLE PAIN. Most aches and cramps in children and adults result from physical exertion and pass within one to two days, or accompany illnesses such as influenza. Pregnant women are particularly susceptible to cramps because of the extra weight they must carry and the posture they must maintain to balance it.

- **Cramps of leg muscles,** common during the second half of pregnancy, usually disappear within a few minutes. They most often occur after sleep and while lying down. To prevent them, avoid stretching the legs with toes pointed out to the sides. To relieve cramps, rub and knead the muscle while gently stretching with the toes pointed up toward the head. Apply a heating pad. Avoid the use of painkilling drugs. Consult a physician if cramps recur frequently.

NASAL CONGESTION. Sniffles or a runny nose are symptoms of the COMMON COLD, which afflicts children more frequently than adults. Children have an average of two or three colds each year. The same symptoms can also warn of other illnesses.

If nasal congestion interferes with an infant's breathing, gently suction out the mucus with a rubber bulb aspirator. Provide a room vaporizer to increase the moisture in the air. Administer decongestants only on the advice of a physician.

If a child's nasal congestion is associated with white spots on the insides of the cheeks and a red rash on the face, the cause may be MEASLES, a viral illness that also causes other cold symptoms. The cheek spots appear about a day after the cold signs, and the rash starts about two days later. Isolate the child for one week after the rash begins; consult a physician if symptoms are severe.

If a child's nasal congestion and other cold symptoms are followed 10 to 14 days later by episodes of violent coughing punctuated by a deep, high-pitched gasping breath, the cause may be WHOOPING COUGH, a bacterial infection also known as PERTUSSIS. Consult a physician immediately.

NAUSEA AND VOMITING. Nausea and vomiting are among the body's first responses to any physical or emotional disorder and they are especially common among children and pregnant women. To counter them, avoid solid foods but do drink liquids.

• **Nausea upon awakening** is an early sign of pregnancy. However, this MORNING SICKNESS can occur at any time of the day. To control it, eat small, frequent meals, avoiding foods that are difficult to digest. Eating a cracker or dry toast a half hour before getting out of bed in the morning may help. Consult a physician if vomiting is frequent or severe or causes a loss of weight.

• **Nausea in children,** although usually brought on by the same causes that affect adults, may indicate potentially serious diseases.

If a child's nausea occurs with vomiting, a rash, sore throat and swollen glands in the neck, the cause may be SCARLET FEVER, a streptococcus infection. Consult a physician immediately.

If vomiting in a child is accompanied by violent coughing that is followed by gasping for air and a bluish face, the cause may be WHOOPING COUGH. Consult a physician immediately.

If nausea in a child is accompanied by difficulty in swallowing and breathing as well as fever, headache and severe sore throat, the cause may be DIPHTHERIA. Consult a physician immediately.

If vomiting in a child under six months of age is accompanied by fever, see a physician immediately. Vomiting causes dangerous DEHYDRATION in infants.

• **Nausea in children** often occurs when they are riding in a vehicle. This is probably MOTION SICKNESS, caused by oversensitivity of the balance system. Those who are susceptible can avoid an attack by resolutely keeping the eyes fixed on the horizon, by sitting in the front seat of the car or by concentrating on distractions such as games. If none of these methods helps, consult a physician.

RASH. Infants and children are quite prone to illnesses that produce rashes, and the rash may be the first or only symptom. Many can be relieved by home remedies and disappear when the underlying cause is eliminated. Consult a physician for any rash that persists for more than a week or if associated symptoms are severe.

If a young child develops pinhead-sized red bumps with yellow centers, the cause may be PRICKLY HEAT, a rash due to blocked sweat glands that swell when the baby is overheated. The rash appears on the face, neck and chest, and it usually clears after removal of excess clothing, a cool-water sponge bath and increased ventilation. Do not put ointments on this rash, since they make things worse by trapping body heat.

If a diapered child develops a rash on the lower abdomen, groin or buttocks, it is probably DIAPER RASH, irritation caused by heat, moisture and bacteria. Keep the area clean, dry and exposed to air. Leave diapers off for as long as possible, and avoid plastic pants or disposable diapers with heavy plastic liners, as these retain heat and moisture. Change diapers frequently. Do not use preventive ointments, such as zinc oxide or petroleum jelly, until the rash has cleared up. Consult a physician if the rash spreads beyond the diaper area or if fluid-filled blisters appear.

If an infant develops pink or red dry, rough and scaly patches on the cheeks, the cause may be ECZEMA, a skin disorder. Consult a physician within the day.

If an intensely itchy rash appears as numerous welts, it may be HIVES, a skin disorder caused by an allergy. Apply cold compresses or soak in a lukewarm bath to relieve itching. Nonprescription antihistamines can also help. Consult a physician if hives recur or if there is difficulty breathing.

If a rash on the scalp or body begins as small, round red spots that have raised, scaly edges, the cause may be RINGWORM, a fungal infection that has nothing to do with worms. The round spots get progressively larger and the centers begin to heal first. Apply nonprescription medicine containing tolnaftate. Consult a physician if there is no improvement after a week or so.

If an itchy rash begins as small red bumps, then forms blisters that ooze yellow liquid, it may be IMPETIGO, a bacterial skin infection. This rash can be spread to other parts of the body as well as to other children. Consult a physician within a day.

If a young child develops a blotchy red rash after suffering a very high fever, irritability and appetite loss, the cause is probably ROSEOLA, a virus infection. The rash does not require treatment. Consult a physician if symptoms are severe or if the ailment lasts longer than five days.

If a child develops an intensely itchy rash about a day after a mild fever and headache, the cause may be CHICKEN POX, a very contagious and common virus infection. The rash begins as small red bumps that blister, break open and then crust over. The first lesions start on the scalp and face, with later crops spreading to the rest of the body for about a week. Treat the itching with baths in water containing baking soda or oatmeal. Keep the child's fingernails trimmed to prevent skin damage from scratching. Consult a physician if symptoms are severe. Acetaminophen may be used to reduce fever; aspirin is not recommended for children because of its suspected link with a serious brain ailment, Reye's syndrome.

If a child develops white spots inside the cheeks, followed by a fine red rash on the face, neck and trunk—particularly after exhibiting symptoms of a cold—the cause may be MEASLES, a virus infection. Isolate the child for a week after the rash appears; keep the lights dimmed if the child's eyes are sensitive and use a room vaporizer to help minimize cough symptoms.

If a child develops a rash like measles (above) but white spots do not appear inside the cheeks, the cause may be GERMAN MEASLES, a virus infection also called RUBELLA. The illness lasts only for about three days. However, a pregnant woman who is exposed to children with rubella should consult a physician within 24 hours, for this disease can harm a growing fetus.

If a child develops a scarlet rash on the chest several days after suffering a sore throat along with fever, painful swallowing and enlarged lymph nodes in the neck, the cause may be SCARLET FEVER, a streptococcus infection. This illness can be treated with antibiotics and is not the dread disease it once was. Consult a physician immediately.

If a facial rash in an adolescent appears as pimples and blackheads, it is probably ACNE. It is often a source of emotional distress and can leave permanent scars on the skin. To control it, wash the face thoroughly several times a day with warm water and soap. Nonprescription medicines that contain benzoyl peroxide, sulfur or salicylic acid may help. If home remedies do not work, consult a dermatologist.

If an infant develops pimples and blackheads resembling acne, the cause may be ACNE NEONATORUM. Do not use nonprescription acne medicines. Treat only by washing with mild soap and water. It usually disappears by itself.

If a rash appears as red swelling and then turns into blisters, the cause may be POISON IVY, POISON OAK or POISON SUMAC. The rash usually begins within 48 hours of touching the plants or contaminated pets or clothing. Wash thoroughly with strong soap to rid the skin of the irritating plant secretion and prevent the spread of the ailment to other parts of the victim's body; the rash itself will not spread from person to person. Wash all contaminated clothing. Apply cool compresses containing Burow's solution, which is available without a prescription. A hot bath or shower may also provide relief from the itching. Consult a physician if home treatment does not alleviate the itching or fails to make the rash disappear in a week or so.

RED EYES. Most eye redness is harmless, caused by lack of sleep or minor irritation, but in children it sometimes warns of illness.

If red eyes, particularly in a child, are accompanied by itching and thick, sticky discharge that sticks the eyelids together, the cause may be BACTERIAL CONJUNCTIVITIS, an infection commonly known as pinkeye. It is highly contagious. Consult a physician if it does not disappear within a few days.

If red eyes in a child are accompanied by pain, sensitivity to light and impairment of vision, the cause may be INFANTILE GLAUCOMA, increased pressure within the eye; KERATITIS, infection of the cornea; or UVEITIS, infection of the iris. Any of these ailments can lead to blindness. Consult a physician immediately.

SCROTAL LUMP. Any lump that can be felt in the scrotum should be reported immediately to a physician. The lumps often cause no pain, but those arising in the testicle are usually cancerous; those arising inside the scrotum but outside the testicle are usually not cancerous.

SCROTAL PAIN. Scrotal pain may be caused by injury but it may also warn of illness. It is frequently accompanied by swelling of the scrotum. Bed rest, application of ice packs to the injured part, and scrotal support relieve the pain, but medical treatment may also be necessary.

If scrotal or penis pain is caused by sores that become fluid-filled blisters, then break open and scab over before healing, the cause may be GENITAL HERPES, a disease that is usually sexually transmitted and is caused by the herpes simplex virus. The painful blisters may be preceded by groin itching, tingling or burning. Consult a physician within 24 hours, and avoid sexual contact during an attack.

If scrotal pain is accompanied by itching and discharge from the penis, it may be due to URETHRITIS, an inflammation of the urethra. Consult a physician within 24 hours.

If scrotal pain is accompanied by swelling, chills, fever and swollen salivary glands, it may be due to MUMPS ORCHITIS, an inflammation of the testicles that can accompany a case of mumps in men or teenage boys. Mumps orchitis can cause sterility. Consult a physician immediately.

If a dull ache in the scrotum is accompanied by a mass that can be felt, the cause may be CANCER OF THE TESTICLES. Consult a physician immediately.

If scrotal pain radiates from the lower abdomen, it may be an INGUINAL HERNIA. A lump may be felt behind the pubic hairs. It may be very small or as large as an egg. It may disappear on lying down. Surgery is usually necessary to prevent complications. Consult a physician in a day or so.

If scrotal pain is accompanied by swelling, chills and fever, it may be EPIDIDYMITIS, an inflammation of the spermatic cord and tissues. Consult a physician immediately.

SORE THROAT. Sore throats are one of the more common symptoms of childhood illness. They can be caused by simple irritation from yelling, but they are more often the result of an upper-respiratory infection. In children, there is no reliable way to distinguish between the symptoms of a relatively minor viral illness and those of the more serious bacterial infections, which require antibiotic treatment. For this reason, all sore throats in children should be diagnosed by a doctor, who will swab material that can be analyzed by a laboratory.

Whatever the cause of the sore throat, the sufferer may obtain some relief from its symptoms by using a room vaporizer to increase the moisture in the air, sucking on hard candy or lozenges, gargling with salt water (¼ teaspoon salt in one cup warm water) and taking acetaminophen.

• **A sore throat accompanied by sneezing and a runny or stuffed-up nose** suggests a COMMON COLD. Have a throat culture done and follow the sore-throat treatment outlined above.

• **A sore throat accompanied by cough, fever, headache and body aches** suggests INFLUENZA, a viral illness. Obtain a throat culture, follow the steps described above and consult a physician if symptoms are severe or if fever goes over 103° F.

• **A sore throat accompanied by fever, painful swallowing, swollen glands in the neck, fatigue, nausea, vomiting or a rash,** may indicate STREP THROAT, a bacterial infection that can lead to heart or kidney disease if left untreated.

URINATION DIFFICULTY. Increased frequency of urination, if not accompanied by other symptoms, is most often caused by excess ingestions of fluids, especially alcoholic or caffeine-containing beverages. It may also be an early sign of pregnancy, and can occur again later in pregnancy when the enlarged uterus presses against the bladder.

• **Pain and burning on urination** most often suggests an infection of the urinary system.

If frequent, painful urination in a girl or woman is associated with turbid, foul-smelling or bloody urine, it may be a sign of CYSTITIS, a bladder infection. In women, this can be the result of sexual intercourse (and has been called HONEYMOON CYSTITIS). Drink plenty of water and cranberry juice—at least 10 glasses a day—avoid caffeine, alcohol and spices, and consult a physician within several hours.

If frequent, painful urination in a man is associated with a thick discharge from the penis, it may suggest GONORRHEA, a venereal infection. Consult a physician within several hours.

If frequent, painful urination in a man is associated with fever, pain between the penis and anus, or discharge from the penis, the cause may be PROSTATITIS, an infected prostate gland. Consult a physician within a few hours.

Difficulty in starting urination in a man, combined with reduced force of the urinary stream and frequent nighttime urination, may be due to PROSTATISM, enlargement of the prostate gland. This is an extremely common ailment after middle age. Consult a physician within a few days.

Frequent urination, combined with unusual thirst, may signal DIABETES, a disorder of carbohydrate metabolism that can occur in children or adults. It may also cause loss of weight despite normal or increased appetite. Consult a doctor within a few days.

VAGINAL BLEEDING. Vaginal bleeding is part of menstruation, but bleeding that is excessively heavy or starts between periods, during pregnancy or after menopause should be brought to the attention of a physician.

• **Heavy bleeding during an otherwise normal menstrual cycle** may indicate only the hormonal changes often associated with the onset of menopause; but it can also be caused by FIBROIDS (muscular growths in the womb) or POLYPS (tissue growths in the womb). Consult a physician if menstrual periods involve heavier flow than is normal for you.

• **Vaginal bleeding between periods** may be a normal sign of ovulation—rupture of the egg cell from the ovary and stimulation of the uterus. Such bleeding will be manifested as a single episode of "spotting," and can also be accompanied by the lower-abdomen pain called MITTELSCHMERZ. However, if vaginal bleeding between periods is more than spotting, producing an actual flow of blood, the cause may be CANCER OF THE CERVIX or UTERUS. Consult a physician within 24 hours.

• **Vaginal bleeding that occurs suddenly** and is accompanied by one-sided lower-abdomen pain may suggest ECTOPIC PREGNANCY, the development of a fertilized egg outside the uterus, usually in one of the Fallopian tubes. Consult a physician immediately.

• **Vaginal bleeding during the first 20 weeks of pregnancy** may be an indication of an impending MISCARRIAGE. Consult a physician immediately.

• **Vaginal bleeding during late pregnancy** may be caused by PLACENTA PREVIA, a condition in which the placenta (afterbirth) partially covers the opening to the birth canal. For any bleeding, consult a physician immediately.

• **Vaginal bleeding after menopause** may be due to ATROPHIC VAGINITIS, drying of the vaginal tissues due to lowered levels of the hormone estrogen, but it can also be a sign of CANCER OF THE UTERUS or CERVIX. Report all such postmenopausal bleeding to a physician immediately.

VAGINAL PAIN. This ailment is often accompanied by burning or itching. It may be caused by any of a number of infections, growths or anatomical changes.

If vaginal pain is caused by sores that become fluid-filled blisters, then break open and scab over before healing, the cause may be GENITAL HERPES, a disease that is usually sexually transmitted and is caused by the herpes simplex virus. The painful blisters may be preceded by itching, tingling or burning. Consult a physician within 24 hours and avoid sexual contact during an attack.

If vaginal pain or pressure is accompanied by discharge and itching, burning or redness, it probably is VAGINITIS, inflammation of the vagina. Consult a physician within 24 hours.

If vaginal pain or pressure is accompanied by difficulty urinating and loss of bladder control when sneezing, laughing, coughing or climbing stairs, it may be due to CYSTOCELE, a condition in which the bladder sags and presses down on the roof of the vagina. Consult a physician within a few days.

If vaginal pain or pressure is accompanied by difficult bowel movements, the cause may be RECTOCELE, a condition in which the rectum presses up into the floor of the vagina. Consult a physician within a few days.

If vaginal pain is accompanied by bladder pain and very heavy menstrual bleeding, the cause may be FIBROIDS or POLYPS, abnormal but noncancerous growths in the uterus or cervix. Consult a doctor if your periods begin to involve heavier flow than is normal for you.

If vaginal pain is accompanied by bleeding following sexual intercourse, by a watery discharge, by urinary difficulty or by painful bowel movements, the cause may be CANCER OF THE VAGINA. Consult a physician immediately.

If vaginal pain occurs during or just after sexual intercourse, the cause may be ENDOMETRIOSIS, an abnormal growth of tissue in various locations within the abdomen. This type of pain can also be caused by PELVIC INFLAMMATORY DISEASE, an infection of the genital system. Consult a physician within a few days.

WEIGHT CHANGE. Fluctuations in weight are common indications of illness in children and of problems in pregnancy. Consult a physician about any weight reduction or weight gain that occurs without ready explanation.

If a child's weight loss is accompanied by persistent loss of appetite and there is a perceptible abdominal mass, the cause may be WILM'S TUMOR, a rare cancer of the kidney that occurs in children under six years of age. Consult a physician.

- **Weight gain,** almost always the result of overeating, can also suggest an accumulation of excess fluid, called edema, which may indicate heart, liver or kidney disease.

If weight gain occurs periodically, during the week before menstruation, it suggests PREMENSTRUAL SYNDROME, a condition that generally includes swelling of the legs or hands, headache, irritability or breast swelling and tenderness. A low-salt diet helps reduce the fluid build-up. Consult a physician if symptoms are bothersome.

If weight gain, swelling of the legs or face, dizziness or headache occurs during the later stages of pregnancy, it may be due to PRE-ECLAMPSIA, a condition characterized by an abnormal elevation of blood pressure. Consult a physician immediately.

Bibliography

BOOKS

A Baby is Born: The Picture Story of Everyman's Beginning. Maternity Center Association, 1978.

Bash, Deborah Blumenthal, and Winifred Atlas Gold, *The Nurse and the Childbearing Family*. Wiley, 1981.

Benson, Ralph C., et al., *Current Obstetric & Gynecologic Diagnosis & Treatment*. Lange Medical Publications, 1980.

The Boston Children's Medical Center and Richard I. Feinbloom, *Child Health Encyclopedia: The Complete Guide for Parents*. Dell, 1975.

Brazelton, T. Berry:
Doctor and Child. Dell, 1976.
Toddlers and Parents: A Declaration of Independence. Dell, 1974.

Caplan, Frank, ed.:
The First Twelve Months of Life: Your Baby's Growth Month by Month. Bantam/Grosset & Dunlap, 1973.
The Parenting Advisor. Anchor/Doubleday, 1978.

Carrera, Michael, *Sex: The Facts, the Acts and Your Feelings*. Crown, 1981.

Cherry, Sheldon H., *For Women of All Ages: A Gynecologist's Guide to Modern Female Health Care*. Macmillan, 1979.

Chinn, Peggy L., *Child Health Maintenance*. C. V. Mosby, 1979.

Decker, Albert, and Suzanne Loebl, *Why Can't We Have a Baby?* Dial, 1978.

Dick-Read, Grantly, *Childbirth Without Fear: The Original Approach to Natural Childbirth*. Harper & Row, 1972.

Drillien, C. M., ed., *Neurodevelopmental Problems in Early Childhood: Assessment and Management*. Blackwell Scientific Publications, 1977.

Eiger, Marvin S., and Sally Wendkos Olds, *The Complete Book of Breastfeeding*. Bantam/Workman, 1972.

Ewy, Rodger and Donna, *Preparation for Childbirth*. Pruett, 1976.

Gesell, Arnold, et al., *The First Five Years of Life: A Guide to the Study of the Preschool Child*. Harper & Brothers, 1940.

Green, Maurice R., ed., *Violence and the Family*. Westview, 1980.

Guttmacher, Alan F., *Pregnancy, Birth and Family Planning: A Guide for Expectant Parents in the 1970's*. New American Library, 1973.

Guyton, Arthur C., *Textbook of Medical Physiology*. W. B. Saunders, 1981.

Hamilton, Persis Mary, *Basic Pediatric Nursing*. C. V. Mosby, 1982.

Hatcher, Robert A., Gary K. Stewart, Felicia Stewart, Felicia Guest, Nancy Josephs, Janet Dale, *Contraceptive Technology 1982-1983*. Irvington, 1982.

Heslin, Jo-Ann, et al., *No-Nonsense Nutrition for Your Baby's First Year*. CBI, 1978.

Kellerman, Jonathan, *Helping the Fearful Child*. Norton, 1981.

Kerr, Charlotte H., and A. Lois Scully, *The American Medical Association Book of WomanCare*. Random House, 1982.

Leach, Penelope, *Your Baby & Child: From Birth to Age Five*. Alfred A. Knopf, 1978.

Pantell, Robert H., et al., *Taking Care of Your Child: A Parent's Guide to Medical Care*. Addison-Wesley, 1977.

Pillitteri, Adele:
Child Health Nursing: Care of the Growing Family. Little, Brown, 1981.
Maternal-Newborn Nursing: Care of the Growing Family. Little, Brown, 1981.

Pipes, Peggy L., *Nutrition in Infancy and Childhood*. C. V. Mosby, 1981.

Pomeranz, Virginia E., *The First Five Years*. Doubleday & Company, 1973.

Pritchard, Jack A., and Paul C. MacDonald, *Williams Obstetrics*. Appleton-Century-Crofts, 1980.

Russell, Keith P., *Eastman's Expectant Motherhood*. Little, Brown, 1977.

Shiller, Jack G., *Childhood Illness*. Stein and Day, 1972.

Silber, Sherman J.:
How to Get Pregnant. Warner, 1980.
The Male: From Infancy to Old Age. Charles Scribner's Sons, 1981.

Spock, Benjamin, *Baby and Child Care*. Simon & Schuster, 1976.

Stewart, Felicia Hance, et al., *My Body, My Health: The Concerned Woman's Guide to Gynecology*. Wiley, 1979.

Vaughan, Victor C., III, et al., *Nelson Textbook of Pediatrics*. W. B. Saunders, 1979.

Vickery, Donald M., and James F. Fries, *Take Care of Yourself: A Consumer's Guide to Medical Care*. Addison-Wesley, 1977.

Whitson, Betty Jo, and Judith M. McFarlane, *The Pediatric Nursing Skills Manual*. Wiley, 1980.

PERIODICALS

Cadden, Vivian, ''The Miracle of the Smiling Face: How Babies Know Their Mothers—for Sure.'' *Working Mother*, April 1982.

Cooper, Julie, ''Bathing Your Baby.'' *Parents*, April 1980.

Davis, Clara M., ''Self Selection of Diet by Newly Weaned Infants.'' *American Journal of Diseases of Children*, Vol. 36, No. 4, October 1928.

Drummond, A. H., Jr., ''Motion Sickness.'' *Sea Frontiers*, January/February 1979.

''How Sex Scientists Masters and Johnson Saved Our Marriage.'' *Ladies' Home Journal*, July 1969.

''Lending a Hand to the Young and Old.'' *The Healing Arts*, Vol. XII, No. 1, 1982.

McCall, Robert B., ''Sudden Infant Death.'' *Parents*, October 1981.

Martin, Lori, ''Your Child's Sex—Can You Choose?'' *Parents*, October 1981.

''Next to Mother's Milk, There's Infant Formula.'' *FDA Consumer*, July-August 1980.

Restak, Richard M., ''Newborn Knowledge.'' *Science 82*, January/February 1982.

Schuman, Wendy, ''Tonsillectomy.'' *Parents*, November 1981.

''TV Report on DTP Galvanizes U.S. Pediatricians.'' *JAMA*, July 2, 1982.

Van Thiel, David H., and Arnold Wald, ''Evidence Refuting a Role for Increased Abdominal Pressure in the Pathogenesis of the Heartburn Associated with Pregnancy.'' *American Journal of Obstetrics and Gynecology*, Vol. 140, No. 4, June 15, 1981.

Wessel, Morris A., ''Tonsils and Adenoids: When Should They Be Removed?'' *Parents*, November 1981.

Whelan, Elizabeth M., ''Dr. Elizabeth Whelan Discusses the After-Baby Blues.'' *American Baby*, April 1982.

OTHER PUBLICATIONS

''Accident Facts.'' National Safety Council, 1981.

''Care of Children's Teeth.'' American Dental Association, 1976.

''Consensus Development Conference Summaries.'' National Institutes of Health, Vol. 3, 1980.

''Do Your Gums Bleed When You Brush Your Teeth?'' American Dental Association, 1980.

''Good Teeth for You and Your Baby.'' National Institutes of Health, June 1979.

''A Parent's Safety Guide to Kid Stuff.'' National Safety Council, 1976.

''Preparation for Childbearing.'' Maternity Center Association, 1977.

''Tooth Decay.'' National Institutes of Health, 1982.

''Your Child's Teeth.'' American Dental Association, 1981.

Picture credits

The sources for the illustrations that appear in this book are listed below. Credits for the illustrations from left to right are separated by semicolons, from top to bottom by dashes.

Cover: John Senzer. 7: The Granger Collection. 12, 13: Drawings by Trudy Nicholson. 15: Prabodh K. Gupta, M.D., Johns Hopkins University. 17: © 1974 Lennart Nilsson from *Behold Man,* Little, Brown and Co. 21: Leonard McCombe for *Life*. 22, 23: © 1974 Lennart Nilsson from *Behold Man,* Little, Brown and Co. 24: Junichiro Takeda, Cine Science, Tokyo. 25: © 1974 Lennart Nilsson from *Behold Man,* Little, Brown and Co.—Drawing by Trudy Nicholson. 26, 27: © 1974 Lennart Nilsson from *Behold Man,* Little, Brown and Co.—Drawing by Trudy Nicholson; Junichiro Takeda, Cine Science, Tokyo. 28: Junichiro Takeda, Cine Science, Tokyo. 29: Junichiro Takeda, Cine Science, Tokyo—Drawing by Trudy Nicholson. 31: Joseph Baker/F. P. G. 34: © 1976 Edward Lettau. 36: © 1981 Ken Spencer. 38: © 1981 Howard Sochurek from Woodfin Camp & Associates. 40, 41: Drawings by Trudy Nicholson. 42: © 1981 John Marmaras from Woodfin Camp & Associates. 44-51: Drawings by Lois Sloan. 53: Suzanne Szasz. 58, 59: Drawings by Trudy Nicholson. 61-63: Linda Bartlett. 65: Gabe Palmer/The Image Bank. 66-79: Linda Bartlett. 83-86: R. J. Cass Jr. 90-91: Barbara Campbell. 94: John Senzer. 98, 99: Linda Bartlett. 100: Fil Hunter. 101-105: Barbara Campbell. 106, 107: Fil Hunter. 109: Barbara Campbell. 112: Walter Hilmers Jr. from H J Commercial Art. 113: Drawing by Cynthia Richardson. 115-118: Linda Bartlett. 120: Foto Archivo Salmer/J. Bellapart Murillo, Barcelona. 122: Barbara Kreye/The Image Bank. 125: Marlis Müller. 128-137: Linda Bartlett. 139: John Senzer. 141: © Nubar Alexanian Visions. 142-149: From the Studio of Kathryn D. Rebeiz. 152-159: Fil Hunter.

Acknowledgments

The index for this book was prepared by B. L. Klein. For their help in the preparation of this volume, the editors wish to thank the following: Fran and Rich Becker, Vienna, Va.; Dr. Jason Birnholz, Harvard Medical School, Cambridge, Ma.; Dr. William H. Bowen, National Institute of Dental Research, Bethesda, Md.; Diane and Tom Brimijoin, Lynchburg, Va.; Dr. Paul Burka, Falls Church, Va.; Mary Byers, The Little Acorn Patch, Springfield, Va.; Dr. Michael Carrera, New York, N.Y.; Betty Ann Chaze, Fairfax Hospital, Falls Church, Va.; Dr. Andrew Christopher, Georgetown University School of Dentistry, Washington, D.C.; Dr. Patricia Cole, Austin Speech, Language and Hearing Center, Austin, Tx.; Dr. Hugh de Fries, Georgetown University Medical Center, Washington, D.C.; Dr. Samuel Fomon, University of Iowa College of Medicine, Iowa City, Iowa; Betsy Gipson, Columbia Medical Plan, Columbia, Md.; Freda Greenebaum, Columbia Medical Plan, Columbia, Md.; Debra Haffner, Planned Parenthood, Washington, D.C.; Laurie Hall, American College of Obstetricians and Gynecologists, Washington, D.C.; Dr. Robert A. Hatcher, Emory University Family Planning Program, Atlanta, Georgia; Dr. Edward Hindman Jr., Fairfax, Va.; Barbara Kaplan, The Little Acorn Patch, Springfield, Va.; Dr. Robert Kim-Farley, Center for Disease Control, Atlanta, Georgia; Dr. John Kraft, George Washington University Hospital, Washington, D.C.; Morton Lebow, American College of Obstetricians and Gynecologists, Washington, D.C.; Eileen McCarthy, National Center for Health Statistics, Hyattsville, Md.; Dr. Laurence Miller, Bethesda, Md.; Niall O'Connor, Dublin, Ireland; Nancy O'Sheay, Fairfax Hospital, Falls Church, Va.; Dr. Dorothy A. Richmond, Georgetown University School of Medicine, Washington, D.C.; Dr. Martha Rogers, Center for Disease Control, Atlanta, Georgia; Dr. Albert Spiegel, Fairfax, Va.; Dr. Steele F. Stewart Jr., Columbia Hospital for Women, Washington, D.C.; Dr. Robert Stillman, George Washington University Hospital, Washington, D.C.; Sally Tom, American College of Nurse-Midwives, Washington, D.C.; Dr. Maria Turner, George Washington University Medical School, Washington, D.C.; Vernon C. Urich, Michigan State University, Lansing, Michigan; Dr. Victor C. Vaughan III, Temple University School of Medicine, Philadelphia, Pa.; Day Waterman, U.S. Department of Transportation, Washington, D.C.

Index

Page numbers in italics indicate an illustration of the subject mentioned.